CARE OF THE CRITICALLY ILL MEDICAL PATIENT

To RCS.

Commissioning Editor: Michael Parkinson
Development Editor: Janice Urquhart
Project Manager: Joannah Duncan
Senior Designer: Erik Bigland
Illustrator: Cactus and Chartwell Illustrators

CARE OF THE CRITICALLY ILL MEDICAL PATIENT

Edited by

Stephen Bonner MRCP FRCA
Consultant in Anaesthesia specialising in Intensive Care Medicine,
The James Cook University Hospital,
Middlesbrough, UK

Co-edited by

Mark Carpenter BSc MRCP FRCA
Consultant in Anaesthesia and Intensive Care Medicine,
City Hospitals Sunderland NHS Foundation Trust,
Sunderland, UK

Emilio Garcia FRCA
Consultant in Anaesthesia specialising in Intensive Care Medicine,
The James Cook University Hospital,
Middlesbrough, UK

Foreword by

Professor Mike Bramble MD FRCP
Medical Director, South Tees Hospitals NHS Trust, Middlesbrough, UK

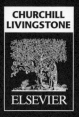

CHURCHILL
LIVINGSTONE

ELSEVIER

EDINBURGH LONDON NEW YORK OXFORD PHILADELPHIA ST LOUIS SYDNEY
TORONTO 2007

CHURCHILL LIVINGSTONE
ELSEVIER

© 2007, Elsevier Limited. All rights reserved.

The right of Stephen Bonner, Mark Carpenter and Emilio Garcia to be identified as editors of this work has been asserted by them in accordance with the Copyright, Designs and Patents Act 1988

First published 2007

ISBN-13: 978 0 443 10011 6
ISBN-10: 0 443 10011 X

British Library Cataloguing in Publication Data
A catalogue record for this book is available from the British Library

Library of Congress Cataloging in Publication Data
A catalog record for this book is available from the Library of Congress

Notice

Knowledge and best practice in this field are constantly changing. As new research and experience broaden our knowledge, changes in practice, treatment and drug therapy may become necessary or appropriate. Readers are advised to check the most current information provided (i) on procedures featured or (ii) by the manufacturer of each product to be administered, to verify the recommended dose or formula, the method and duration of administration, and contraindications. It is the responsibility of the practitioner, relying on their own experience and knowledge of the patient, to make diagnoses, to determine dosages and the best treatment for each individual patient, and to take all appropriate safety precautions. To the fullest extent of the law, neither the Publisher nor the Editors assume any liability for any injury and/or damage to persons or property arising out of or related to any use of the material contained in this book.

The Publisher

Printed in China

Foreword

Changes in the way that junior hospital doctors are trained have necessitated the development of courses such as CCrISP (care of the critically ill surgical patient) and CRIMP, which is the medical equivalent. At the time of writing the traditional SHO medical rotation is soon to be replaced by a second foundation year, followed by the first years of speciality training and a further reduction in working hours. This means that there is now an over-whelming need for junior doctors dealing with acutely ill medical patients to understand the pathophysiology and management of patients with conditions that they may have never seen before. Foundation year and specialist training doctors will increasingly find themselves in situations where they have little or no experience but where they should have some theoretical knowledge. This book bridges the gap between theory and practice by giving practical guidance on assessing such patients and initiating both investigations and treatment.

CRIMP is also very much geared to the acutely ill patient who might appear in the medical assessment unit just after midnight. The accurate assessment and appropriate investigation of such a patient is vital to effective management and treatment. Specific chapters deal with all the common medical emergencies in addition to excellent chapters on oxygen, fluid balance and sepsis. Ethical dilemmas are covered in a further chapter which I consider to be essential reading.

In my view this is a book that every junior doctor should read before they finish their foundation years.

Professor Mike Bramble MD FRCP
Medical Director, South Tees Hospitals NHS Trust,
Middlesbrough, UK

Preface

Over recent years it has been clearly demonstrated that the early recognition and treatment of critically ill patients improves outcome. This understanding had led to the development of services such as outreach, extending critical care skills out of critical care units to the ward environment. Such demands reinforce the requirement that hospital doctors of all grades and all specialities will need to have an understanding of critical care principles and the skills that may be transferred to the ward, high dependency or A&E environment to direct and guide management, particularly in the early hours and days of a patient's presentation where treatment may improve outcome, and indeed may remove the need for subsequent ventilation or admission to a critical care unit at all. This book aims to teach the principles of recognizing, approaching and treating the critically ill patient, together with practical advice, tips, how to perform common practical procedures in critically ill patients, ethical principles involved to guide decision making and self assessment clinical scenarios.

This book was written for all doctors in training grades in any acute hospital speciality who may be called upon to treat patients on the ward who develop life-threatening emergencies. It will also be useful for final year medical students approaching critical care attachments. In particular it should be invaluable reading for foundation year doctors who will rotate through a broad mix of acute hospital specialities, often involving critical care, where it should give them invaluable insight into approaching the critically ill patient and transferring these skills to the rest of their training. The acquisition of these vital skills is particularly important as the reduction in hours and patterns of work have reduced significantly the exposure of hospital medical trainees to medical emergencies and critically ill patients.

Topics include how to establish patients on non-invasive ventilation, understanding arterial blood gases, stabilising a patient in shock, oxygen and fluid resuscitation, principles of inotropic support, how to approach an unconscious patient, how to manage a tracheostomy on the ward and how to insert chest drains, perform lumbar punctures and different routes of central venous access, including use of ultrasound. In addition, chapters cover how to manage medical emergencies in cardiology, respiratory medicine, gastroenterology, metabolic disorders and neurology as well as the ethical principles involved in caring for the critically ill and recognizing futility, such as DNAR orders and advance directives.

This is a practical book aimed at transferring skills and principles for critical care, where patients often initially require urgent, potentially life-saving treatment, which may initially be directed more at stabilization than diagnosis. However, the topics covered also represent an essential knowledge base for any postgraduate medical examination where the principles of caring for the acutely ill patient are increasingly recognized as vital in examinations such as the MRCP, FRCS and FRCA. The book also contains numerous algorithms and updated national guidelines and we hope it will provide useful reading in acute medical wards, emergency units and high-dependency areas and for nurse practitioners and allied professions involved in treating acutely ill patients.

S. B.
M. C.
E. G.
2007

Contributors

Stephen Bonner MRCP FRCA
Consultant in Anaesthesia specialising in Intensive Care Medicine,
The James Cook University Hospital, Middlesbrough, UK

Kaye Cantlay BA MRCP FRCA
Specialist Registrar in Anaesthesia and Intensive Care Medicine,
Northern Region, c/o Royal Victoria Infirmary, Newcastle upon Tyne, UK

Mark Carpenter BSc MRCP FRCA
Consultant in Anaesthesia and Intensive Care Medicine,
City Hospitals Sunderland NHS Foundation Trust, Sunderland, UK

Nicky Cree FRCA
Specialist Registrar in Anaesthesia and Intensive Care Medicine,
The James Cook University Hospital, Middlesborough,
UK

Andrew Fisher BMedSci MRCP PhD
Senior Lecturer in Respiratory Medicine, University of Newcastle upon
Tyne, Newcastle upon Tyne, UK

Emilio Garcia FRCA
Consultant in Anaesthesia specialising in Intensive Care Medicine,
The James Cook University Hospital, Middlesbrough,
UK

Kyee Han FRCS FFAEM
Consultant in Accident and Emergency Medicine, The James Cook
University Hospital, Middlesbrough, UK

Richard Harrison MD FRCP
Consultant Physician in Respiratory Medicine, University Hospital of
North Tees, Stockton-on-Tees, UK

Emma Johns MD MRCP
Specialist Registrar in Gastroenterology, The Freeman Hospital,
Newcastle upon Tyne, UK

Jonathan Louden FRCP
Consultant Renal Physician, The James Cook University Hospital,
Middlesbrough, UK

Diane Monkhouse MRCP FRCA
Consultant in Anaesthesia specialising in Intensive Care Medicine,
The James Cook University Hospital, Middlesbrough, UK

Nick Pace FRCA
Consultant in Anaesthesia specialising in Intensive Care Medicine,
Western Infirmary, Glasgow, UK

Sean Parker BA MRCP
Clinical Research Associate/Specialist Registrar in Respiratory Medicine,
Freeman Hospital, Newcastle upon Tyne, UK

Richard Parris BSc MRCP FFAEM
Consultant in Accident and Emergency Medicine, Royal Bolton Hospital,
Bolton, UK

Jon Sturman MRCP FRCA
Specialist Registrar in Anaesthesia, Alder Hay Hospital, Liverpool, UK

Andrew Turley MRCP (UK) BMedSci(Hons) CertClinEd
Cardiology Specialist Registrar, University Hospital of North Tees,
Stockton on Tees, UK

Contents

An approach to the critically ill medical patient

Mark Carpenter

OBJECTIVES

After reading this chapter you should be able to:

- Understand the rationale behind the airway, breathing and circulation (ABC) approach to the critically ill patient

- Recognize and treat airway compromise

- Recognize severe respiratory compromise, and situations in which urgent treatment is required

- Understand the need to administer oxygen to all critically ill patients

- Recognize the presence of shock, and understand the principles behind its treatment

INTRODUCTION

Classical medical teaching tells us to treat patients according to the model in Figure 1.1. This model works well when establishing that the correct diagnosis is the major problem and when there is no urgency in starting treatment. It works less well when dealing with critically ill patients. The purpose of the modified approach (below) is two-fold: firstly, to recognize acutely ill patients as it is only through timely recognition of the patient who is acutely unwell that we can start resuscitation, and secondly, to start resuscitation at the same time as proceeding towards a diagnosis.

KEY POINTS IN APPROACHING THE CRITICALLY ILL PATIENT
- Management of the airway, breathing and circulation (ABC) can be done at the same time as progress towards a diagnosis.
- Assessment and treatment should occur simultaneously.
- Do not move on until the previous system is stable or being stabilized.
- Continual reassessment of the ABC is vital.

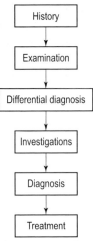

Figure 1.1 The classical approach to treatment of medical patients.

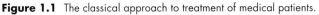

THE ABC APPROACH

The use of the ABC approach in patient assessment is widespread on resuscitation courses. The rationale is that problems that more quickly lead to patient death are dealt with and stabilized first. The fact that the abbreviation for the approach consists of the first three letters of the alphabet is fortuitous.

Airway

KEY POINTS: COMMON CAUSES OF AIRWAY COMPROMISE
- Altered level of consciousness
- Foreign body
- Inflammation
- Infection

In the presence of a completely obstructed airway, cardiorespiratory arrest will follow within minutes. Airway compromise makes breathing inadequate and the circulation pointless.

Airway assessment should be done first. A pragmatic approach is to address the patient. If a fluent answer follows it is reasonable to assume that the airway is open and the breathing adequate whilst formal assessment is performed. Airway assessment and resuscitation can be divided into four parts: look, listen, feel and act.

Look for evidence of obstruction: cyanosis, accessory muscle use, tracheal tug, tachypnoea, paradoxical breathing and reduced level of consciousness.

Listen for noisy breathing, and the phase of respiration in which it occurs. Inspiratory noise is common in large airway obstruction, whereas expiratory noise is more common with small distal airway obstruction, e.g. asthma.

Airway obstruction can be partial or complete. Partial obstruction is noisy with inspiratory or expiratory noise. Complete airway obstruction is silent but is accompanied by signs of respiratory difficulty.

Feel for movement of air.

Act: in the presence of airway obstruction open the airway immediately. Call for help but stay with the patient.

KEY POINT
- A patient with signs of airway obstruction should never be left alone.

Treatment follows a logical sequence progressing from simple measures that should be within the capabilities of the competent first-aider to complex airway manoeuvres requiring trained input. After every airway manoeuvre the airway should be reassessed. If the airway remains obstructed the next manoeuvre should be followed.

Basic life support measures

In the conscious patient, airway patency is maintained by muscle tone in the mouth and pharynx. This is lost in the unconscious patient. Basic life support measures are:

- Look in the mouth to exclude a large object (blind finger sweeping is no longer recommended as it can push obstructing objects further into the airway).
- Extend the neck and lift the chin. This has the effect of lifting the tongue off the back of the pharyngeal wall. This should not be done if there is a history of cervical instability, either because of trauma or arthritis.
- Perform a jaw thrust. This brings the jaw forward without moving the neck and is both a useful way of opening the airway in cases of suspected cervical spine disease, and a useful way of ensuring the position of an oropharyngeal airway following insertion.

Nebulized adrenaline (epinephrine)

Nebulised adrenaline (5 mg nebulized in oxygen) is of use with inflammatory and infectious causes of airway obstruction. Classically these would present as stridor in a conscious patient. The use of basic life support and airway adjunct methods in these patients is to be avoided as it can convert partial airway obstruction into total airway obstruction. Such patients should be allowed to sit erect and often forwards; laying them flat may precipitate total airway obstruction and cardiorespiratory arrest.

Oropharyngeal/nasopharyngeal airway insertion

If simple airway manoeuvres fail to open the airway, then an oropharyngeal or nasopharyngeal airway should be used. These work by bringing the tongue forward from the back of the pharyngeal wall. However, they are stimulating and can precipitate vomiting and laryngospasm in a partially conscious patient. The nasopharyngeal airway is less stimulating and can be used if the patient will not tolerate an oropharyngeal airway.

Oropharyngeal airways are sized in length from the incisors to the angle of the jaw. They are inserted concave side upwards and then rotated into position. A jaw thrust is often required to bring the tongue forward and allow it to sit properly. Once the airway is in place it may need to be kept there using a chin lift or jaw thrust.

Nasopharyngeal airways are sized from the tip of the nose to the tragus of the ear. They should be lubricated (with lidocaine (lignocaine) jelly in the conscious patient), and inserted backwards along the floor of the nose.

Definitive airway manoeuvres

Basic life support measures allow the opening of the airway and resuscitation by staff trained in basic life support. With an open airway, the patient may recover consciousness and the airway may improve. If this is not the case the airway may need to be secured to prevent aspiration of gastric contents. This is especially the case in patients who are sufficiently obtunded to tolerate an oropharyngeal airway. A definitive airway prevents aspiration of gastric contents and allows prolonged ventilation of the patient's lungs. This means tracheal intubation or tracheostomy insertion:

- Tracheal intubation: in the non-cardiac arrest patient this will require sedation and muscle relaxation. These skills are beyond the scope of this book. Call an anaesthetist.
- Tracheostomy: this can be carried out under local anaesthesia but is usually done in theatre under general anaesthesia. It is rarely performed as a first line measure in the emergency situation unless tracheal intubation is thought to be difficult, in which circumstances it is usually performed under local anaesthesia in theatre or occasionally in accident and emergency (A&E). It is more commonly carried out on an elective basis after a few days in intensive care and after the upper airway has been secured with tracheal intubation.

Breathing and oxygen

Once the airway has been opened and kept open the breathing should be assessed. Assessment should be by:

Look

- Rate
- Pattern
- Inequalities of the two sides of the chest
- Confusion.

Listen

- Adequacy of air entry bilaterally
- Presence of added sounds.

Feel

- Trachea
- Tidal volume.

This examination is aimed at resuscitation and finding immediately life-threatening situations. It should therefore be brief. This is not the time to, for example, elicit tactile vocal fremitus; such detailed examination is best left until after patient stability is assured.

Signs of severe respiratory compromise

- Tachypnoea > 25 bpm
- Bradypnoea < 10 bpm
- Accessory muscles of respiration
- Unable to complete sentences
- Confusion
- Cyanosis
- PaO_2 < 8 kPa despite high flow oxygen (patients with longstanding respiratory disease may have low PaO_2 and appear completely well; in these patients the clinical features above should be looked for instead of blindly looking at values of arterial blood gases (ABGs))
- $PaCO_2$ > 6 kPa (in patients with longstanding chronic obstructive pulmonary disorder (COPD) this figure should be revised in light of their normal figures).

Act

In the face of features of severe respiratory compromise act with:

- oxygen administration
- emergency measures appropriate for the patient.

Oxygen

This should be high concentration in the majority of patients (see chapter on oxygen).

Emergency measures

- Decompression of pneumothorax if tensioning (simple pneumothorax will rarely cause severe respiratory compromise in the previously well patient).
- Administration of salbutamol to patients with acute severe asthma.

- Nebulized adrenaline (epinephrine) or Heliox to patients with acute upper airway obstruction.
- Preparing nitrates/opioids/diuretics in severe pulmonary oedema.

These should be administered as soon as such conditions are diagnosed and delays in establishing such treatments should be avoided.

KEY POINT
- Oxygen and fluids will benefit the vast majority of critically ill medical patients.

High concentration oxygen and patients with COPD

All critically ill patients should receive oxygen. The incidence of hypoxic drive in a small proportion of patients with COPD should not deprive the hypoxic patient with pneumonia, asthma, or pulmonary oedema of high flow oxygen.

Deterioration due to failure of hypoxic drive producing a rising CO_2 is a gradual phenomenon which should be monitored and the patient regularly assessed by arterial blood gases and clinical status. Most patients who do rely on a hypoxic drive have severe limiting respiratory disease and often are known to have an established hypoxic drive. If in doubt give oxygen and review. Hypoxia kills rapidly.

Aim to get the oxygen saturation > 90% in all patients, using as much oxygen as is required to achieve this. Be observant in all patients and monitor blood gases, particularly if the patient appears to be hypoventilating or is becoming drowsy. Hypercarbia usually represents exhaustion and is a predictor of potential for respiratory arrest. In most patients the appropriate action is to institute artificial ventilation, either invasive or non-invasive rather than reduce the inspired oxygen concentration.

Circulation

The circulation should then be assessed, and treated.

KEY POINTS
- Shock is a failure of organ perfusion.
- Hypotension is a late and often (if untreated) premorbid sign in all forms of shock.

Assessment

Look

- Sweating
- Pallor
- Tachypnoea (a sign of metabolic acidosis).

Feel

- Cold peripheries
- Capillary refill time > 2 s
- Tachycardia
- Narrow pulse pressure
- Hypotension.

Act

IV access

IV access should be established in all critically ill patients; this should be large bore cannulae (16 or 14G). In cases of shock it is advisable to site two cannulae for rapid infusion of fluids and in case one becomes dislodged.

Fluid therapy

Fluid therapy is appropriate for all cases of shock with the exception of some cases of cardiogenic shock. This is best administered as fluid boluses of 250–500 mL with reassessment of the patient between successive boluses. Optimization of fluid status is essential if inotropes are being considered. Inappropriate use of inotropes without adequate filling can lead to increased myocardial oxygen consumption, and too great a degree of vasoconstriction with diversion of blood flow away from the gut.

Inotropes/vasodilators

Inotropes should be used following adequate fluid resuscitation. Usually central venous access will have been established both for monitoring of cardiac filling and administration of the inotropes.

Monitoring

Arterial lines: allow beat to beat measurement of blood pressure and repeated measurement of blood gases.

Central lines: it is often difficult to determine fluid status of a critically ill patient using clinical signs alone (Table 1.1). Central lines and the administration of inotropes are useful for this. It is usually more appropriate to insert

Table 1.1 Clinical signs

	Hypovolaemia	Hypervolaemia
Pulse	→ or ↑	→ or ↑
Blood pressure	→ or ↓	→ or ↑
Respiratory rate	↑	↑
Oedema	+/−	+/−
Urine output	↓	↓ or → or ↑

The ABC approach

Table 1.2   Hypovolaemic shock

	Class I	Class II	Class III	Class IV
Blood loss	< 750 mL	750–1500 mL	1500–2000 mL	> 2000 mL
Blood loss as a percentage of total blood volume	< 15%	15–30%	30–40%	> 40%
Pulse rate	< 100	> 100	> 120	> 140
Blood pressure	Normal	Normal	Decreased	Decreased
Pulse pressure	Normal or increased	Decreased	Decreased	Decreased
Respiratory rate	14–20	20–30	30–40	> 35

a central line to optimize fluid filling in a shocked patient in order to achieve stability, before carrying on to secure a diagnosis with either detailed physical examination or investigations. Fluid resuscitation can therefore be ongoing as such investigations are happening.

Hypotension is a particularly late and dangerous sign in patients with hypovolaemic shock. Table 1.2 shows the response to shock in a patient with a normal cardiovascular response. The elderly and those on drugs that prevent a tachycardic response to hypovolaemia may exhibit Class IV shock without passing through the tachycardic stage. Children and adolescents maintain blood pressure until very late in shocked states.

Disability/brief neurological assessment

Assessment of level of consciousness is the last part of the initial assessment. Again this is not a thorough neurological examination but a brief assessment with which to guide immediate resuscitative therapy.

The AVPU scale combined with assessment of the pupils is sufficient at this stage.

AVPU

A Alert
V Responds to verbal stimuli
P Responds to painful stimuli
U Unresponsive

The presence of P or U is consistent with a diagnosis of coma and requires urgent attention to protection of the airway before any transfer is considered. More in-depth measurement of coma should be considered once the patient has been initially assessed. This should be done using the Glasgow Coma Score (see Ch. 9 for central nervous system emergencies).

Pupils

Are the pupils equal, what size are they, and do they respond to light?

Inequality should alert you to the possibility of intracranial space-occupying lesions. Small pupils should alert you to the possibility of opiate abuse or brain stem stroke. It is important not to become too focused on the neurological status of the patient too early. This assessment and investigation and treatment of the underlying pathology (e.g. computed tomography (CT) scan, lumbar puncture) should always be delayed until the patient is stabilized.

Seek diagnosis

Once the patient has been stabilized move on to seeking a definitive diagnosis, but be aware that deterioration can occur and it may be necessary to reassess and treat the ABC. Diagnosis takes the form of:

- history
- examination
- chart review.

Definitive treatment

Instigate appropriate treatment.

Referral

Determine the appropriate place to care for the patient. This will depend largely on the patient's physiological status and the amount of continuing resuscitation that will be required. It is also important to consider whether there is a possibility of subsequent deterioration after your initial assessment. Examples include patients after tricyclic antidepressant overdoses and those having taken large quantities of slowly absorbed opioids. These patients should be kept under continuous observation.

Seek help

Patients quite reasonably expect to be treated by appropriately trained personnel. Get help if you feel that you need it. This can be from senior people in your own speciality or from fellow trainees in an emergency. If you feel that you might be out of your depth then you almost certainly are.

KEY POINTS
At all times:
- Recognize the severity of illness and call for appropriate personnel and equipment.
- Reassess ABC informally or formally.
- Monitor the patient.
- Do not leave the patient alone.
- Ensure ECG, pulse oximetry, and non-invasive blood pressure (NIBP) as a minimum standard of monitoring.
- Do not get out of your depth: ask for the help of seniors, fellow trainees and other specialities.

Scoring systems

Various scoring systems exist to define the severity of patient illness and to predict mortality. Most of these are not designed to be used on individual patients, but as statistical tools for research and audit.

Acute Physiology and Chronic Health Evaluation II (APACHE II) is widely used to measure the severity of illness of patients admitted to critical care units, and can be used to predict the mortality of patients admitted to different units with different case mixes. It combines two main components, 12 Acute Physiology markers (weighted and the worst result in the first 24 h of the patient's admission), points for age and points for severe comorbidity. It is widely used to measure the differences between critical care units' case mix and to compare mortality in different years. Scores range from 0–59.

MEWS (modified early warning system) exists in many different forms throughout the UK. It is used differently to APACHE in that it is used on an individual patient basis to define the severity of a patient's physiological response to illness. It can be easily applied on the ward and used as part of ward observations. It relies on observations that can be made easily by the most junior member of ward staff. In addition it can be used as part of a track and trigger approach to critical care outreach services (see below).

An example of a typical MEWS scoring system is shown in Table 1.3.

Levels of dependency

Comprehensive Critical Care (Department of Health) defined different levels of care that can be delivered in different parts of the acute hospital. Care was defined from level 0 to level 3 (Table 1.4). Increasingly, level 2 and 3 beds are being grouped together as part of integrated critical care units, allowing more flexibility.

Critical care outreach

Comprehensive Critical Care (Department of Health) suggested a hospital-wide integrated approach to critical care: 'critical care without walls'. Part of the recommendations was to establish critical care outreach teams in every

Table 1.3 Typical MEWS scoring system

	3	2	1	0	1	2	3
Heart rate		< 40	41–50	51–100	101–110	111–130	>130
Systolic blood pressure	< 70	71–80	81–100	101–160	161–200	> 200	
Respiratory rate		< 8		9–14	15–20	21–29	> 30
Temperature		< 35	35.1–36.0	36.1	37.5	> 37.5	
Neurological response	Unconscious	To pain	To voice	Alert			

In this example a patient score varies from 0–14. Typical scores to trigger response from critical care outreach are in the order of 5–6 depending on the clinical situation.

Table 1.4 Levels of dependency

Level 0 Patients whose needs can be met through ward care in an acute hospital
Level 1 Patients at risk of their condition deteriorating or those recently relocated from higher levels of care, whose needs can be met on an acute ward with additional advice and support from the critical care team
Level 2 Patients requiring more observation or intervention including support for a single failing organ system or postoperative care and those 'stepping down' from higher levels of care
Level 3 Patients requiring advanced respiratory support alone or basic respiratory support together with support for at least two organ systems. This level includes all complex patients requiring support for multiorgan failure

hospital. These teams have different names and operational policies in different hospitals, but have similar goals to:

- avert admissions to intensive care through early recognition and treatment of the critically ill
- enable discharge from intensive care, by supporting the care of patients on the ward following a critical care unit stay
- share critical care skills with ward staff.

Outreach staff have the ability to support staff on the ward with the sickest patients, either to prevent their admission to higher levels of care or to facilitate their stabilization prior to transfer to the appropriate place of care.

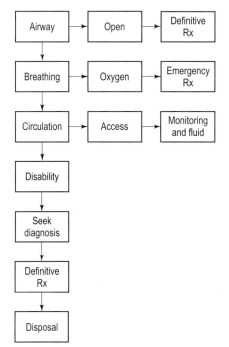

Figure 1.2 The CCrIMP approach to treatment of medical patients.

The ABC approach

SUMMARY

Effective treatment of medical emergencies relies on treating what is most important first. Whilst a social history may be vital to the effective rehabilitation of an elderly stroke patient, a young asthmatic about to have a respiratory arrest in A&E requires immediate treatment before a detailed history and examination are undertaken. In such circumstances, questions and examinations should be limited to those areas relevant to the patient's immediate treatment, e.g. are theophyllines or steroids being taken and what treatment has been received before presentation? The rest of the history and examination may be gathered as treatment is ongoing. Following this approach to the critically ill patient will allow you to assess and treat the critically ill in a more logical manner (Fig. 1.2).

FURTHER READING

Department of Health 2000 Comprehensive Critical Care. Online. Available: http://www.dh.gov.uk/assetRoot/04/08/28/72/04082872.pdf

Knaus W A, Draper E A, Wagner D P et al 1985 APACHE II: a severity of disease classification system. Critical Care Medicine 13(10):818–829

Murphy R, Mackway-Jones K, Sammy I et al 2001 Emergency oxygen therapy for the breathless patient. Guidelines prepared by North West Oxygen Group. Emergency Medicine Journal 18:421–423

National Confidential Enquiry into Patient Outcome and Death (NCEPOD). An acute problem. Online. Available: http://www.ncepod.org.uk/2005report/NCEPOD_Report_2005.pdf

Stenhouse C, Coates S, Tivey M et al 2000 Prospective evaluation of a modified Early Warning Score to aid early detection of patients developing critical illness on a general surgical ward. British Journal of Anaesthesia 84:663

AN APPROACH TO THE CRITICALLY ILL MEDICAL PATIENT

Oxygen delivery

Emilio Garcia

2

OBJECTIVES

After reading this chapter you should have an understanding of:

- *Oxygen cascade*

- *Means of oxygen storage*

- *Means of oxygen delivery*

- *Oxygen measurement*

- *Practical tips*

> **KEY POINTS**
> - Hypoxia kills.
> - All critically ill patients are at risk of hypoxia.
> - Do not wait for the results of investigations before treating with oxygen.

THE OXYGEN CASCADE

Oxygen is essential for maintenance of cellular function and stability. The main objective of treating any patient is ensuring adequate oxygen delivery. The transfer of oxygen from the atmosphere to the tissues involves a number of steps called the oxygen cascade (Fig. 2.1).

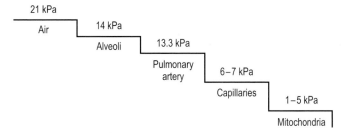

Figure 2.1 Oxygen cascade.

Table 2.1 Altitude

Altitude (feet)	BP (mmHg)	PO_2 in air (mmHg)	PO_2 alveoli (mmHg)	Sats (%)
0	760	159	104	97
10 000	523	110	67	90
20 000	349	73	40	70
30 000	226	47	21	20
40 000	141	29	8	5
50 000	87	18	1	1

Dry atmospheric gas contains a partial pressure of 21 kPa of oxygen (21%). This is dependent mainly on atmospheric pressure. Consequently, at altitude this will be less (see Table 2.1). This is what we breathe. As atmospheric gas is inhaled the gas is humidified and mixed with exhaled carbon dioxide; hence the partial pressure of oxygen is decreased to 14 kPa at alveolar level.

Airplanes normally fly at 36 000 feet but are pressurised between 5000–8000 feet resulting in an inspired PO_2 of 125 mmHg ($\div$ 17 kPa).

Oxygen then will diffuse into lung capillaries down a concentration gradient, and in arterial blood in the normal individual the partial pressure of oxygen is around 13.3 kPa. By the time oxygen reaches the peripheral capillaries, partial pressure of oxygen is only 6–7 kPa. Oxygen diffuses into mitochondria where the oxygen content varies between 1 and 5 kPa.

Any abnormalities at any step of the oxygen cascade will cause hypoxia at mitochondrial level. Hypoxia can be classified into a number of types as follows.

CLASSIFICATION OF HYPOXIA

Hypoxic hypoxia: this occurs in situations where the arterial partial pressure of oxygen PaO_2 is reduced. In other words the arterial oxygen content is low despite normal haemoglobin. This could be due to reduced inspired oxygen (aircrafts, fires, altitude, etc.), shunt (any situation where ventilation/perfusion mismatch occurs, e.g. pneumonia) and limited lung diffusion capacity (e.g. pulmonary fibrosis).

Anaemic hypoxia: despite adequate inspired oxygen, the oxygen cannot be delivered to peripheral tissues due to reduced haemoglobin. This occurs in anaemia or due to abnormally functioning haemoglobin, e.g. in carbon monoxide (CO) poisoning resulting in impaired oxygen carriage.

Stagnant hypoxia: this is due to reduced tissue blood flow owing to either poor cardiac output, e.g. in the case of congestive cardiac failure (CCF) or to local flow interruption, e.g. in the case of myocardial infarction (MI).

Histotoxic hypoxia: this is where, despite adequate oxygen delivery to mitochondria, the organelles cannot make use of it due to abnormally or non-functioning enzymes, e.g. cyanide poisoning. This results in conversion to anaerobic metabolism and cellular dysfunction, which may lead to death if not corrected.

CONTROL OF RESPIRATION

Respiratory rate and depth varies from person to person. In general, normal respiratory rate varies between 12 and 20 breaths per minute (bpm). Through respiration we aim to maintain oxygen, carbon dioxide and pH homeostasis.

The elements involved are the cortex (voluntary control), brain stem (automatic control) and mechano- and chemoreceptors, which all modify the action of respiratory muscles.

- Chemoreceptors respond to changes in CO_2, O_2 and pH.
- Mechanoreceptors respond to changes in the compliance of respiratory muscles and lung.

  Involuntary breathing originates from three centres in the brainstem:

- Medullary respiratory centre, which is divided into two parts:
    - dorsal, which is involved in inspiration, with output through the phrenic nerve
    - ventral, which is involved in expiration; it is inactive in normal respiration.
- Apneustic centre, which is located in the lower pons.
- Pneumotaxic centre, which is located in the upper pons.

By complex interaction they regulate breathing in response to signals obtained from mechano- and baroreceptors. This is a feedback system.

Chemoreceptors are responsible for the regulation of normal quiet breathing. They are located in the ventrolateral medulla in close proximity to cerebrospinal fluid (CSF) and in the carotid and aortic bodies. These respond to changes in $PaCO_2$ which alter CSF [H^+] concentration.

Central chemoreceptors only respond to changes in $PaCO_2$. Peripheral chemoreceptors also respond to PaO_2 and dissolved oxygen content.

Response to hypercarbia

This is the most important mechanism in the control of respiration. Hypercarbia is sensed by chemoreceptors in proximity to CSF. Changes in $PaCO_2$ result in changes in the concentration of H^+ in CSF, which is not significantly buffered and therefore is dependent only on respiratory changes in $PaCO_2$ to maintain normal CSF pH. Changing pH in the CSF is detected by chemoreceptors on the ventral surface of the medulla. The changes in ventilation in relation to $PaCO_2$ are linear. This means if we halve ventilation (minute volume) we will double $PaCO_2$, hence the importance of this mechanism. When $PaCO_2$ values are above 12 kPa CO_2, narcosis occurs, eventually rendering the patient unconscious and depressing ventilatory drive.

Response to hypoxia

The response to hypoxia is mediated by carotid bodies. It is less important than the response to hypercarbia, however in some types of chest disease (CO_2 retainers) it can overcome the importance of the response to hypercarbia.

The response to hypoxia is non-linear. In fact it is negligible until the PaO_2 is less than 12 kPa and then increases dramatically when the PaO_2 is below 7 kPa.

Response to acidaemia

Metabolic acidosis will exacerbate the normal response to an increase of $PaCO_2$ and metabolic alkalosis will decrease the response to hypercarbia.

It is important to note that acidosis will be compensated for by other mechanisms over a few days, making this response only temporary once the main abnormality is compensated for.

SYMPTOMS AND SIGNS OF HYPOXIA

Hypoxia can cause very mild symptoms that are initially difficult to interpret and may not be apparent until very late in the disease process, by which time irreversible damage may have occurred.

Common symptoms and signs of hypoxia are:

• cyanosis
• hyperventilation
• confusion
• altered level of consciousness
• hypertension
• tachycardia
• convulsions.

MEANS OF OXYGEN STORAGE

Cylinders

Oxygen cylinders in the UK are universally marked with a black body and white shoulder. Any other cylinder with different colour coding will not contain oxygen (Fig. 2.2).

Oxygen content and outlet connectors of most common cylinders vary according to cylinder size and it is vital to ensure that the appropriate connections are available. In order to choose the appropriate cylinder size for oxygen treatment away from a wall connector, e.g. for a journey, whether this is to another hospital or the X-ray department, it is necessary to know the oxygen content of each cylinder and the oxygen flow required together with an estimate of the duration of the oxygen therapy required. It is then possible to calculate the total amount of oxygen required and therefore the number of cylinders required. The content of the most popular cylinders and fittings are listed in Table 2.2.

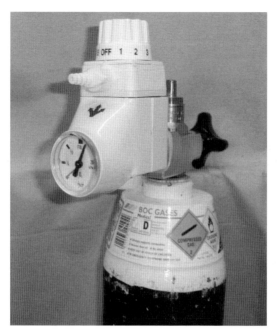

Figure 2.2 Oxygen cylinder.

Table 2.2 Oxygen content and outlet fittings in different cylinder sizes

Cylinder size	Valve outlet connection	Content in litres
C	Yoke fitting	170
SD	Yoke fitting	300
D	Yoke fitting	340
AD	6 mm firtree	460
RD	6 mm firtree + yoke fitting	460
CD	6 mm firtree + yoke fitting	460
DD	6 mm firtree	460
E	Yoke fitting	680
F	BSP	1360
G	BSP	3400

CASE 2.1

A 62-year-old man on 4 L/min of oxygen requires a V/Q scan. You estimate the maximum time for the transfer plus the scan amounts to 2 h. How much oxygen is required and which cylinder is required?

4 L/min × (120 + 30 min) = 600 L

It is always recommended that at least an additional 30 min of oxygen is taken to overcome unexpected events = 720 L.

Therefore a size E cylinder or 2 × D (or AD/CD/RD/DD) would be required for transfer.

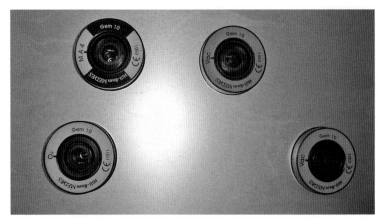

Figure 2.3   Schraeder connectors from a wall outlet.

Liquid oxygen

Smaller hospitals supply oxygen using a bank of oxygen cylinders. However, large hospitals find it more convenient and economic to store oxygen in a liquid state. This is stored in a large container situated outside the hospital and looks like a fuel tank with a frozen pipe coming out of it.

Nonetheless, whatever oxygen supply your hospital has, the common wall outlet is a universal Schraeder connector, which is not only colour coded white but is also key coded so that only an oxygen connector can be attached, for example, either an oxygen flowmeter or a male Schraeder connector is used to connect to a ventilator (Fig. 2.3).

Oxygen concentrators

Small hospitals and some patients at home will have oxygen concentrators. These pass compressed air through a series of zeolites to eliminate nitrogen and deliver 99.8% oxygen. This is very economic although dependent on electrical supply.

Oxygen concentrators are very reliable but require servicing every 5000 h of use. Home devices produce flows up to 8 L/min.

Commonly, where there is any oxygen use, no smoking is allowed near concentrators or oxygen tubing.

MEANS OF OXYGEN DELIVERY

Once you have decided to administer oxygen to a patient you must decide on the concentration to be delivered and therefore the appropriate means of delivery. There are plenty of different commercial devices available and for simplicity we can classify them as:

- fixed performance devices
- variable performance devices
- devices that will allow intermittent positive pressure ventilation (IPPV).

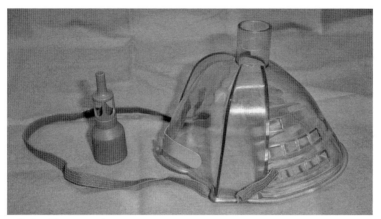

Figure 2.4 Venturi mask.

Fixed performance devices

These are based on the Bernouilli effect. When a fluid or gas increases velocity through a constriction, this causes an increase in kinetic energy, and as total energy must remain the same, this is compensated for by a drop in pressure which may be used to entrain a second fluid (Venturi principle).

As the masks in Figure 2.4 use the Venturi principle they are commonly called Venturi masks. They consist of a fixed orifice through which oxygen passes, increasing velocity and hence causing a drop in pressure, which determines air entrainment to a fixed percentage.

The fixed orifice is also colour coded and the amount of oxygen needed for the mask to function is marked on the side.

These masks are very accurate and have the capacity to deliver a high flow of oxygen. Their main disadvantages are that they deliver a high flow of dry gas which in turn will dry the patient's upper airway and secretions, and that some patients find this high flow of gas (30–60 L/m) claustrophobic.

Variable performance devices

Variable performance devices (VPDs) deliver an approximate concentration of oxygen which is dependent on many other factors and can only be roughly estimated. VPDs in common use include:

Nasal prongs

These are commonly referred to as nasal specs (Fig. 2.5). This is a very simple device that consists of a clear plastic tube that adapts to the face with two exits, one for each nostril. It is connected to an oxygen flow of 2–4 L/min to deliver between 24–35% oxygen. The oxygen can be humidified.

Nasal prongs are well tolerated by patients, but very ineffective as most patients breathe through their mouth, particularly at times of distress and also because peak inspiratory flow rate (60 L/min) will greatly exceed the maximal flow administered. Such a high flow is very difficult to match and it

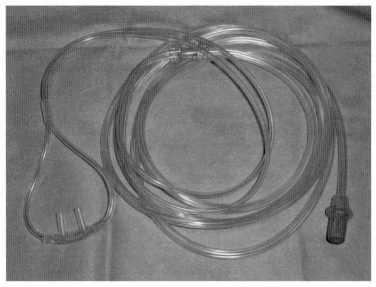

Figure 2.5 Nasal prongs.

is certainly not feasible to do this without specialized devices, bearing in mind that maximum flow from a flowmeter is 15 L/min.

Nasal sponge

This device is very similar to the nasal prongs. It consists of a plastic tube with an open end surrounded by sponge that fixes the tube to one of the nostrils. The nasal sponge suffers from the same pitfalls as the nasal prongs. This device is particularly useful during the performance of a bronchoscopy.

Hudson mask

This is the most common device used in clinical practice (Fig. 2.6). It consists of a face mask which is attached to oxygen tubing and has side vents for air entrance and exhaled gases.

When attached to an oxygen flow of 12 L/min it delivers approximately 50–60% oxygen. This will vary a lot depending on the patient's breathing pattern. When used with lower flows the percentage of oxygen delivered is also decreased, for example if we attach it to a 4 L/min flow the concentration of oxygen delivered will be between 35 and 40% depending again on the patient's inspiratory flow rate.

This mask is well tolerated by patients and oxygen can easily be humidified, however it does not allow close control of inspired oxygen.

Hudson mask with reservoir (Fig. 2.7)

This is a modification of the Hudson mask that consists of the addition of a reservoir bag attached to the mask through an orifice that is bigger than the

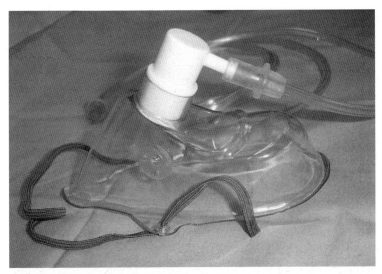

Figure 2.6 Hudson mask.

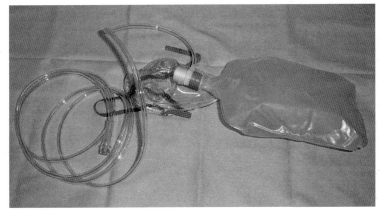

Figure 2.7 Hudson mask with reservoir bag to deliver high percentage of oxygen.

side vents of the mask. In this way, during inspiration, gas will be drawn preferentially from the mask rather than from the atmosphere.

When connected to an oxygen flow greater than 12 L/min it delivers approximately 90% oxygen. It is important to fill the reservoir bag before connecting it to the patient. This can be done easily by occluding the mask from the inside with your thumb or finger.

New models of this device have a ball attached in a side tube to allow easy monitoring of respiratory rate.

Devices that will allow continuous positive airways pressure (CPAP) or intermittent positive pressure ventilation (IPPV)

These devices are mostly used by anaesthetists in theatre although physicians may use them during resuscitation. We will only discuss two of the most commonly used devices, the Ambu bag and the Water's circuit.

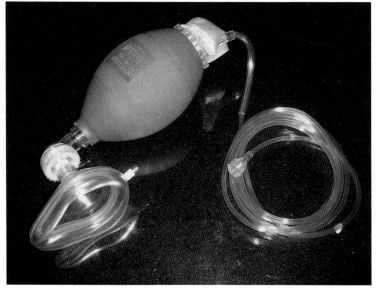

Figure 2.8 Ambu bag.

Ambu bag (Fig. 2.8)

This device consists of a semirigid bag into which oxygen is administered and two one-way valves to prevent mixing of inspired and exhaled gases. This device will allow spontaneous breathing but it will also allow assisted breathing by squeezing the bag. The oxygen mixture can be enriched by attaching oxygen to the bag and it is possible to get close to 100% oxygen by adding a reservoir bag to the system and ensuring that oxygen flow is more than 12 L/min.

This device can function independently of oxygen supply, however in this scenario it will only provide air.

Water's circuit

This is also known as a rebreath bag. It consists of a reservoir bag, oxygen inlet and a variable pressure relief valve.

The oxygen inlet is connected to an oxygen flowmeter through oxygen tubing and is set at 10–15 L/min. When the variable pressure relief valve is opened it allows spontaneous breathing, but when it is closed it allows artificial ventilation. As there is no one-way valve this apparatus allows the mixing of inspired and expired gases, hence allowing rebreathing (rebreath bag) and limiting its inspired oxygen concentration to approximately 90%. It is however a very versatile device (and a favourite of anaesthetists) as it allows the patient to breathe spontaneously. Because of the reservoir bag in the circuit it also allows observation of respiration and performance of CPAP.

Whatever method is selected requires an understanding of the ability of each device to deliver different percentages of oxygen as may be demonstrated in Table 2.3.

Table 2.3 Approximate oxygen delivery using different delivery devices

Oxygen flow rate	L/min	FiO$_2$
Nasal cannulae	2	0.28
	4	0.36
	6	0.44
Hudson mask	5–6	0.40
	6–7	0.50
	7–8	0.60
Hudson mask with	6	0.60
reservoir	8	0.80
	10	> 0.80

FiO$_2$, fraction of inspired oxygen

OXYGEN MEASUREMENT

In order to determine which patients may benefit from oxygen therapy we need to have a means of assessing oxygenation.

These must include clinical signs. If the patient is pink and cerebrating normally one may assume that the patient's brain is receiving sufficient oxygen. As was mentioned before the clinical signs of hypoxia can be very subtle and range from mild confusion or inappropriate behaviour to cyanosis, convulsions and death.

Another means of assessing the patient's oxygenation must then be used. In particular we will look at pulse oximetry and arterial blood gases.

Pulse oximetry

Pulse oximetry gives an indication of oxygen saturation through the measurement of radiation absorption. The pulse oximeter relies on measuring the different absorption of oxyhaemoglobin and deoxyhaemoglobin at two wavelengths, 940 nanometers (nm) (oxyhaemoglobin) and 660 nm (deoxyhaemoglobin), and then calculating the amount of oxyhaemoglobin as a percentage (Fig. 2.9).

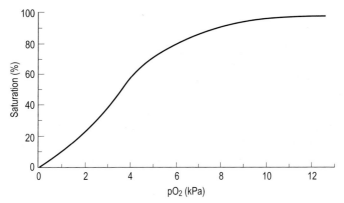

Figure 2.9 Oxygen dissociation curve.

Because of the sigmoid shape of the oxygen dissociation curve we must try to keep oxygen saturation above 90–92%, as from there, any further drop in saturation will correspond to a greater drop in arterial oxygen content and therefore oxygen delivery to the tissues, as indicated in Fig. 2.9.

The amount of O_2 carried by haemoglobin is not directly dependent on the PO_2. This is due to positive cooperativity, which means once haemoglobin binds the first oxygen molecule it is easier for others to do so, hence the sigmoid shape of the dissociation curve.

The oxygen dissociation curve can shift to the right or to the left depending on circumstances. A right shift indicates decreased oxygen affinity, so the haemoglobin molecule is more likely to release O_2. This potentially allows more oxygen to be released to the tissues in times of stress. A right shift will be caused by an increase of four factors:

- temperature
- (H$^+$)
- PCO_2
- red cell 2–3 DPG level.

This is, for example, what happens in tissues during exercise, whereas a decrease in the four factors listed above causes a deviation to the left.

The Bohr Effect plays an important role in the oxygen dissociation curve. Carbon dioxide diffuses into alveoli when the blood passes through the lungs; this results in a decrease in both blood PCO_2 and hydrogen ion concentration. This shifts the dissociation curve to the left. The amount of oxygen that binds with haemoglobin at any given alveolar PO_2 increases and provides for greater O_2 transport to the tissues. When the blood reaches tissue capillaries, CO_2 enters the blood and shifts the curve to the right, thus displacing oxygen from haemoglobin and oxygen delivery occurs at a higher PO_2.

Shortcomings of a pulse oximeter

- Low pulse pressure, hypotension, vasoconstriction, irregular heart rate and venous pulsation make it harder for the instrument to define the points of maximum and minimum absorption. This may be overcome by the use of the c-lock mode with which the measurements are synchronized with the QRS of the ECG. C-lock is also useful during transfers of critically ill patients as vibrations from movement interfere with the signal.
- Abnormal haemoglobin cannot be detected:
  - carboxyhaemoglobin – falsely high reading
  - methaemoglobin – 85% reading.
- High bilirubin levels – falsely low reading.
- Pulse oximetry does not imply any assessment of CO_2, which may rise to dangerous levels in the presence of adequate pulse oximeter readings.

Arterial blood gas monitoring

This is the gold standard for the measurement of arterial oxygen. An arterial blood sample is obtained and transported in a heparinized syringe. This blood sample will be analyzed by the blood gas machine that has a Clarke electrode and will indicate the arterial oxygen content.

Other information obtained from an arterial blood gas that is of utmost relevance to the physician is pH, PCO_2 and BE. All these factors are necessary for the correct interpretation of blood gas (see Ch. 4).

Tip

Very little heparin is necessary for a blood gas. If using a prefilled syringe simply expel any excess heparin but if using a normal 2 mL syringe, aspirate 0.5 mL of 1:1000 heparin (red one) and expel it completely. The amount left in the syringe will suffice. Do not use 1 : 5000 heparin (blue one) as the result will be affected by its acidity.

PRACTICAL TIPS

Oxygen is rarely detrimental to patients, whatever underlying pathology they may have, hence as a rule you should administer oxygen to anyone who appears unwell. A good starting point will be the administration of 12 L/min of oxygen via a Hudson mask. One must remember that hypoxia kills faster than hypercarbia. In patients with known severe chronic obstructive pulmonary disease (COPD), start with sufficient oxygen to increase the SpO_2 to > 90%, but be prepared to alter this depending on the blood gas results (see Ch. 8).

Hypoxic drive is rare and is usually only seen in patients with severe COPD and usually prolonged raised CO_2. In this group of patients, normal respiratory drive is no longer determined by hypercarbia as their respiratory centres have become accustomed to hypercarbia and only respond to hypoxia, a much more primitive stimuli of the respiratory centres.

Early use of pulse oximetry will be a helpful tool in the assessment of response, however this will need to be matched to an arterial blood gas for accuracy and carbon dioxide assessment.

In patients with COPD, previous history and previous arterial blood gases, particularly at the time of discharge, will be of paramount importance at the time of choosing the type of oxygen therapy. Equally, in patients who have been discharged from the critical care unit, the blood gas on discharge for comparison will be of utmost importance for any subsequent deterioration on the ward.

Patients who will require long-term oxygen therapy must have their oxygen humidified. Dried gases will result in dried secretions and abnormal ciliary function with both resulting in sputum retention and worsening of the initial problem.

Remember to involve the critical care unit team and physiotherapists early, as both can give you helpful tips in the administration of oxygen therapy and will continue to assess the patient in order to decide whether critical care unit admission is appropriate or not.

CASE 2.2

A 65-year-old epileptic woman is admitted to accident and emergency after having been involved in a chip pan fire at home. Other past medical history includes a subarachnoid haemorrhage three years previously resulting in good recovery other than epilepsy.

The casualty officer calls you to review her due to the lack of control of her epilepsy but he is happy with her as there are no signs of inhalation injury and her oxygen saturation is 99% on air.

What are your preliminary thoughts?

There should be a few initial concerns with the management of this patient, as follows.

The patient should be administered high flow oxygen despite her saturation as there is a high chance that she has carboxyhaemoglobinaemia. Carbon monoxide binds to haemoglobin with an affinity 240 times greater than oxygen and only reverses in the presence of high fraction of inspired oxygen (FiO_2). The pulse oximeter will not differentiate between oxyhaemoglobin and carboxyhaemoglobin, hence the reading of 99% is not informative. The only way of identifying abnormal haemoglobin is the use of a co-oximeter. Carboxyhaemoglobin levels should be checked using a co-oximeter and if there is severe poisoning, hyperbaric oxygen should be considered.

CASE 2.3

A 45-year-old man is admitted to your ward with community-acquired bronchopneumonia which is confirmed clinically, radiologically and is awaiting microbiology results.

The nurses are concerned because he does not look as well now as he did originally. They show you three sets of blood gases. What is your interpretation of them?

	On admission	3 hours later	Current
FiO_2	Air	60%	60%
pH	7.31	7.30	7.18
PO_2	6.7	15.8	14.9
PCO_2	4.3	4.8	8.7
BE	−1.2	−2.0	−3.7

The most important issue that these blood gases highlight is the fact that PO_2 is the best marker of oxygenation; however it is not a good marker for ventilation. PCO_2, on the contrary, is and this gentleman's PCO_2 has continued to rise despite adequate oxygenation, demonstrating type II respiratory failure. This patient is getting tired and will probably need respiratory support of some form, either invasive or non-invasive ventilation.

APPENDIX: OXYGEN CALCULATIONS

Oxygen cylinder contents

Oxygen is carried as a compressed gas in oxygen cylinders. To calculate the amount of oxygen present in a cylinder you must know:

- the cylinder size
- the cylinder gauge pressure
- Boyle's law.

Boyle's law

At constant temperature the volume (V) of a fixed mass of a perfect gas varies inversely with pressure (P).

i.e: $P \times V = constant$
and: $P1 \times V1 = P2 \times V2$

> **Example**
> A full oxygen cylinder size E has a gauge pressure of 137 bar and a volume of 5 L.
> $137 \times 5 = 685$ L
> This will be the equivalent of 680 L at atmospheric pressure plus 5 L left in the empty oxygen cylinder.

Oxygen requirement calculation

Calculate how much oxygen will be required for the journey, and take TWICE AS MUCH to allow for unexpected delays. An extra 30 min supply of oxygen should be the minimum requirement.

To calculate the amount of oxygen required, you must know:

- present oxygen flow
- expected journey time (min).

> **Example**
> Patient using a Hudson mask with a reservoir: 15 L/min
> Journey time 50 min
> Journey time = 50 + 30 = 80 min
> Gas required = $15 \times 80 = 1200$
> Size E cylinders required = 1200/680 = 1.76 = 2 cylinders

Oxygen calculations

In the UK, oxygen cylinders are black with white shoulders.

D size   340 L
E size   680 L
F size   1360 L (F size cylinders may have bull nose valve fittings instead of pin index fittings; appropriate connections must be available.)

FURTHER READING

Al-Shaikh B, Stacey S 1995 Essentials of anaesthetic equipment. Churchill Livingstone, Edinburgh

American Thoracic Society/European Respiratory Society Task Force 2004 (updated 8 September 2005) Standards for the diagnosis and management of patients with COPD. Version 1.2. New York: American Thoracic Society. Online. Available: http://www.thoracic.org/copd/

Davis P, Parbrook G, Kenny G 1995 Basic physics and measurement in anaesthesia, 4th edn. Butterworth Heineman, Oxford

Guyton A C, Hall J E 2006 Textbook of medical physiology, 11th edn. W B Saunders, Philadelphia

Halpin D 2004 NICE guidelines on COPD. Thorax 59:181–182

MacNee W, Calverley P M 2003 Chronic obstructive pulmonary disease. 7: Management of COPD. Thorax 58(3):261–265

Moyle J 2002 Pulse oximetry, 2nd edn. BMJ Books, London

Perren A, Marone C 2005 Remember a posterior diagnosis of carbon monoxide poisoning. European Journal of Emergency Medicine 12(5):259–260

Safe use of oxygen cylinders. http://www.hse.gov.uk/pubns/hse8.pdf

West J B 2004 Respiratory physiology: the essentials, 7th edn. Williams and Wilkins, Baltimore

Fluid balance

Jon Sturman, Emilio Garcia

3

OBJECTIVES

After reading this chapter you should be able to:

- *Understand the basic principles of normal body fluid homeostasis*
- *Understand the effects of illness on fluid balance*
- *Estimate the fluid status of a patient*
- *Prioritize and rationally prescribe intravenous fluids*
- *Integrate fluid balance with other aspects of critical care management*

INTRODUCTION

Fluid balance in the critically ill patient may be complicated. Frequently the disease process itself causes abnormalities in fluid homeostasis (i.e. by fluid loss, redistribution or retention). In addition, inappropriate treatment can worsen such biochemical disturbances and significantly affect morbidity and even mortality. It is essential to have an understanding of the patho-physiological processes in fluid shifts, together with an understanding of the consequences of administration of different intravenous fluids to aid the clinician in selecting appropriate fluid therapy. Indeed, severe biochemical derangement and the need for accurate fluid balance management may itself be an indication to upgrade a patient's level of care.

CONSEQUENCES OF BAD FLUID BALANCE MANAGEMENT

Dehydration

Dehydration can lead to hypovolaemia, pre-renal failure and gut ischaemia. There is an increased incidence of later multi-organ failure.

Overhydration

Overhydration can lead to pulmonaty and peripheral oedema, delayed wean-ing from ventilation and delayed mobilization. There may be worsening of cerebral oedema and there is possibly a worse outcome in acute respiratory distress syndrome (ARDS).

Poorly selected fluid

Administration of incorrect fluids can produce life-threatening electrolyte disturbance, e.g. cardiac arrhythmias or profound muscle weakness.

APPLIED PHYSIOLOGY

Body compartments

An understanding of the partition of fluid and electrolytes in the body is required to appreciate the effect of prescribed IV fluids.

Two-thirds of body mass is water: of this two-thirds is intracellular fluid (ICF) and one-third extracellular fluid (ECF) (Fig. 3.1). With regard to ECF, two-thirds is extravascular and one-third intravascular. ECF sodium is high whilst ICF sodium is low – the converse applies to potassium. This relationship is maintained by the sodium–potassium pump at the expense of energy. Water and electrolytes move freely.

Between the intra- and extravascular ECF, however, by virtue of the capillary basement membrane, large molecules and blood cells are prevented from moving out of the extravascular space.

Most fluid losses occur from the ECF and therefore high sodium fluids are required for replacement. Administration of low sodium fluids, e.g. dextrose, expands the ECF poorly as most of the water will pass intracellularly.

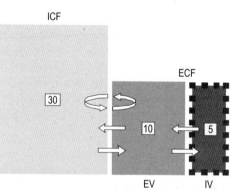

Figure 3.1   Representation of body fluid compartments. EV, extravascular; IV, intravascular.

Tip

Serum electrolyte results represent the ECF and therefore reflect body sodium accurately in the absence of oedema, but are only the tip of the iceberg with regard to other important ions, particularly total body potassium.

Normal requirements

Water is lost in urine and stool as well as through 'insensible' loss from respiratory vapour and sweat. These losses are normally controlled by the body in the context of intake, ambient conditions and activity, such that body water remains tightly regulated. Sodium and potassium losses occur alongside these, but the kidneys, under the control of the pituitary–adrenal hormone axis, regulate these. Normal fluid requirement is often quoted as 2–3 L per day, but should be more accurately determined on an hourly basis guided by the patient's ideal body weight. The following is a guide for the healthy individual:

Daily requirements:

- Water requirement: 1.5 mL/kg/h
- Sodium requirement: 2 mmol/kg/day
- Potassium requirement: 1–2 mmol/kg/day.

Remember urine output needs to be maintained at 0.5 mL/kg/h or more for adequate toxin excretion.

PATHOLOGICAL STATES

Fluid loss

The majority of critically ill patients have intravascular fluid deficit on presentation. Causes include:

- fasting
- intestinal obstruction and vomiting
- diarrhoea
- trauma, burns
- peritonitis
- capillary leak
- sepsis.

Increased capillary leak is common to a number of pathologies, but is particularly prevalent in sepsis. White cell activation causes damage to the capillary basement membrane causing leakage of large molecules into the extravascular space, loss of oncotic pressure and hypovolaemia. Thus the severely ill patient may have much greater fluid requirements than might be expected from measured losses alone. As discussed, these losses should generally be replaced with high-sodium solutions.

The stress response

Hypovolaemia results in activation of the renin–aldosterone–angiotensin system, resulting in renal conservation of salt and water. This forms part of the stress response, which is activated by illness, trauma or surgery. Thus, on presentation, a mild degree of oliguria may be expected as a 'normal' response. This is usually mild and self limiting. Any patient with oliguria warrants meticulous attention to blood pressure and fluid balance status as it may be the only sign of more serious problems of hypoperfusion.

ASSESSMENT OF FLUID BALANCE

When a patient presents de novo, assessment of fluid requirement can be difficult. There is no single clinical or laboratory reading available at the bedside which can accurately determine hydration status (although serial weights may be helpful in the more stable patient where feasible). Therefore assessment should be focussed on answering the following questions:

What is the patient's history?

- This is often the best clue as to the patient's fluid status. Consider the duration of fasting and the magnitude of the insult, e.g. the bigger the operation or area of trauma or inflammation, the greater the fluid losses.

What is the patient's intravascular status – hypovolaemic or otherwise?

- Delayed capillary refill and a core peripheral temperature gradient are early signs. Tachycardia is a late sign, with hypotension more so (see Ch. 1). In 'not sure if full or not' cases, and where the central venous pressure (CVP) is indeterminate, a challenge with fluid boluses shows no or minimal rise if the patient is still hypovolaemic. Urine is concentrated and the patient is oliguric (remember this will take some hours to assess).

If hypovolaemic, where is the loss occurring?

- This may be obvious, e.g. vomiting from intestinal obstruction. If occult, think of occult bleeding or inflammation. Most often, sepsis is the cause, either localized (e.g. abdominal collection) or generalized (e.g. bacteraemia from line infection). Imaging may be required to locate the source.

Is there fluid overload?

- Fluid overload may present with peripheral oedema but in the non-ambulant patient, fluid may accumulate in the trunk and more specifically in the lungs. A steady decline in pulmonary gas exchange is often the clue here, accompanied by fluid balance chart evidence (see below). In the critical care unit, this may present as a cause of delayed weaning from ventilation.

Investigations

- Haematocrit: this may be raised with dehydration. It is important to maintain haemoglobin levels whilst optimizing fluid therapy. It is generally maintained at 8–10 g/dL, although recent evidence implies > 7 g/dL is acceptable in the absence of central nervous system or cardiovascular system disease and haemoglobin is not falling.
- Urea and electrolytes: there may be raised urea with dehydration. It is important to have a baseline for electrolytes whilst commencing IV fluids.
- Blood gases: these may show raised lactate, base deficit and acidosis associated with poor tissue perfusion. Serial lactates and base excess may be a guide to the effects of fluid resuscitation.
- Chest X-ray (if worsening oxygenation): this may show signs of fluid overload (interstitial oedema).

Tip

Remember that investigations can be used to support decision making but may not in themselves reflect total body fluid status accurately.

Tip – how to do a fluid challenge

If fluid status is uncertain, there is evidence of hypovolaemia (e.g. oliguria), and the CVP remains equivocal, consider a CVP fluid challenge.
- Measure accurate CVP.
- Give 250 mL fluid rapidly (saline or low molecular weight colloid).
- Measure CVP.

If the CVP does not rise, or rises slightly after the challenge, but falls within minutes to the pre-test reading, assume that the patient remains hypovolaemic. This is because the capacitance vessels are expanding to accommodate the extra fluid. If the CVP rises with the extra fluid, then the circulation is not dilating to accept the extra fluid and is therefore full. Further fluid may therefore overload the circulation.

PRACTICAL FLUID BALANCE MANAGEMENT

Phases

When calculating fluid replacement always remember to include:

Deficit + Maintenance + Ongoing losses

In calculating fluid requirements in practical terms for the critically ill patient with capillary leak, fluid prescription can be split into the following phases:

1. *A resuscitation phase*, in which rapid boluses of fluid are used to restore tissue perfusion. Appropriate solutions are high-sodium (see crystalloid versus colloid debate below); occasionally blood transfusion may be necessary to prevent extreme haemodilution. Treating the underlying pathology (e.g. fixation of fractures, drainage of abscess) occurs during this phase.

2. *A consolidation phase*, when the patient is adequately filled, as judged clinically, using CVP measurement and blood gas analysis if necessary to support this. At this point ongoing fluid requirements are met in a more calm and leisurely manner, and during this phase fluid intake is reduced to maintenance requirement. Thought should be given to commencing feeding during this phase.

3. *A transition phase*, where resolution of the underlying pathology has occurred. Patients are commonly in a positive fluid balance from phases 1 and 2 as a result of resuscitation fluid, fluid retention as part of the stress response and renal conservation of salt and water. Control of fluid balance should be handed back to the patient and this involves the use of enteral feeding and oral medication where possible. Occasionally it is necessary to use diuretics cautiously during this phase to reduce lung water and improve pulmonary function.

Some patients will develop further sepsis and/or undergo repeat surgery with the reappearance of capillary leak. In this event one may need to go back one or two phases in fluid balance management.

Which fluid to use?

The composition of commonly used IV fluids per L is listed in Table 3.1.

Maintenance fluid requirements can be met initially with 4% dextrose/ 0.18% saline although prolonged use (> 48 h) is undesirable as the patient may become hyponatraemic. Gastrointestinal secretions are sodium-, and to a lesser extent, potassium-rich, so high-sodium crystalloid should be given to cover nasogastric or diarrhoeal loss. Hartmann's solution may be viewed as the ideal replacement fluid as it contains potassium also. If potassium levels are very low (< 3.5) then normal saline can be used and potassium 10–40 mmol/L added. If a central line is placed and profound hypokalaemia exists, high concentrations of potassium may be administered through a central port, e.g. 10–20 mmol/h. If such concentrations are used, regular reassessment of serum potassium should be undertaken every few hours

Table 3.1 Composition of IV fluids per litre

Fluid	Na	K	Ca	Cl	pH
Normal saline	150			150	5.0
7.5% saline	1283	1283		1283	5.0
Dextrosaline	30			30	4.5
Dextrose 5%					4.0
Hartmann's	131	5	2	111	6.5
8.4% bicarbonate	1000			1000	8
Haemacell	145	5.1	6.25	145	7.4
Gelofusine	154	< 0.4	< 0.4	125	7.4
Hetastarch	154			154	5.0
Voluven	154			154	5.0
7.5% saline in dextran	1283			1283	4.5

and each new 50 mL syringe of potassium only prescribed after medical reassessment. Such treatment is usually reserved for critical care areas due to the dangers of inappropriate use of high concentration potassium infusions. High potassium concentration infusions should not be administered peripherally as this may cause skin necrosis.

Remember that all these solutions have little or no calorific value. To avoid swings in blood sugar the fasted diabetic should be maintained on a constant glucose-potassium-insulin (GKI) infusion with normal saline infused separately to cover any shortfall in salt and water requirements.

Colloid versus crystalloid

Colloids differ from crystalloids in that they contain large molecules, e.g. starches, gelatins, and albumin, which tend to remain intravascular. The oncotic effect tends to keep the solutions' water intravascular. This effect is observed in the healthy individual but less so with capillary leak.

Colloids can be classified into two groups: plasma derivatives such as human albumin solutions (4.5% and 20%), FFP and PPF; and semisynthetic preparations such us gelatines, dextrans and starches.

Potential problems with colloid use include allergic reaction (risk ~ 1 in 10 000) and adverse effects on blood coagulation if volumes of more than 30 mL/kg are used. They are more expensive than crystalloids. Crystalloid solutions, however, have little oncotic effect and therefore larger volumes (up to triple) may be required to achieve the same effect.

Little evidence exists as to whether a policy of colloid or crystalloid resuscitation is preferable. A large meta-analysis concluded that the use of albumin on general intensive care patients was associated with no significant benefit: the results of further large prospective studies are awaited. A practical solution, meantime, may be to use colloid to replace blood loss, volume for volume, and crystalloid for all other losses, as well as maintenance.

There is some evidence that pre-hospital resuscitation of trauma patients with hypertonic fluids followed by the use of colloids improves outcome and this may become more common in the future. This is presumably through the maintenance of plasma volume through an osmotic effect. Hypertonic normal saline produces similar effects in fluid expansion to colloids without the risks of anaphylaxis and derangement of coagulation. Further studies are awaited.

The use of albumin has been topical recently. However the SAFE study has proved that compared to normal saline, no significant difference was seen in 28-day all-cause mortality, days in the intensive care unit, days in hospital, days of mechanical ventilation or days of renal replacement therapy.

Albumin preparations contain more than 95% albumin, which is a uniform molecule of approximately 29 000 Kd. Most synthetic colloid preparations contain molecules of a varying size.

Albumin solutions

Human albumin is a naturally occurring colloid. It comes as a salt-poor preparation and at concentrations of 4.5% (normal) or 20% (hypertonic).

During its preparation it is heat treated in order to eliminate the risk of transmission of infections such as HIV and hepatitis.

It is the colloid of choice in situations where the patient is hypo-albuminaemic but waterlogged, e.g. liver failure patients.

Dextrans

Dextrans are synthetic polysaccharides derived from fructose. Two forms are available commercially and their names reflect their molecular weight:

- Dextran 40 (40 000 Kd)
- Dextran 70 (70 000 Kd).

They are very rarely used as a plasma substitute due to the high incidence of anaphylactic reactions and their effect on impaired coagulation. Dextran 40, however, is not uncommonly used in vascular and plastic surgery for its beneficial effects on microcirculation and coagulation.

They can both produce renal failure.

Gelatines

Gelatines are derived from the hydrolysis of bovine collagen. There are two common preparations:

- Haemacell (urea linked)
- Gelofusine (succinylated).

Advantages of these products are their price and stability leading to a prolonged shelf life; however, they have a significant incidence of ana-phylaxis (< 0.5%) and Haemacell contains calcium, making its administra-tion contraindicated contemporaneously with blood. They have a moderate plasma half-life of between 90–120 min and they have little effect on coagulation. As they are formulated in normal saline they have a high chloride content.

Despite their origin they are considered to be safe regarding the spread of spongiform encephalopathy.

Starches

Starches are derived from amylopectin, a glucose polymer originating from maize or sorghum. This product is then synthetically modified by hydroxy-ethyl substitution of the amylopectin. This substitution makes it resistant to enzymatic attack and hence improves its half-life. However, this is also a disadvantage as these molecules can be found in reticuloendothelial cells many years after their administration, with uncertain long-term effects. The molecular weight of starches is varied and, owing to this fact, they have to be represented by two values. These are the range of molecular weight and the mean molecular weight or a mean molecular weight and a substitution index.

These products can be formulated in normal saline or low sodium preparations that avoid the risk of hyperchloraemic metabolic acidosis.

Side effects of these products are risk of anaphylaxis (although smaller than in gelatines), derangement of coagulation (if administered in excess of 25 mL/kg/day) mostly due to interference with factor VIII, and itching. The effect of their presence in reticuloendothelial cells for several years after their administration is not clear and has been implicated in itching and immunosuppression but without clear evidence for either.

Different starches are:

- Hespan
- Haesteril (6 or 10%)
- Elo-Hes
- Pentaspan
- Voluven (6%).

Voluven with its molecular weight of 130 000 Kd is said to have the lesser incidence of coagulopathy.

Hypertonic saline

Hypertonic saline includes 1.8%, 3%, 5%, 7.5%, and 10% sodium chloride solutions. The osmolality of these solutions exceeds that of intracellular water and because Na and Cl cannot freely cross membranes, hypertonic solutions increase the intravascular volume more than would the same volume of a balanced salt solution but at the expense of intracellular volume. Volumes used must be very low, otherwise there is a risk of sodium overload and hypernatraemia.

Hypertonic saline (7.5% saline or hypertonic saline in dextran 70%) is currently used for initial resuscitation. This is due to its effect of drawing fluid intravascularly without the side effects of colloids such as anaphylaxis and alteration of coagulation, resulting in increased plasma volume. Other effects of this preparation have been described such as decreased intracranial pressure (ICP), vasodilatation, increased myocardial contractility and increased tissue blood flow.

Other uses for hypertonic saline include: management of head injuries, burns and nebulization in patients with fibrosing alveolitis, and with caution in the treatment of hyponatraemia.

Correction of hyponatraemia needs to be done carefully in order to avoid the risk of cerebral oedema. As a rule of thumb it is safe to correct hyponatraemia at the same speed as it has occurred. For example, if hyponatraemia has developed over a few hours it can be corrected rapidly (1 mmol/L/h). Insidious hyponatraemia needs to be corrected more carefully (< 0.5 mmol/L/h), at typically 10 mmol/L/day. Like the treatment of hypernatraemia, hyponatraemia must be corrected slowly and with the underlying diagnosis in mind (see Ch. 11).

Hypotonic saline

This is used mostly during the treatment of hypernatremia. The treatment of hypernatremia is two-fold. On one hand we must treat the underlying cause and on the other we have to reduce the sodium concentration.

When oral fluids (water nasogastrically can be useful) are not appropriate, 0.2% sodium chloride (commonly referred to as one-quarter normal saline) or 0.45% normal saline (half normal saline) can be used. The more hypotonic the infusion used, the lower the rate of infusion will be required.

There are different formulas to calculate the reduction in sodium and one of them is:

$$\frac{(Na^+\ infused) - (Na^+\ serum)}{Total\ body\ water} = Na^+\ change$$

Another potential use of hypotonic saline is in the management of diabetic ketoacidosis (DKA). Patients with DKA are often severely dehydrated (5–7 L) and require intense fluid replacement. If sodium chloride alone is used the patient is at risk of developing a secondary hyperchloraemic metabolic acidosis due to the excess chloride administered in conjunction with the sodium.

A SYSTEM OF FLUID BALANCE MANAGEMENT

Resuscitate first

Go back to 'ABC': this is not the time to be assessing hourly maintenance but rather to give boluses of fluid (10–20 mL/kg of sodium-containing fluid) rapidly to restore intravascular volume and therefore tissue perfusion. This may require use of a central line to assess intravascular filling. Stop when vital signs are improving and move to the next step.

Note: Recent evidence implies that in patients with ruptured abdominal aortic aneurysms, fluid resuscitation should be limited to aiming for a blood pressure of 90 mmHg or a good radial pulse. Achieving a higher blood pressure may only promote increased blood loss and worsen outcome. The same logic may not necessarily be extended to other patient groups, such as non-penetrating trauma or gastrointestinal haemorrhage, as these represent different pathophysiological states that do not necessarily involve imminent surgical procedure to terminate ongoing loss.

Start a record

It is important to document the intake of all fluids immediately, both enteral and parenteral, and this includes drugs where these are given with significant fluid load. Similarly, all losses should be recorded where possible: urine, nasogastric (NG) losses and drain losses. Make records hourly.

Make some calculations

Estimate the patient's hourly maintenance volume based on the patient's weight in mL/h. Then estimate the fluid requirement to replace losses hitherto. This involves a degree of guesswork based on history (fasting time, severity of illness, etc.). Take the volume of resuscitation fluid used from this. Aim to give this fluid over the next 24 h in addition to maintenance. Assess net fluid balance daily or twice daily.

Check the investigations

By this time results of blood tests should be available. Unless potassium is high (> 5) then this should prompt the use of potassium in replacement fluid. If magnesium is low and the patient is critically ill, consider replacing magnesium (e.g. 40 mmol by IV infusion over 6 h). Seek specialist advice for major abnormalities in serum sodium, urea and creatinine.

Frequently reassess

After 1–2 h the urine output becomes a useful guide to adequacy of resuscitation. If fluid requirement remains high, consider whether the underlying pathology has been correctly diagnosed or adequately treated.

Tip

Remember to clinically assess the response to fluid therapy frequently. Every patient should be assessed for fluid status daily; in critically ill patients this may need to be hourly.

   Include drug administration, which may not only include considerable amounts of water, but also salt in particular, and even calories.

Consolidate

Cut back intake to maintenance level only when ongoing losses have abated. Consider the need to provide caloric support (enteral and/or parenteral). Aim to keep total intake to a set hourly figure: include drugs and feed in this. Drug solutions may need to be concentrated to achieve the desired caloric intake or fluid targets. This phase is particularly important where fluid overload has major adverse effects (cerebral oedema, lung injury and ARDS, and established renal failure with anuria). With anuric renal failure, fluid should be cut by one-third to allow for the lack of renal water loss. Seek specialist advice in the management of these patients.

Diurese

Most patients will achieve a negative balance (remember insensible losses again) as they mobilize. Consider cautious use of diuretics (e.g. furosemide) if lung water is impairing gas exchange and serial fluid balances show accumulation. Only do this if the patient is intravascularly stable.

A system of fluid balance management

Tips
- Replace fluid losses with equal fluids (like with like).
- In non-haemorrhagic shock, use crystalloid first.
- In pre-hospital care do not over-resuscitate as this may worsen blood loss.
- Do not use starches in excess of 25 mL/kg/day (1750 mL for a 70 kg person).
- Be aware of hyperchloraemic metabolic acidosis.
- Continually reassess the fluid status of any critically ill patient.

CASE 3.1

A 60-year-old man of average build (70 kg) presents in septic shock with a tender lower abdomen. He is resuscitated with boluses of Hartmann's solution and, despite 3 L, remains tachycardic. A central line is therefore inserted and further fluid boluses given (resuscitate first).

He is then taken to theatre where a diverticular abscess is drained and an ileostomy is performed. Antibiotics are started. On arrival in the critical care unit he is ventilated and warmed peripherally. Hourly fluid balance recording is commenced. Maintenance is calculated at 70(kg) × 1.5 mL/h = 105 mL/h. Dextrose/saline is started for this. Drain and NG losses are replaced with Hartmann's mL for mL (make some calculations).

Bloods show a potassium of 4.0 so potassium is added to his maintenance fluid (check the investigations).

His urine output falls 6 h later accompanied by cooling of his peripheries. A further bolus of fluid is therefore given (frequently reassess) with subsequent improvement.

24 h later his FiO_2 has increased to 60% from 40% and he has peripheral oedema. A check on his fluid balance reveals a net positive balance of > 3 L. Further investigation reveals the origin of this to be IV antibiotics, sedatives and the addition of total parenteral nutrition (TPN). The hourly fluid total is therefore reduced to 80% maintenance and now includes these items. Small doses of furosemide are given to speed a diuresis and the patient is subsequently weaned. Total fluid intake now comprises TPN. Oral fluids are slowly introduced, and once absorbed these are included in the fluid balance calculation and the patient is weaned off TPN (consolidate and diurese).

FURTHER READING

American Thoracic Society 2004 Evidence-based colloid use in the critically ill: American Thoracic Society Consensus Statement. American Journal of Respiratory and Critical Care Medicine 170:1247–1259

Cochrane Injuries Group Albumin Reviewers 1998 Human albumin administration in critically ill patients: systematic review of randomised controlled trials. BMJ 317:235–240

Choi P T, Yip G, Quinonez L G et al 1999 Crystalloids vs. colloids in fluid resuscitation: a systematic review. Critical Care Medicine 27:200–210

Finley T 2004 Intravenous therapy. Blackwell Publishing, UK

Lewis C A, Martin G S 2004 Understanding and managing fluid balance in patients with acute lung injury. Current Opinion in Critical Care 10:13–17

Preston R E 1997 Acid-base, fluids and electrolytes made ridiculously simple. Medmaster Inc US, USA

SAFE Study Investigators 2004 A comparison of albumin and saline for fluid resuscitation in the intensive care unit. New England Journal of Medicine 350:2247–2256

Schierhout G, Roberts I, Alderson P 1999 Colloids versus crystalloids for fluid resuscitation in critically ill patients (Cochrane Review). The Cochrane Library, Issue 1, Oxford

Stephens R, Mythen M 2003 Resuscitation fluids and hyperchloraemic metabolic acidosis. Trauma 5(2):141–147

Traylor R J, Pearl R G 1996 Crystalloid versus colloid versus colloid: All colloids are not created equal. Anaesthesia and Analgesia 83:209–212

Further reading

Arterial blood gas interpretation

Stephen Bonner, Diane Monkhouse

4

OBJECTIVES

After reading this chapter you should be able to:

● *Understand mechanisms of normal acid base homeostasis*

● *Interpret acid base disturbances and relate them to clinical practice*

● *Understand the techniques for blood gas analysis and recognize their limitations*

INTRODUCTION

Arterial blood gas analysis gives rapid and crucial information on disturbances in gas exchange and acid base homeostasis. The interpretation of acid base disturbance is central to the management of the critically ill as it conveys crucial information about the underlying pathological process, the degree of adaptation by the body's compensatory mechanisms and response to therapy. In order to interpret such data correctly, it is important to establish basic definitions, understand the homeostatic mechanisms involved and appreciate how the measurements are derived.

DEFINITIONS AND TERMINOLOGY

pH: (normal range 7.35–7.45). Tight biochemical control of the hydrogen ion concentration (H^+) is necessary to maintain normal cellular enzyme activity. pH is defined as the negative logarithm of hydrogen ion concentration. It is a measure of the degree of acidity or alkalinity of the blood sample. A normal pH value of 7.4 equates to a H^+ concentration of 40 nanomoles per litre. A decrease in pH from 7.4 to 7.1 represents a doubling of the H^+ ion concentration.

Acidaemia: results when blood pH is less than 7.35.

Acidosis: describes an abnormal process that tends to lower blood pH.

Alkalaemia: results when blood pH is greater than 7.45.

Alkalosis: describes an abnormal process that tends to raise blood pH.

Compensation: occurs in an attempt to restore normal pH.

Standard bicarbonate: a measure of the metabolic component of any acid–base disturbance. It can be defined as the bicarbonate concentration when $PaCO_2$ is corrected to 5.3 kPa and temperature is 37°C. The normal range is 22–26 mmol/L.

Base excess: the amount of acid or base required to titrate 1 L of blood back to pH 7.4 at a $PaCO_2$ of 5.3 kPa and temperature of 37°C. Because the respiratory component is corrected, this is a measure of the metabolic component of any acid–base disturbance.

(normal range is –2 to +2 mmol/L)

Anion gap: the difference between major plasma cations and major plasma anions.

Anion gap = $[Na^+] + [K^+] - ([Cl^-] + [HCO_3^-])$
(normal range is 8–16 mmol/L)

PaO_2: the partial pressure of oxygen in arterial blood.

(normal range is 11.0–13.3 kPa)

$PaCO_2$: the partial pressure of carbon dioxide in arterial blood.

(normal range is 4.5–6.0 kPa)

ANALYSIS OF ACID BASE DISTURBANCE

All enzyme systems have an optimal working pH. Disturbances in pH lead to disruption of metabolism, which may have life-threatening consequences.
Other affected processes include:

- molecular ionization (e.g. hypocalcaemia in alkalosis)
- distribution of drugs and metabolites
- distribution of ions across cell membranes, most commonly potassium
- shifts of the oxygen haemoglobin dissociation curve.

Changes in pH are therefore minimized by the body with a sophisticated system of buffers (mainly bicarbonate, phosphates, proteins and haemoglobin). Other regulatory systems include the lungs altering $PaCO_2$ by adjusting alveolar ventilation. Longer-term measures involve excretion of acids or bases by the kidneys.

Maintenance of H+ homeostasis

Maintenance of H^+ homeostasis involves:

1. Chemical buffering by intracellular and extracellular buffers
2. Elimination of CO_2 by respiration
3. Renal regeneration of bicarbonate and excretion of H^+.

The main buffers in the body are the carbonic acid/bicarbonate system, phosphates and proteins. Of these the carbonic acid/bicarbonate system is the most clinically useful because it accounts for over 60% of the blood buffering capacity and is involved in both renal and respiratory compensatory mechanisms:

$$H^+ + HCO_3^- \Leftrightarrow H_2CO_3 \Leftrightarrow CO_2 + H_2O$$
ionic dissociation   carbonic anhydrase

Disturbances in acid–base balance can be modified by respiratory control over CO_2 and renal regulation of HCO_3^-, ammonia and titratable acid. If the primary disturbance is respiratory, the compensatory response will be metabolic via the kidneys. That is, if the $PaCO_2$ rises, the kidneys excrete the excess H^+ and also chronically retain HCO_3^- to bring pH back to normal. This is a slow process, taking hours to days and is rarely complete. If the primary disturbance is metabolic, the compensatory response is respiratory. That is, if acid accumulates, more CO_2 is produced and exhaled. This process is rapid and often incomplete, although if prolonged the patient may become exhausted and unable to continue to maintain a low PCO_2.

The Henderson-Hasselbach equation may be rewritten as follows:

$$[H^+] \, \alpha \, \frac{PCO_2}{[HCO_3^-]}$$

Plasma bicarbonate can be plotted against pH [H^+] for differing levels of $PaCO_2$ and abnormalities of acid–base disturbance described in relation to

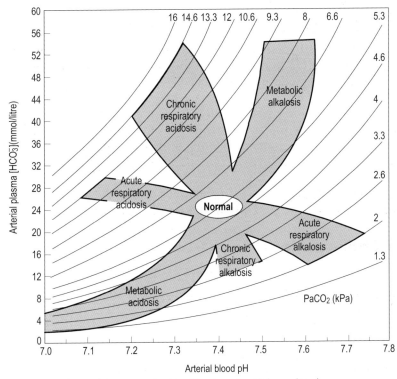

Figure 4.1   The acid–base map for identification of acid–base disturbance.

this. This may be conveniently described in a nomogram which helps determine acid–base disorders clinically by simply plotting bicarbonate against pH and $PaCO_2$ (Fig. 4.1).

It is important to remember that the function of acid–base homeostasis is to attempt to restore normal pH and that pH is proportional to the bicarbonate to CO_2 ratio.

$$pH \; \alpha \; \frac{HCO_3^-}{CO_2}$$

Respiratory acidosis

Hypoventilation leads to a rise in PCO_2, which is followed by a rise in [H^+]. In the acute phase there may be a small rise in bicarbonate levels due to the dissociation curve (see above). In chronic states, renal retention of bicarbonate brings pH and [H^+] to normal over 2–5 days. In these circumstances the primary abnormality is a respiratory acidosis with a compensatory metabolic alkalosis. The most common cause for this is chronic obstructive pulmonary disease (COPD).

$$pH \downarrow \alpha \; \frac{HCO_3^- \Uparrow}{CO_2 \uparrow}$$

($\Uparrow$ indicates compensatory change)
($\uparrow$ indicates primary disturbance)

Respiratory alkalosis

Hyperventilation leads to a fall in PCO_2 and [H^+]. In the acute phase, the bicarbonate concentration may fall slightly. However, if the hyperventilation becomes chronic (an uncommon clinical problem), renal compensation occurs which may produce a mild metabolic acidosis. Complete correction of acidosis is unusual in this situation. Acute hyperventilation is commonly due to anxiety but chronic hyperventilation is more unusual and may be due to chronic hypoxaemia, e.g. as a consequence of altitude. Type 1 respiratory failure is occasionally produced during artificial ventilation in the critical care unit.

$$pH \uparrow \alpha \; \frac{HCO_3^- \Downarrow}{CO_2 \downarrow}$$

($\Downarrow$ indicates compensatory change)
($\downarrow$ indicates primary disturbance)

Metabolic acidosis

Metabolic acidosis results from excess production of endogenous acids (e.g. lactic acid, keto-acids), loss of alkali (e.g. renal tubular acidosis) or from exogenous acid (e.g. methanol, salicylates). Compensatory respiratory alkalosis develops once the brain has sensed the rise in [H^+] and hyperventilation is stimulated.

Lactic acidosis most commonly occurs as a consequence of anaerobic metabolism due to tissue hypoxia in a shocked hypotensive patient.

Diabetic ketoacidosis is characterized by a triad of hyperglycaemia, metabolic acidosis and ketosis. Compensatory hyperventilation (Kussmaul respiration) is typically seen.

$$pH \downarrow \alpha \frac{HCO_3^- \downarrow}{CO_2 \Downarrow}$$

($\downarrow$ indicates primary disturbance)
($\Downarrow$ indicates compensatory change)

The anion gap

The anion gap (AG) is the difference between the sum of bicarbonate and chloride and the sum of sodium and potassium. It is useful in determining the cause of metabolic acidosis as it estimates the unmeasured anions (e.g. sulphates, phosphates). If the acidosis is due to loss of base, then the AG will be normal, but a raised AG implies the presence of acid. This may be due to ketoacids, renal failure, lactic acid or the presence of exogenous (ingested) acids.

Care must be exercised in clinical interpretation of the AG. The reported normal range in the literature varies from 6–20 mmol/L and several other factors influence the AG. The major contributor to the normal AG is albumin, which is invariably low in critical illness, giving a falsely low reading when other acids are present. Indeed the calculated AG is normal in 50% of cases of lactic acidosis. Causes of metabolic acidosis with an increased anion gap include diabetic ketoacidosis, lactic acidosis, salicylate overdose, methanol or ethylene glycol poisoning.

Metabolic alkalosis

This may be caused by loss of acid (commonly from the gastrointestinal tract) or exogenous administration of alkali (e.g. milk-alkali syndrome). If the cause is unclear, a high urinary chloride may suggest hyperaldosteronism, Cushing's syndrome or severe potassium deficiency. A decrease in the extracellular fluid compartment results in the loss of hydrogen ions in preference to sodium re-absorption and total body potassium deficiency results in loss of hydrogen ions in exchange for potassium. Respiratory compensation is severely limited and a PCO_2 over 6.5 kPa is rare, even in profound metabolic alkalosis. Once underlying factors are corrected, acetazolamide may be considered.

$$pH \uparrow \alpha \frac{HCO_3^- \uparrow}{CO_2 \Uparrow}$$

($\uparrow$ indicates primary disturbance)
($\Uparrow$ indicates compensatory change)

Biochemical features of acid–base disturbance are summarized in Table 4.1.

STEPWISE APPROACH FOR INTERPRETATION OF ARTERIAL BLOOD GASES

Any interpretation of arterial blood gases must be performed in the clinical context in order to ascertain the primary abnormality. In critically ill patients

Table 4.1 Biochemical features of acid–base disturbance

Acid–base imbalance	pH	Primary disturbance	Compensation	Example
Metabolic acidosis	Low	Decreased HCO_3^-	Hyperventilation with resulting decrease in $PaCO_2$	Acute renal failure Diabetic ketoacidosis Severe liver disease
Metabolic alkalosis	High	Increased HCO_3^-	Hypoventilation with resulting increase in $PaCO_2$	Prolonged vomiting Potassium depletion Exogenous alkali
Respiratory acidosis	Low	Increased $PaCO_2$	Increased renal excretion of H^+ resulting in increased serum HCO_3^-	COPD Neuromuscular causes of respiratory failure
Respiratory alkalosis	High	Decreased $PaCO_2$	Decreased renal excretion of H^+ resulting in decreased serum HCO_3^-	Hyperventilation due to any cause

who are dehydrated, acidotic, or severely hypokalaemic with respiratory failure, there may be many processes occurring simultaneously.

1. Assess oxygenation

Is the patient hypoxic?

2. Determine acid–base status

pH < 7.35 acidaemia
pH > 7.45 alkalaemia

3. Determine whether the primary disturbance is respiratory or metabolic

A primary respiratory disturbance alters $PaCO_2$
A primary metabolic disturbance alters HCO_3^-
That is, if the $PaCO_2$ is low, the patient must either be compensating for a metabolic acidosis, in which case the pH and bicarbonate will be low, or it is a primary hyperventilation, in which case the pH will be high. Compensatory mechanisms will attempt to restore pH over time, but the primary acidosis/alkalosis will not be fully compensated. Plot numbers are on the graph in Figure 4.1.

4. Determine whether there is compensation for the primary disturbance

For a respiratory disturbance, is there metabolic compensation by the kidneys?

For a metabolic disturbance, is there respiratory compensation by increasing or decreasing alveolar ventilation?

5. For a metabolic acidosis determine the anion gap

$$\text{Anion gap} = [Na^+] + [K^+] - ([Cl^-] + [HCO_3^-])$$

This may be particularly useful if there is no obvious cause for the acidosis, however bear in mind the cautions described above.

6. Aim to identify the underlying cause

This involves thorough history taking, clinical examination and analysis of other laboratory investigations. Lactate measurements are particularly valuable in a metabolic acidosis.

The blood gas machine

Blood gas interpretation should always be performed with an understanding of how such values are derived from the blood gas machine and co-oximeter.

Measured variables

In the blood gas machine, pH (or $[H^+]$ in nmol/L) is measured by the generation of a potential across a pH sensitive glass membrane. Common causes of error include coating of the pH electrode with blood proteins and excess heparin in the sample syringe. PO_2 is measured directly using the reduction of oxygen between a platinum cathode and a silver anode which generates a small current. Oxygen electrodes often under-read slightly since oxygen is consumed around the cathode tip. This inaccuracy increases with increasing oxygen tensions. PCO_2 measurements are achieved by allowing CO_2 to diffuse through a Teflon membrane altering the pH of a test solution. These measurements are usually accurate although the CO_2 electrode needs frequent changes owing to holes appearing in the Teflon membrane or loss of silver coating on the reference electrode. Such frequent changes often do not allow blood protein coating of the electrode to become a problem.

Haemoglobin (Hb) estimation is usually performed photometrically, but may be more accurately measured using a co-oximeter. In a co-oximeter blood is haemolyzed and subjected to absorption spectroscopy to give an accurate measurement of total Hb, fetal Hb, oxyhaemoglobin, carboxyhaemoglobin, methaemoglobin and sulphaemoglobin. The principle of using absorption spectroscopy is the same as is used in a pulse oximeter. In pulse oximetry, only two wavelengths of light are used to distinguish between oxy- and deoxyhaemoglobin. In contrast, the co-oximeter uses 14 different wavelengths allowing identification of abnormal forms of haemoglobin. If there is suspicion of a dyshaemoglobinaemia, co-oximetric analysis is essential.

Although co-oximeters are increasingly often found in critical care units, emergency departments and acute medical wards, they are not universally available.

These values are the only directly measured values from the blood gas machine. All other variables are derived and therefore open to more error and require careful interpretation.

Derived variables

Total or actual bicarbonate concentration is calculated by the blood gas machine using the Henderson-Hasselbach equation:

$$pH = 6.1 + \log_{10} \frac{\text{arterial } [HCO_3^-]}{PaCO_2 \times 0.03}$$

This includes bicarbonate, carbonate and carbamate concentrations. Standard bicarbonate can be derived to assess the contribution of metabolic factors and ignore the contribution of CO_2. It does this by estimating the bicarbonate concentration that would be present if the PCO_2 was 5.3 kPa (40 mmHg), PO_2 13.3 kPa [100 mmHg] and temperature 37°C. The base deficit is a way of quantifying the metabolic component of an acidosis as the amount of base that would have to be added to or subtracted from a litre of extracellular fluid to return the pH to a value of 7.4 at a PCO_2 of 5.3 kPa at 37°C. Standard base excess is calculated to an in vivo state.

Most blood gas machines also give the oxygen saturation. This is a derived variable calculated on the assumption that the oxygen haemoglobin dissociation curve is normal. Some machines also calculate oxygen content which may be more clinically relevant than PO_2. Such calculations are of limited value since they assume that the Hb is normal and do not take into account the presence of abnormal haemoglobins such as carboxyhaemoglobin.

CASE 4.1

A 68-year-old woman had a massive haematemesis followed by cardiorespiratory arrest. She was intubated and ventilated by the attending anaesthetist who noted evidence of aspiration. Cardiac output was restored after 6 min of cardiac massage and fluid resuscitation. The following arterial blood gases were taken 10 min later:

pH	6.924
PCO_2	9.1 kPa
PO_2	5.6 kPa
Bicarbonate	14 mmol/L

Base excess	−12 mmol/L
Lactate	10 mmol/L
Haemoglobin	4.6 g/dL

The arterial blood gases demonstrate that the patient is hypoxic with a profound mixed metabolic and respiratory acidaemia. The metabolic component can be attributed to a combination of tissue hypoxia, hypotension and hypovolaemia, whilst the respiratory component is due to inadequate alveolar ventilation and shunting. When there is an imbalance between systemic oxygen supply and demand, cells rely on anaerobic metabolism producing lactate. Normal levels are ≤ 2 mmol/L. Initial resuscitation should begin with airway assessment. In view of her hypoxic state, it is necessary to confirm the position of the endotracheal tube and exclude intubation of the oesophagus or right main bronchus. Given that there is clear evidence of aspiration of blood, tracheobronchial toilet (which may involve fibreoptic bronchoscopy) should then be performed to improve oxygenation and decrease shunt. Ventilatory support (either manual or mechanical) should be continued in an attempt to correct hypoxia and hypercarbia.

Fluid resuscitation with crystalloids/colloids and blood in order to restore tissue perfusion is fundamental in this patient. Serial lactate measurements are useful in following the response to therapy.

KEY POINTS: CAUSES OF LACTIC ACIDOSIS

Type A (tissue hypoxia present)	Type B (tissue hypoxia absent)
Severe hypoxia	Renal failure
Severe anaemia	Diabetes mellitus
Severe hypotension	Liver failure
Hypovolaemia	Leukaemia, lymphoma
Cardiac failure	Salicylate overdose
Septic shock	Methanol/ethylene glycol ingestion

CASE 4.2

A 76-year-old man with a history of hypertension and peptic ulcer disease was admitted to the medical admissions unit with a 3-day history of vomiting. His medication included atenolol and bendroflumethiazide. On examination he was mildly dehydrated, normotensive with epigastric tenderness but had no signs of peritonism. An arterial blood gas sample was subsequently taken on air:

pH	7.49
PCO_2	6.1 kPa
PO_2	10.2 kPa
Bicarbonate	34 mmol/L
Base excess	+6 mmol/L
K^+	2.6 mmol/L
Cl^-	93 mmol/L

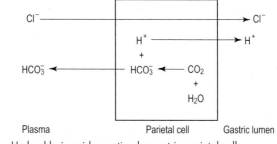

Figure 4.2 Hydrochloric acid secretion by gastric parietal cells.

The blood gas shows that this patient has a hypochloraemic metabolic alkalaemia presumed secondary to persistent vomiting. Hypokalaemia is also present as a consequence of gastric losses and thiazide diuretic use. The PCO_2 value is high/normal suggesting there is a degree of respiratory compensation.

In this case, metabolic alkalosis is generated by loss of gastric secretions rich in acid and a net gain in bicarbonate.

Secretion of hydrochloric acid into the gastric lumen is accompanied by generation of equivalent amounts of bicarbonate by the gastric parietal cells. Bicarbonate is then transported out of parietal cells in exchange for chloride (Fig. 4.2). Under normal circumstances, gastric acid stimulates pancreatic secretion of bicarbonate into the duodenum. During vomiting, the stimulus for pancreatic bicarbonate secretion is lost and there is an increase in plasma bicarbonate which drives the metabolic alkalosis.

The kidneys normally have a large capacity to excrete bicarbonate and return the plasma level to normal. Maintaining factors such as potassium, chloride and ECF depletion with reduced glomerular filtration contribute to the persistent alkalotic state.

Thiazide diuretics act mainly on the distal convoluted tubule where they inhibit sodium and chloride reabsorption. The increased sodium load in the

KEY POINTS: CAUSES OF METABOLIC ALKALOSIS
Inappropriate loss of acid from gut or kidneys
- Potassium depletion
  - Hyperaldosteronism (usually secondary)
  - Cushing's syndrome
  - Bartter's syndrome
  - Kaliuretic diuretics
- Chloride depletion
  - loss of gastric acid
  - diuretics
  - villous adenoma

Ingestion or infusion of alkali in excess of excretory capacity
- Milk-alkali syndrome
- Excessive bicarbonate intake
- Massive blood transfusion due to metabolism of citrate
- Recovery phase from metabolic acidosis due to excess regeneration of bicarbonate

distal tubule stimulates sodium exchange for potassium and hydrogen, increasing their excretion and causing hypokalaemia and metabolic alkalosis.

Management involves fluid resuscitation with saline, correction of hypokalaemia, stopping the diuretics and treating the underlying pathology (pre-pyloric ulcers).

CASE 4.3

A 46-year-old man with recently diagnosed motor neuron disease and moderate impairment of mobility was admitted to hospital with a 3-day history of increasing shortness of breath, productive cough and fever. He was given 15 L/min of oxygen via mask with reservoir bag during transfer to hospital. On arrival he was confused, febrile and tachypnoeic with clinical signs consistent with a right basal pneumonia. The following blood gases were obtained:

pH	7.16
PCO_2	10.7 kPa
PO_2	12.8 kPa
Bicarbonate	24 mmol/L
Base excess	−1 mmol/L
Glucose	6.6 mmol/L
Lactate	1.4 mmol/L

This gentleman has respiratory failure with uncompensated respiratory acidaemia secondary to pneumonia and neuromuscular weakness.

KEY POINTS: CAUSES OF RESPIRATORY ACIDOSIS
Respiratory tract disease
- Chronic obstructive pulmonary disease
- Chest wall disease
- Ankylosing spondylitis
- Severe kyphoscoliosis
- Flail chest

Neuromuscular disease
- Myasthenia gravis
- Poliomyelitis
- Guillain-Barré
- Muscular dystrophy
- Myotonic dystrophy
- Motor neurone disease

Obstructive sleep apnoea
CNS depression
- Drugs
- Raised intracranial pressure
- Trauma
- Encephalitis
- Brainstem ischaemia/infarct
- Central sleep apnoea

Hypoventilation during assisted ventilation

Stepwise approach for interpretation of blood gases

In patients with motor neurone disease, significant bulbar and respiratory muscle weakness occurs in approximately 50% and in a few cases respiratory failure can be the presenting complaint. Respiratory compromise is due to impairment of the muscle groups essential for normal ventilation (internal and external intercostals and those controlling the upper airway). Bulbar dysfunction, poor cough and atelectasis increase the risk of aspiration and infection. Increasing respiratory demands cannot be met and hypoxia and acidosis ensue. This further impairs diaphragmatic function. Treatment involves assisted ventilation, protection from aspiration and appropriate management of the underlying pneumonia. Weaning from ventilatory support is likely to be prolonged and difficult. Decisions about long-term management need to be addressed with the patient and his family at an appropriate time.

CASE 4.4

An 18-year-old girl was admitted to the ward with drowsiness, disorientation, vague abdominal pain and tinnitus. She was febrile, tachypnoeic, tachycardic and normotensive with a Glasgow Coma Score (GCS) of 11. Abdominal and neurological examinations were unremarkable. A head CT was reported as normal. Her blood results were as follows:

Na	142 mmol/L
K	3.1 mmol/L
Cl	101 mmol/L
Urea	7.8 mmol/L
Creatinine	126 μmol/L
pH	7.26
PCO_2	3.4 kPa
PO_2	10.8 kPa
Bicarbonate	18 mmol/L
Base excess	9.1 mmol/L
Glucose	6.6 mmol/L
Lactate	1.1 mmol/L

This patient has a metabolic acidaemia with either respiratory compensation or a co-existing respiratory alkalosis.

The anion gap is markedly elevated at 26 $[(Na^+ + K^+] - (Cl^- + HCO_3^-)]$. The normal range is approximately 8–16 mmol/L. Renal failure and diabetic ketoacidosis can be excluded on the basis of results and lactate is only mildly elevated. Therefore the possibility of exogenous acid ingestion should be considered (salicylate, ethylene glycol, methanol). The clinical presentation and co-existing respiratory alkalosis would be consistent with a diagnosis of salicylate overdose.

In overdose, salicylate directly stimulates the medullary respiratory centres leading to hyperventilation and respiratory alkalosis. Later, it also causes uncoupling of oxidative phosphorylation with impairment of aerobic pathways and accumulation of lactate and pyruvate producing a metabolic acidosis. In addition, high levels of salicylate interfere with carbohydrate, fat and protein metabolism giving rise to gluconeogenesis with production of ketoacids. Dehydration and uraemia may also contribute to the acidosis.

Management should include aspiration of gastric contents, administration of activated charcoal (if the airway is protected), rehydration and correction of pH with bicarbonate infusions if there is severe poisoning to promote drug excretion. In severe cases, forced alkaline diuresis or haemodialysis should be considered, ideally in a critical care area.

KEY POINTS: CAUSES OF METABOLIC ACIDOSIS
High anion gap
- Uraemia
- Ketoacidosis
- Lactic acidosis
- Salicylate overdose
- Ethylene glycol poisoning
- Methanol poisoning
- Paraldehyde poisoning

Normal anion gap
- GI loss of bicarbonate
  - Diarrhoea
  - Enterocutaneous fistula
  - Enteric diversion of urine
- Renal loss of bicarbonate
  - Proximal renal tubular acidosis
- Failure of renal H^+ secretion
  - Distal renal tubular acidosis
- Rapid volume expansion with normal saline

CASE 4.5

A 19-year-old student presented to the emergency department with a history of headaches and irritability for several days and, more recently, shortness of breath. Despite this he looked pink, had a pulse of 90 bpm, BP 135/86 and oxygen saturation 98% on room air. His chest was clear to auscultation. His blood gas results (on air) were as follows:

pH	7.48
PO_2	9.2 kPa
PCO_2	3.9 kPa
Bicarbonate	21 mmol/L
Base excess	−4.4 mmol/L
Co-oximeter	oxygen saturation 76%

This man has a mild respiratory alkalaemia. There is hyperventilation and a marked discrepancy between the oxygen saturation on pulse oximetry, measured PaO_2 with a blood gas machine and oxygen saturation measured by a co-oximeter, implying low oxygen carriage. The diagnosis is carbon monoxide (CO) poisoning.

Carbon monoxide has a 240 × greater affinity for haemoglobin than oxygen and forms carboxyhaemoglobin (CoHb), which does not release oxygen in the tissues. The absorption spectrum for CoHb is similar to oxyhaemoglobin so currently available pulse oximeters that use two wavelengths of light for analysis cannot distinguish between them. Conventional arterial blood gas machines calculate SpO_2 from the PaO_2 and therefore will also be inaccurate in the presence of significant CoHb. Consequently the PaO_2 of 9.2 is a significant overestimate, revealed only when the co-oximeter confirms the true saturation of 76%, implying a 'true' PaO_2 of around 5.5 kPa.

Significant levels of CoHb occur in smokers (up to 10%), in fires in confined spaces, in inhalational injuries and from poorly maintained vehicles or domestic gas appliances. This student might live in a house with a poorly maintained gas fire, which is well known to produce CO poisoning. Both pulse oximetry and arterial blood gas analysis will overestimate circulating blood oxygen content in such patients and a blood gas machine using a co-oximeter should always be used.

Symptoms usually arise from tissue hypoxia and this is the cause of his shortness of breath, not centrally sensed hypoxia. The aortic chemosensors respond to partial pressure of oxygen, not content. Partial pressure may be normal in his case as this is largely due to dissolved oxygen rather than total carriage which relies on haemoglobin. Other symptoms include headache, dizziness, confusion, abdominal and chest pain, nausea and vomiting and in severe poisoning, coma, convulsions and cardiac arrest. Symptoms generally start at levels greater than 15% CoHb. His case is mild and will settle with administration of oxygen. Severe poisoning occurs with levels greater than 40%, and with levels greater than 50% mortality may be as high as 50%. Treatment is based on the administration of 100% oxygen and supportive measures. The half-life of CoHb in room air (FiO_2 0.21) is 240 min and this decreases to 90 min on 100% oxygen. The use of hyperbaric oxygen is controversial. Although the half-life of CoHb falls to only 20 min at 2 atmospheres, there are logistical problems as well as potential problems with oxygen toxicity. Hyperbaric chambers are rarely close to emergency departments and by the time patients are transferred, CoHb levels will often be within safe limits. However, some authorities believe that neurological recovery is better if hyperbaric oxygen is administered. In moderate to severe poisoning, the risk/benefit ratio should be discussed with the regional hyperbaric centre.

FURTHER READING

Goldberg M et al 1973 Computer based instruction and diagnosis of acid-base disorders. JAMA 223:269–275

Nutrition in the critically ill

5

Diane Monkhouse

OBJECTIVES

After reading this chapter you should be able to:

● Recognize the metabolic and nutritional changes during critical illness

● Understand how to measure nutritional status and estimate nutritional requirements

● Compare enteral and parenteral routes of administration

● Consider the role of immunonutrition during critical illness

● Explore nutritional support in specific diseases

INTRODUCTION

Nutritional support is a fundamental component of standard supportive care in the management of the critically ill patient. However, it is not without inherent risk. Enteral nutrition can increase the risk of aspiration pneumonia while parenteral nutrition has been associated with gut mucosal atrophy, hyperglycaemia and catheter-related infections. So why do we bother?

By detecting and correcting pre-existing malnutrition, providing appropriate nutritional support and optimizing the patient's metabolic state, we aim to improve wound healing, decrease the catabolic response to injury, restore gut mucosal integrity and reduce complication rates.

METABOLIC AND NUTRITIONAL CHANGES DURING CRITICAL ILLNESS

It is well recognized that patients deteriorate nutritionally long before hospital admission. Studies suggest that up to 27% of patients admitted to general medical, general surgical, orthopaedic, respiratory or elderly care wards showed evidence of moderate or severe malnutrition. Further nutritional deterioration in hospital occurs in two-thirds of patients. They continue to lose an average of 7% of their residual weight during their stay (see Key points: causes of malnutrition).

KEY POINTS: CAUSES OF MALNUTRITION PRE-HOSPITAL ADMISSION

Inability to eat
- Neurological disorders
- Swallowing dysfunction

Gastrointestinal disease
- Inflammatory bowel disease
- Radiation enteritis
- Gluten enteropathy
- Short bowel syndrome

Anorexia
- Malignancy
- Chronic disease
- Depression

Inflammatory response to infection

The consequences of malnutrition can be profound. Muscle weakness, reduced hypoxic ventilatory drive and early fatiguability are commonly found in malnourished patients. These have major implications for weaning from ventilatory support and subsequent mobilization. Similarly, cardiac muscle size and function may be impaired. Malnutrition adversely affects immune function with atrophy of lymphoid tissue (including gut-associated lymphoid tissue), depletion of IgA and a reduction in T-lymphocytes. Intestinal barrier function can be compromised and pancreatic exocrine function impaired. Both are potentially reversible with the introduction of enteral nutrition.

Malnutrition not only refers to protein-energy malnutrition but also micronutrient deficiency and altered antioxidant status, which can influence the extent of tissue injury in the context of critical illness. Other adverse effects of malnutrition include delayed wound healing, altered thermoregulation and peripheral oedema (due to hypoalbuminaemia and reduced colloid osmotic pressure).

The acute phase response to infection or injury is a primitive response designed to limit tissue damage and facilitate repair. It is characterized by three phases (Fig. 5.1):

1. A brief shock or ebb phase during which the metabolic rate is reduced.
2. A catabolic or flow phase in which the metabolic rate rises and substrates are mobilized in order to mount inflammatory and immune responses (Table 5.1). The magnitude of the response is proportional to the extent of the injury. In addition, there is accelerated gluconeogenesis, mobilization of glycogen, lipolysis and breakdown of muscle proteins. The major gluconeogenic precursors are amino acids derived from muscle protein. The consequence is that the catabolic phase results in accelerated loss of

muscle mass. In critical illness, protein breakdown may result in a 30 g nitrogen loss per day. This equates to a loss of 1 lb of skeletal muscle mass with potential for functional impairment.

Changes in cytokines and hormones occur as part of the catabolic phase. Cytokines such as interleukin-1, interleukin-6 and tumour necrosis factor are released by cells at the site of injury. They act locally to initiate the inflammatory response, systemically to enhance the neuroendocrine responses and at the level of the hypothalamus to induce fever. Release of catecholamines, adrenocorticotrophic hormone (ACTH), cortisol, glucagon and growth hormone produce a state of hyperglycaemia and insulin resistance.

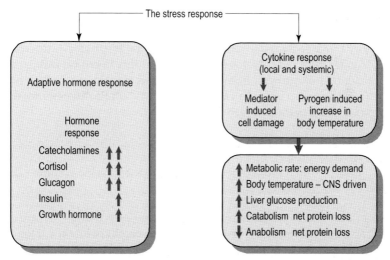

Figure 5.1 The stress response to infection or injury.

Table 5.1 A comparison of the metabolic effects of starvation and catabolism seen in critical illness

Starvation	Catabolic response to critical illness
Reduced metabolic rate and calorie requirements	Increased metabolic rate and calorie
Fat is the main non-carbohydrate energy source	Neuroendocrine and cytokine response
Increased lipolysis	Protein is the major energy source
Reduced insulin levels	Limited use of fat or carbohydrate as energy source
Protein levels and lean body mass relatively well preserved until late into the period of starvation	Massive nitrogen loss from muscle protein
Anabolism occurs when nutritional support is restored	Catabolic state is not reversed by restoration of nutritional support

3. An anabolic or convalescent phase during which glycogen and proteins are resynthesized, enabling lost tissue to be restored.

ASSESSMENT OF NUTRITIONAL STATUS

Critically ill patients are a heterogeneous group. Consequently, there are no definitive tests of nutritional status or universal formulae for feeding.

Assessment involves taking a detailed history looking for estimated weight loss, changes in appetite or food intake and severity of illness.

Clinical examination with measurement of body mass index is quick and simple but of limited value. Estimation of daily weight is more helpful in determining fluctuations in fluid balance than loss of lean body mass.

Measurements of skinfold thickness and midarm circumference have been used as markers of muscle mass but these are of limited value in oedematous patients. Measurements of hand grip strength by dynamometry and respiratory muscle strength by assessing maximum inspiratory force require patient cooperation and therefore have limited utility in critical care.

A calculation of nitrogen balance can be used to estimate the severity of the catabolic response but it has no value in renal failure and assumes that a steady state exists in the nitrogen pool (Fig. 5.2).

Nitrogen balance = intake – loss/24 h
Intake = protein/6.25   *g/24 h*
Loss or urinary nitrogen = urinary urea × 24 h urine volume × 0.028
      g/24 h   *mmol/L*   *litre*

Serum albumin is often inappropriately used as a marker of nutrition. During acute illness, albumin leaks out from the capillary into the interstitial space ten times more rapidly than it is synthesized. Hence serum albumin levels are more indicative of redistribution than nutritional state. It is further

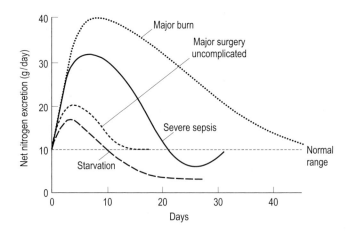

Figure 5.2 Nitrogen excretion in critical illness.

handicapped by its long half-life of 20 days. The synthesis of acute phase proteins occurs preferentially over that of visceral proteins regardless of the nutritional state. Concentration of acute phase proteins such as C-reactive protein (CRP) and fibrinogen rise while levels of albumin, pre-albumin and transferrin all fall. An index of inflammation and nutrition can be derived from:

$$\frac{CRP \times \alpha1\text{-acid glycoprotein}}{albumin \times pre\text{-albumin}}$$

NUTRITIONAL REQUIREMENTS (Table 5.2)

Balanced feeds in the proportion of 15% protein, 30–40% fat and 55–60% carbohydrate are widely available. The total calorie intake should be equivalent to normal resting energy expenditure. Approximately 150 kcal of non-protein energy source are required per gram of nitrogen to permit adequate protein synthesis. Non-protein calorie to nitrogen ratios should be in the order of 125–150 in the critically ill patient.

It is common practice to commence feeding with a total energy intake which equals the resting energy expenditure calculated by either the Harris-Benedict or Schofield equations (Table 5.3) and to increase delivery by × 1.2–1.3 during the first week, depending upon tolerance and the clinical condition of the patient.

Although the Harris-Benedict and Schofield equations are commonly used in clinical practice, it must be emphasized that estimated and measured resting energy requirements may differ by 30–50%. Under ideal circumstances, daily measurement by indirect calorimetry would be more efficient. Unfortunately, this is technically demanding and is not routinely available.

Giving excess calories, particularly in the form of carbohydrate, increases fat synthesis, liver deposition of fat and carbon dioxide production. Increased carbon dioxide production can impair weaning from ventilatory support or increase the work of breathing for ward patients. However underfeeding is a more common problem, particularly in enterally-fed patients. On average, they receive only 75% of their estimated requirements.

Table 5.2 Adult daily nutritional requirements

Protein	1.5 g/kg
Carbohydrate	20–25 kcal/kg
Lipid	4% of kcal
Sodium	70–100 mmol
Potassium	70–100 mmol
Chloride	40–100 mmol
Calcium	5–10 mmol
Phosphate	20–30 mmol
Magnesium	7.5–10 mmol
+ Vitamins and trace elements	

Table 5.3   Methods for estimating energy requirements

Harris-Benedict equation (estimates resting energy expenditure (REE))

Male: $13.75W + 5H − 6.76A + 66.47$
Female: $9.56W + 1.85H − 4.68A + 655.1$

W= weight in kilograms
H= height in centimeters
A= age in years

To predict total energy expenditure, add an injury/acuity factor of 1.2–1.8 depending upon the nature or severity of the illness.

Schofield equation

Age	REE (male)	REE (female)
15–18	$17.6 \times W + 656$	$13.3 \times W + 690$
18–30	$15.0 \times W + 690$	$14.8 \times W + 485$
30–60	$11.4 \times W + 870$	$8.1 \times W + 842$
> 60	$11.7 \times W + 585$	$9.0 \times W + 656$

Adjust calculated REE according to pathology.
Add a combined factor for activity and diet-induced thermogenesis.
If an increase in energy stores is required, add 400–1000 kcal/day.

ENTERAL NUTRITION

All critically ill patients should be enterally fed if the gastrointestinal tract is functional. The major benefits are that it is cheap and physiological. It stimulates intestinal and biliary motility and provides a greater range of nutrients (particularly glutamine and short chain fatty acids). In addition, it has been shown to preserve intestinal mucosal integrity, decrease the hypermetabolic response to injury, augment cellular anti-oxidant status and improve immune function and wound healing. Without enteral nutrient delivery, gut mucosal atrophy occurs with the increased risk of bacterial colonization and translocation leading to sepsis. The risks associated with enteral feeding are outlined in the 'Key points: complications associated with enteral nutrition' box.

Enteral feed is most commonly delivered by the nasogastric route because of its relative ease. Large bore nasogastric tubes allow manual aspiration of gastric contents but can encourage reflux. Siting a fine bore tube may help resolve this problem. Nursing the patient in a semirecumbent position can reduce the risk of aspiration and nosocomial pneumonia. Sedated and ventilated patients can have normal gastric emptying in the absence of active bowel sounds. Consequently, initiation of feeding should not be delayed until bowel sounds are present or flatus is passed. Delayed gastric emptying can occur as part of the stress response. Other contributing factors include opioid analgesia, sepsis, burns, head injury and hyperglycaemia. Introduction of a prokinetic agent such as metoclopramide may improve the chances of successful feeding.

KEY POINTS: COMPLICATIONS ASSOCIATED WITH ENTERAL NUTRITION

RELATED TO FEEDING TUBES
- Complications of insertion
- Failed insertion
- Tube displacement
- Erosion of nares
- Sinusitis
- Tube blockage
- Aerophagy
- Patient discomfort

RELATED TO ENTERAL FEEDING
- Nausea, abdominal discomfort or distension
- Regurgitation or vomiting
- Pulmonary aspiration of feed
- Diarrhoea
- Interaction with medication

RELATED TO FEED CONTENTS
- Hyperglycaemia
- Uraemia
- Hypercarbia
- Electrolyte abnormalities
- Deficiencies of vitamins or trace elements with long term therapy

If gastric stasis persists, post-pyloric feeding should be considered. A nasojejunal tube can be sited blindly with varying degrees of success and several are commercially available for this specific purpose. Endoscopic or fluoroscopic placement is much more reliable but requires input from other specialists which may incur delay. For surgical patients, placement of a percutaneous jejunostomy should be considered at the time of initial surgery if problems with gastric feeding are anticipated. Percutaneous tubes are preferable when long-term feeding (> 4 weeks) is envisaged, particularly in patients with chronic neurological disease.

Enteral feeding preparations are usually iso-osmolar (to prevent diarrhoea) and lactose free (because of relative lactase deficiency in malnourished patients). The use of oligosaccharides allows an increase in the carbohydrate content of feed without increase in osmolality. Current recommendations are for the use of whole-protein (polymeric) formulae. Lipids allow a reduction in osmolality of feed but provide a substantial amount of energy in a small volume. Insoluble fibre increases faecal mass through water absorption and can help in reducing diarrhoea. Adjustment of electrolyte composition may be required particularly with renal or hepatic dysfunction. Vitamins and trace elements are essential constituents of enteral feed.

Immune-enhancing feeds supplemented with glutamine, arginine, omega-3 fatty acids and nucleotides have been formulated for nutritional support in the critically ill. The putative benefits include reducing infection

KEY POINTS: AN OVERVIEW OF IMMUNONUTRITION

GLUTAMINE

- Conditionally essential amino acid
- Decreased levels during critical illness
- Acts as an inter-organ nitrogen and carbon transporter for intracellular glutamate
- Fundamental for synthesis of purines, pyrimidines and nucleotides
- Important for T-helper and monocyte function

Current evidence suggests that enteral glutamine should be considered in trauma and burns patients. However, when parenteral nutrition is used in the critically ill supplementation with glutamine is recommended.

ARGININE

- Conditionally essential amino acid
- Substrate for the synthesis of proteins, creatine and nitric oxide
- Improves wound healing and has T-cell immunostimulatory effects

Currently there is no evidence to support the routine use of arginine-enriched feed.

FISH OILS

- Fatty acids may influence the ability of cells to produce cytokines and the ability of target tissues to respond to them

Current evidence suggests that enteral formulae containing fish oils, borage oils and antioxidants should be considered in patients with acute respiratory distress syndrome (ARDS).

NUCLEOTIDES

- Dietary RNA increases protein synthesis and regulates T-cell mediated immune responses.

Currently there is no evidence to support the routine use of nucleotides in enteral feed.

and inflammation and boosting antioxidant status. The balance of evidence does not currently favour the routine use of these feeds. However, there is evidence to support the use of immune-enhancing feed in specific disease states (see Key points: an overview of immunonutrition).

PARENTERAL NUTRITION

There are no nutritional advantages of parenteral over enteral nutrition. In view of its expense and higher risk profile (see Key points box on p. 65), parenteral nutrition should only be considered when the enteral route has failed or is contraindicated. The major indication for its use is functional or mechanical obstruction of the upper gastrointestinal tract which cannot be bypassed by a feeding tube. Under such circumstances it is an ideal way of delivering adequate amounts of nutrients until the enteral route is available. Careful monitoring is required to avoid lipaemia, hyperglycaemia, electrolyte disturbance and overfeeding. It is important to remember that if the patient is sedated with propofol and receiving total parenteral nutrition (TPN), there is a risk of hypertriglyceridaemia. Propofol is supplied as a 10%

KEY POINTS: COMPLICATIONS ASSOCIATED WITH PARENTERAL NUTRITION

Catheter related
- Complications related to insertion or residence
- Local infection at skin entry site
- Septicaemia

Intestinal mucosal atrophy

Metabolic
- Hyperglycaemia
- Lipaemia
- Electrolyte imbalance
- Metabolic acidosis
- Hypophosphataemia
- Micronutrient deficiencies
- Refeeding syndrome

Hepatobiliary complications
- Steatosis
- Acalculous cholecystitis
- Deranged liver function tests (LFTs)

lipid emulsion and provides 1.1 kcal/mL. Intravenous fat supplementation in the form of TPN needs to be decreased accordingly during propofol administration.

Parenteral nutrition can be administered via a peripheral vein for short-term feeding provided that the osmolarity is less than 900 mOsmol/L. Peripheral cannulae avoid the risks of central venous cannulation but the hypertonic nature of the nutrient solution frequently leads to phlebitis and loss of access. Pharmacies are often able to prepare less hypertonic solutions for peripheral delivery. Central veins can be approached from the periphery with a long line or a peripherally inserted central catheter (PICC). They are particularly useful in patients with clotting diatheses but can cause axillary or subclavian vein thrombosis. In critically ill patients central venous access is recommended. If multi-lumen catheters are used, a lumen is dedicated to TPN delivery. Meticulous aseptic technique is required when connecting and disconnecting infusions. A tunnelled feeding line in the subclavian vein minimizes the risk of infective complications and is preferred for longer-term use.

The nutrient solutions can be either pre-prepared commercial solutions or specialist formulations manufactured in the pharmacy under sterile conditions. The latter can be 'tailor-made' according to the needs of the patient. The solution contains amino acids, glucose, lipid, electrolytes, vitamins, minerals and trace elements in a volume of 2–3 L. Nitrogen provision is 0.2–0.3g/kg in a combination of essential and non-essential amino acids. It is difficult to include all non-essential amino acids because of the stability of the solution. Glutamine becomes essential in critical illness and supplementation of TPN with glutamine has been associated with a reduction in mortality in critical care unit patients.

Energy provision is a combination of glucose and fat with fat making up approximately 30–40% of the total calorie intake. It has a higher calorific

Parenteral nutrition

Table 5.4 Functions of essential trace elements

Trace element	Function
Zinc	Cofactor for > 100 enzymes such as carbonic anhydrase
	Essential for competent immune system
Copper	Important in erythrocyte maturation and lipid metabolism
Iron	Essential for haemoglobin synthesis
Selenium	Needed to maintain antioxidant status
Cobalt	Essential constituent of vitamin B_{12}
Iodine	Required for thyroxine synthesis
Manganese	Needed for calcium/phophorus metabolism

value than glucose and is particularly useful when fluid restriction is needed. IV lipids are available as emulsions with egg yolk or phospholipids. Glucose is the carbohydrate of choice and concentrated solutions are necessary to provide adequate calories. Dextrose administration should not exceed 1.5 g/kg/day as excessive amounts can produce glucose intolerance, abnormal liver function tests and fatty infiltration of the liver. Bio-chemical monitoring is therefore mandatory. Water- and fat-soluble vitamins should be added to the solution. Provision of micronutrients in standard feeds may be inadequate in critically ill patents with depleted reserves. Deficiency states can occur without overt symptoms within a few weeks of initiating TPN. The most commonly recognized deficiencies are folic acid presenting with pancytopaenia, thiamine with encephalopathy and vitamin K with hypothrombinaemia. Trace element deficiency states are not uncommon in the critically ill. Zinc, an essential constituent of many enzymes, is prone to deficiency because of increased loss in critical illness. The functions of essential trace elements are outlined in Table 5.4.

NUTRITION IN SPECIFIC DISEASE STATES

Acute renal failure

As patients in acute renal failure are often extremely catabolic, implementation of enteral feeding should be considered early.

Nutritional support should be directed towards correcting deficiencies. Adequate calories should be provided in a low volume, reduced electrolyte solution. Provision of optimal dialysis offers greater nutritional flexibility but it must be remembered that extra protein losses occur with peritoneal dialysis and amino acid losses with haemofiltration. This should be taken into account when planning the feeding regimen. The B-group of vitamins are water soluble and can be removed during dialysis and haemofiltration. They should be supplemented regularly.

Acute hepatic failure

Enteral feed is encouraged providing there is no bleeding from the gastro-intestinal tract. Protein may need to be restricted in encephalopathic patients but normal intakes may be tolerated during continuous feeding. Lipid clearance is usually normal in jaundiced patients but may be reduced in hepatic failure. Because of failure of gluconeogenesis, adequate carbohydrate should be provided. Sodium restriction and vitamin supplementation should also be considered.

Pancreatitis

The role of enteral nutrition in pancreatitis has been extensively debated. Advocates of parenteral nutrition feel that delivery of nutrients into the stomach stimulates pancreatic secretions and creates a further burden on the severely inflamed pancreas. However, jejunal feeding can be implemented without pancreatic stimulation and this has been shown to be beneficial in terms of reduction in septic complications. The feeding regimen is typically high in carbohydrate and low in fat.

Cardiac failure

Low sodium and water intake is essential. For patients on high dose diuretics, magnesium, potassium and thiamine losses may be excessive.

OTHER CONSIDERATIONS

Insulin

Insulin has been used in critical care not only to correct hyperglycaemia but also for its protein-sparing effects and its effect on cell membrane function. A recent study has demonstrated that maintenance of tight glycaemic control in post-operative cardiac patients reduced infection rates, mortality, time spent on a ventilator and length of hospital stay. These effects have been attributed to the preservation of normoglycaemia and normal triglyceride concentrations but other effects of insulin may be beneficial. The maintenance of normoglycaemia has extended into widespread practice in intensive care patients, particularly in the management of severe sepsis.

Gastric protection

The incidence of acute stress ulceration in the critical care unit varies from 8–45%. Recognized risk factors include ventilatory support, advanced age, coagulopathy, lack of enteral feeding, sepsis, burns, polytrauma, spinal injury, head injury, renal failure and liver failure. Gastric hypoperfusion with resulting mucosal ischaemia predisposes to ulceration in these patients. Improvement in end-organ perfusion and enteral nutritional support can help reduce the risk. Prophylactic protection with proton pump inhibitors or H_2 blockers is routinely undertaken in the critically ill at-risk population.

Prokinetics

Successful enteral nutrition relies upon intact gastric motility which is frequently impaired in the critically ill. Prokinetic agents such as metoclopramide and erythromycin have valuable roles in improving gut transit and feeding tolerance, reducing the risk of gastro-oesophageal reflux and promoting the placement of post-pyloric tubes. Cautious use of erythromycin is essential given the increasing incidence of antibiotic resistance.

CASE 5.1

A 44-year-old man presented with a history of acute confusion, fever and dysuria. He was a known alcoholic who consumed 2 bottles of sherry per day. His partner reported that he had had poor dietary intake for several weeks and had lost approximately a stone in weight in the previous 2 months. Examination revealed a cachectic man with a body mass index (BMI) of 45. He was confused, febrile and jaundiced with multiple bruises. On abdominal examination, he had hepatomegaly and an enlarged bladder.

Investigations:

Hb	13.5 g/dL
White cell count	14.6×10^9/L
PT`	22 s
Sodium	133 mmol/L
Potassium	4.6 mmol/L
Urea	7.6 mmol/L
Creatinine	78 µmol/L
Glucose	3.2mmol/L
Magnesium	0.48 mmol/L
Albumin	28 g/L
ALT	1506 IU
AST	1227 IU
Bilirubin	88 µmol/L
Urinalysis	protein++, nitrites++, blood +

This gentleman has alcoholic hepatitis causing hypoglycaemia, hypoalbuminaemia, deranged coagulation and elevation of transaminases. Confounding this is a urinary tract infection secondary to bladder outflow obstruction leading to deranged renal function. The infection is the most likely precipitant of hepatic encephalopathy although Wernicke's encephalopathy secondary to thiamine deficiency should be considered.

He is likely to have gross protein energy malnutrition because of his poor oral intake. True weight loss may be masked by oedema and/or ascites. In addition, he may have multiple vitamin deficiencies especially thiamine. His bruising can be accounted for by his prolonged prothrombin time secondary to liver disease. He will have an increased metabolic rate because of his fever and infection.

After IV antibiotics and bladder catheterization, enteral feeding using a standard polymeric feed should be started. In this case 0.2 g nitrogen/kg per day would be a reasonable starting point. The feed should be introduced slowly and increased gradually to meet target nutritional requirements. This should take into account a 10% increase for diet-induced thermogenesis and a 13% increase per °C rise in temperature. Vitamin supplementation with thiamine, vitamin K and a multivitamin preparation should also be prescribed.

Progress: despite starting feed (1 kcal/mL) at 30 mL/h and increasing to 80 mL/h over 3 days, his serum potassium dropped to 2.7 mmol/L, phosphate fell to 0.33 mmol/L and magnesium levels were recorded at 0.42 mmol/L necessitating intravenous supplementation of all three.

The case above is typical of refeeding syndrome.

When a severely malnourished patient is given nutritional support, there is an initial increase in extracellular volume due to positive water and sodium balance. As the patient receives energy and protein supplements, there is a stimulus for glycogen storage and protein synthesis. This promotes movement of water into cells. Carbohydrate administration stimulates insulin secretion leading to enhanced cellular uptake of glucose, potassium, phosphate and magnesium. Rapid refeeding can precipitate cardiac arrhythmias which may be fatal.

The feeding regimen for a malnourished patient needs to take into account the risks of refeeding. Cautious energy, protein and fluid repletion is essential with regular monitoring of potassium, magnesium and phosphate levels, particularly in the first week. Seek help from the dietician.

FURTHER READING

Allison S, Lobo D 2005 Nutritional and metabolic care. In: Brooks A, Girling K, Riley B et al. Critical care for postgraduate trainees. Hodder and Arnold, London

Bennett M J 2001 Nutritional support in critically ill patients: the role of enteral feeding. In: Kaufman L, Ginsburg R. Anaesthesia review. Churchill Livingstone, London

Heyland D K, Dhaliwal R D, Drover J W et al 2003 Canadian clinical practice guidelines for nutritional support in mechanically ventilated, critically ill adult patients. Journal of Parenteral and Enteral Nutrition 27:355–373

Assessment and management of sepsis

6

Emilio Garcia

OBJECTIVES

After reading this chapter you should be able to:

- *Understand the pathophysiology of sepsis*
- *Identify symptoms and signs of sepsis*
- *Assess the septic patient*
- *Organize a septic screen*
- *Manage the septic patient*

INTRODUCTION

Sepsis is a common cause of critical illness, either as the primary diagnosis or as a complication of other diagnoses or hospital management, e.g. as a post-operative complication. Prompt diagnosis and treatment of the condition is paramount as early recognition, fluid resuscitation and antibiotics improve outcome from sepsis, even before the specific source of sepsis has been identified.

DEFINITIONS

Infection: invasion of normally sterile host tissue by organisms determining an inflammatory response.

Bacteraemia: the presence of viable bacteria in the blood stream.

Multiple organ dysfunction syndrome (MODS): presence of altered organ function in an acutely ill patient such that homeostasis cannot be maintained without intervention. It may or may not be due to sepsis.

Systemic inflammatory response syndrome (SIRS): This is defined as two or more of the following:

- Temperature > 38 or < 36
- Heart rate > 90
- Respiratory rate > 20 bpm or $PaCO_2$ < 4.2 kPa
- White blood cell count > 12 or < 4×10^9/L.

71

Sepsis: SIRS in response to infection.

Severe sepsis: this is sepsis in the presence of organ dysfunction and hypotension, defined as blood pressure < 90 mmHg or 40 mmHg reduction from normal blood pressure in the absence of other causes of hypotension.

Septic shock: sepsis-induced hypotension unresponsive to adequate fluid resuscitation along with the presence of perfusion abnormalities that may include, but are not limited to, lactic acidosis, oliguria, or an acute alteration in mental status.

PATHOGENESIS OF SEPSIS

The pathogenesis of sepsis is multifactorial and complex and beyond the scope of this book but it is important to recognize that there are many factors involved, that they can be activated in more than one manner and that it is the imbalance between activators and inhibitors that creates individual responses to the same stimulus. Increasingly it is recognized that genetic factors play an important role in response to, and possibly in survival from, sepsis.

Whereas initially it was thought that sepsis was merely due to the inflammation process it is now clear that other processes are involved, such as coagulation and fibrinolysis as well as endothelial dysfunction. The imbalance between these processes appears to play a very important role by modifying the disease response.

During the process of sepsis a wide variety of cytokines is released, including interleukins, tumour necrosis factor, platelet-activating factor and myocardial depressant factor. All these proinflammatory cytokines damage or are related to damage to the epithelium and intravascular coagulation. This determines increased extravascular permeability and disseminated intravascular coagulation (DIC). The process of fibrinolysis is also altered in sepsis. A decrease of protein C has been noted in patients with sepsis and organ dysfunction.

DIAGNOSIS OF SEPSIS

Early diagnosis and treatment of sepsis is important as it clearly improves outcome. The diagnosis of sepsis is often difficult and a high index of suspicion is required in order not to miss the early warning signs (see Key points box on p. 73). The elderly and immunocompromised patients may in fact display very few or none of the classical signs. Sometimes the only indicator of sepsis could be an unexplained persistent metabolic acidosis. In general, patients tend to have a hyperdynamic circulation.

When examining the septic patient, one must be looking not only for possible sources of sepsis (abdominal pain, infected wound or lines, muco-purulent secretions, etc.) but also to establish the general condition of the patient. A warm patient will be vasodilated and will require fluids to restore

ASSESSMENT AND MANAGEMENT OF SEPSIS

KEY POINTS: SYMPTOMS AND SIGNS OF SEPSIS
- Altered level of consciousness
- Tachypnoea
- Tachycardia
- Hypotension
- Warm peripheries/sweat
- Bounding pulses
- Signs of dehydration
- Decreased urine output
- Elevated white cell count (WCC)
- Elevated fibrinogen
- DIC and signs of DIC
- Nausea/vomiting
- Jaundice

circulating volume and may also require inotropes if fluid resuscitation does not restore perfusion; a cold, shut-down patient is likely to require both.

Patients are likely to be pyrexial and have rigors although some patients may be hypothermic and peripherally shut down, particularly in the later stages of severe sepsis. In the early stages the patient will be vasodilated with a high cardiac output, good capillary refill and bounding pulses. Blood pressure will be normal at first but it will eventually drop if sepsis goes unrecognized. There is high capillary permeability and this will contribute to fluid loss and hypovolemia.

In most septic patients a pulmonary artery catheter (PAC) would reveal an increased cardiac index, normal or reduced pulmonary artery occlusion pressure, normal or reduced central venous pressure (CVP), decreased systemic vascular resistance and increased oxygen delivery. Later on, myocardial depression will occur and the patient will show signs of low cardiac output.

Investigations

Full blood count (FBC): typically, an elevated WCC will be seen. A low white cell count may also indicate sepsis in patients with limited physiological reserve and it is a poor prognostic sign.

Clotting: this may be normal or prolonged. Fibrinogen will also be elevated as are all acute phase proteins.

Serum biochemistry: urea and electrolytes may show dehydration and or signs of renal failure. Potassium abnormalities are common. Liver function tests are likely to be deranged, the most common picture being of cholestasis. Glucose is usually elevated. Other biochemical tests such as serum amylase, lipase, troponin T, CPK, etc. may be necessary as severe sepsis often coexists with other pathology such as pancreatitis, myocardial infarction, etc.

Chest X-ray (CXR): this will provide information, not only regarding the presence of infection, but also in relation to central line and nasogastric tube positioning. Even in the absence of clinical signs a CXR should be performed.

Blood cultures: as above. Other cultures that should be considered depending on clinical suspicion regarding infective source are MSU/CSU, lumbar puncture, sputum culture/bronchoalveolar lavage (BAL), wound swabs, stools cultures, and high vaginal swab.

Interleukin 6 and tumour necrosis factor: these septic markers are still a research tool and their value is uncertain.

Procalcitonin levels: these may be useful as a general marker to support the diagnosis of severe sepsis, however their exact clinical role has not been finally elucidated.

Arterial blood gases: these provide invaluable information regarding respiratory function, acid–base balance and are indicators of physiological reserve and organ perfusion. Also, most modern blood gas machines provide a serum lactate measurement. Sequential lactate may be a useful guide in the evaluation of response to therapy.

Electrocardiogram (ECG): this helps to rule out cardiac causes of hypotension and to differentiate sinus tachycardia from arrhythmia.

MANAGEMENT OF SEPSIS

It is vital that the treatment of the septic patient should be commenced as soon as the diagnosis is suspected and this should not be delayed pending definitive microbiological results, the underlying exact source, or critical care unit bed availability. The reasoning behind this is that goal-directed resuscitation in the septic patient during the first 6 h decreases 28-day mortality (Rivers et al 2001).

Initial management of a critically ill patient starts with resuscitation: immediate assessment of the airway, breathing, oxygen administration and circulation. This is followed by a brief history and a limited examination of the relevant systems of the body.

Airway and breathing

Respiratory failure is common and may develop at any stage so repeated assessments are necessary. A depressed consciousness level is the most common cause of airway obstruction. All seriously ill patients should receive oxygen. Initial oxygen therapy should be guided by pulse oximetry, but its administration should not be delayed due to lack of equipment.

Patients with inadequate airway reflexes should be nursed in the recovery position and assessed by the critical care unit or outreach team to assess the need for airway protection. A clear airway does not indicate effective breathing which can be assessed clinically by assessing other organ

---

Tip

The respiratory rate is one of the most powerful indicators of severity of illness and should be methodically monitored.

dysfunction (like level of consciousness) or by blood gas assessment, looking not only at adequate oxygenation but also at PCO_2 levels.

Respiratory failure is suggested by signs of respiratory distress including dyspnoea, increased respiratory rate, use of accessory muscles, cyanosis, confusion, tachycardia and sweating. The diagnosis is made clinically but may be confirmed by pulse oximetry and arterial blood gases.

Patients with a depressed consciousness level may not react normally to hypoxia and signs of respiratory failure may be difficult to detect. Patients with inadequate ventilation, gas exchange or both require ventilatory support. This usually necessitates intubation and mechanical ventilation, although in some patients gas exchange and oxygenation can be improved by the application of continuous positive airway pressure (CPAP) by face mask or non-invasive ventilation.

A secondary assessment after stabilization of the patient includes a more thorough history, detailed examination by system and appropriate investigations.

Circulation

The management of sepsis should begin as soon as possible and its treatment should not be delayed pending critical care unit admission. Early goal-directed treatment (Figs 6.1, 6.2) should include the following aims:

CVP 8–12 mmHg
MAP > 65 mmHg
Urine output > 0.5 mL/kg
Central venous saturation > 70%.

Initial findings in early sepsis include tachycardia and hypotension. These may not be very obvious in the very early stages and in fit patients, and sometimes will only show if one looks for postural hypotension: lying down and standing or sitting blood pressure. However, in most cases we will find a warm tachycardic patient with a bounding pulse.

After a quick assessment, establishment of IV access and early fluid resuscitation should be commenced. The choice of colloid or crystalloid is well beyond the remit of this chapter, however, at present there is no evidence that one is superior to the other. One has to be pragmatic and practical and choose one or the other depending on availability and fluid to be replaced. Also, in sepsis, one must bear in mind that there is increased capillary permeability and this may outweigh the possible advantages of colloid over crystalloid.

Fluid should be administered fast through a wide bore peripheral cannula. In the young previously fit patient, this could be guided only by clinical response, bearing in mind that several litres of crystalloid may be required to replace intravascular volume. If the patient has other illnesses, in particular cardiac or renal disease where fluid overload may be particularly problematic, fluid resuscitation should be guided by CVP monitoring after the initial administration of 1–2 litres of crystalloid. Although aiming for a

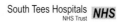

South Tees Hospitals **NHS**
NHS Trust

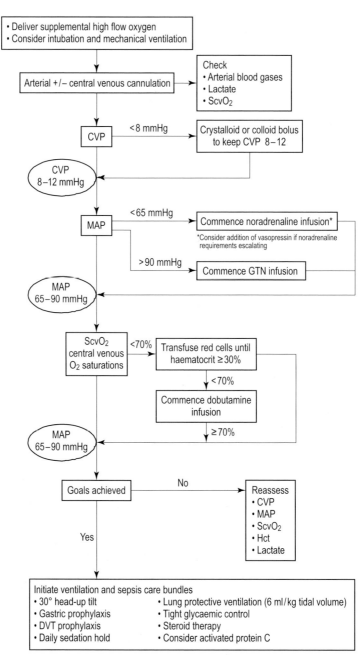

Guidelines for Critical Care Management of Sepsis

- Deliver supplemental high flow oxygen
- Consider intubation and mechanical ventilation

Arterial +/- central venous cannulation

Check
- Arterial blood gases
- Lactate
- $ScvO_2$

CVP → <8 mmHg → Crystalloid or colloid bolus to keep CVP 8–12

CVP 8–12 mmHg

MAP → <65 mmHg → Commence noradrenaline infusion*
*Consider addition of vasopressin if noradrenaline requirements escalating

>90 mmHg → Commence GTN infusion

MAP 65–90 mmHg

$ScvO_2$ central venous O_2 saturations → <70% → Transfuse red cells until haematocrit ≥30%

<70% → Commence dobutamine infusion

≥70%

MAP 65–90 mmHg

Goals achieved → No → Reassess
- CVP
- MAP
- $ScvO_2$
- Hct
- Lactate

Yes

Initiate ventilation and sepsis care bundles
- 30° head-up tilt
- Gastric prophylaxis
- DVT prophylaxis
- Daily sedation hold
- Lung protective ventilation (6 ml/kg tidal volume)
- Tight glycaemic control
- Steroid therapy
- Consider activated protein C

Produced by Dr Diane Monkhouse, Critical Care Directorate, April 2005

Figure 6.1   The James Cook University Hospital goal-directed therapy for patients with sepsis in the ITU. ªNote a CVP > 8 is the appropriate target in ward patients, but this will need to be higher in ventilated patients owing to a higher intrathoracic pressure.

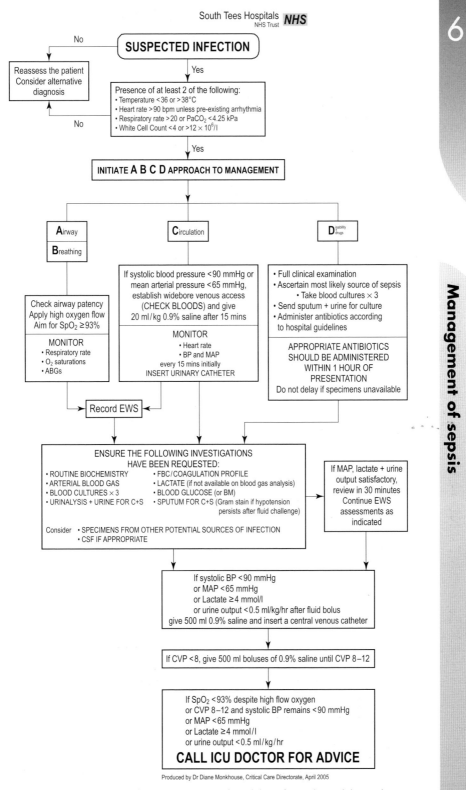

Produced by Dr Diane Monkhouse, Critical Care Directorate, April 2005

Figure 6.2 The James Cook University Hospital guidelines for early goal-directed therapy in sepsis.

Management of sepsis

CVP above 8, the initial reading is less important than what happens to it after fluid challenging. This will allow optimal filling.

Tip
Remember: Fluid challenge should not be confused with maintenance fluid replacement.

If the patient remains hypotensive or there is no improvement in lactate levels following adequate fluid resuscitation, inotropic support will be required. This will require adequate monitoring and includes the use of arterial lines to monitor pressure and a CVP line to ensure adequate filling and to administer inotropes. Blood should be taken from the CVP line and blood gas analyzed to determine central venous saturation. A low mixed venous saturation implies that uptake of oxygen in the tissues exceeds adequate delivery and measures should be taken to improve oxygen delivery.

If central venous saturation is < 70%, one must ensure that haematocrit is at least 30% and if not, transfuse the patient to this level. If despite this there is no improvement in central venous saturation, a dobutamine infusion should be commenced (Fig. 6.1). Paradoxically this may mean running dobutamine and noradrenaline (norepinephrine) infusions simultaneously.

In some cases where the clinical picture is difficult to interpret the use of invasive cardiac output monitoring, such as a pulmonary artery catheter, may be necessary. Although its use is controversial it can be a very useful tool. In particular, the largest randomized trial of pulmonary artery catheterization did not show improved outcome from the use of a catheter. This may be because, although the clinical information obtained may be useful, the incidence of complications associated with insertion may outweigh any benefit gained. Recently the use of less invasive techniques such as cardiac Doppler, LiDCO or PICCO may be superceding the use of the PAC. Such techniques are beyond the remit of this chapter but are well described in other texts.

Tip
A high CVP reading does not indicate adequate filling and a fluid challenge should be considered.

Choice of inotropic drugs

The use of inotropes should not be considered until adequate fluid replacement has been achieved. However, their use may be necessary initially, during fluid challenge, to sustain life in near arrest situations.

The majority of septic patients, at least in the initial stages, will be peripherally vasodilated, so a vasoconstrictor should be considered.

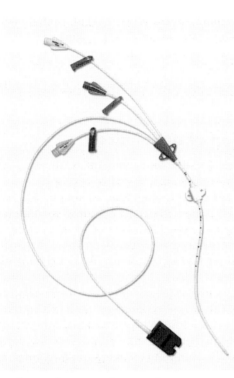

Figure 6.3 Edwards central venous oximetry catheter.

This could be in the form of noradrenaline (norepinephrine) or phenyl-ephrine (Table 6.1).

In patients where myocardial depression is also present, a second inotrope may be required and the use of adrenaline, dobutamine or dopexamine should then be considered.

Table 6.1 Some commonly used inotropic drugs with guiding initial starting doses. Note: these should be administered via central lines, although phenylephrine infusions are useful peripherally for short periods to stabilize a patient whilst more definitive access is obtained. Requirement for inotropes necessitates a critical care bed, i.e. level 2 or 3

Drug	Starting dose
Adrenaline	Make up an infusion with 4 mg of adrenaline diluted to 50 mL with normal saline. The concentration is 80 µg/ mL. Start infusion at 3–5 mL/h
Noradrenaline (norepinephrine)	Make up an infusion with 4 mg of noradrenaline diluted to 40 mL with normal saline. The concentration is 100 µg/mL. Start infusion at 3–5 mL/h
Phenylephrine	Make up an infusion with 10 mg of phenylephrine diluted to 50 mL with normal saline. The concentration is 200 µg/mL. Start infusion at 3 mL/h
Dobutamine	Make up an infusion with 250 mg of dobutamine diluted to 50 mL with normal saline. The concentration is 5 mg/mL. Start infusion at 2 mL/h

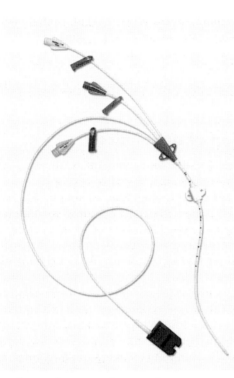

6

Management of sepsis

If, during resuscitation of the septic patient, central venous saturation is below 70% and haematocrit is above 30%, as long as CVP is above 12, dobutamine should be commenced. Central venous saturation can be measured by doing serial venous blood gases taken from the central line or by the use of a continuous oximetric central line such as the Edwards central venous oximetry catheter (Fig. 6.3).

Administration of antibiotics

Current guidelines for the management of severe sepsis include the administration of antibiotic therapy after appropriate cultures have been obtained. This should be achieved within an hour of diagnosis.

In order to identify the pathogenic organism a minimum of two sets of blood cultures should be obtained. One of them must be a peripheral stab and one should be performed from all invasive lines. It is particularly important to consider line sepsis in any patient who is discharged to the ward from critical care units, as lines may have been in situ for several days and this may be forgotten as the patient is new to the ward.

Where possible the source of infection needs to be removed. This may require surgical intervention. When intravascular access devices are suspected of involvement, they need to be removed and replaced if they are still needed. Occasionally, sampling of the source of infection may require aspiration under ultrasound guidance. The performance of complicated tests and investigations requiring transfer to places other than a high dependency area should be carefully considered in order not to delay prompt treatment of the septic patient or put a critically ill patient at risk.

The choice of antibiotic should be based on the suspected pathogen and source of sepsis. The advice of a microbiologist may be helpful. The antibiotic/s or antifungal of choice must also be able to penetrate to the source of infection. Patients' allergies and local pathogens and sensitivities are also important to consider. Initially, a broad spectrum antibiotic should be used, but once the pathogen/s have been identified a narrow spectrum antibiotic to which the pathogen is sensitive should be considered. There is no evidence that combination therapy is superior to monotherapy unless the patient is neutropenic or a pseudomonal infection is suspected. Many guidelines exist for appropriate antimicrobial choice and this will depend partly on hospital policy. Most hospital microbiology departments will have produced hospital antibiotic guidelines and these should be followed.

OTHER ASPECTS OF TREATMENTS OF THE SEPTIC PATIENT

Steroids

Adrenal insufficiency is common in severe sepsis and incidence is quoted at between 25–50% of septic patients. Administration of intravenous corticosteroids in a continuous form or divided doses is recommended in all patients requiring inotropic support: over 1 mg of adrenaline (epinephrine) or noradrenaline (norepinephrine), and in particular, where adrenal insufficiency is suspected (tuberculosis, previous steroid administration, abdominal sepsis with hypotension, etc.). This should be done after a short synacthen test has been performed.

Hydrocortisone regimens

- Hydrocortisone 50 mg IV qds
- Hydrocortisone 200 mg continuous IV infusion over 24 h.

Short synacthen test

- Check baseline cortisol level (U+Es bottle)
- Administer 250 µg of synacthen
- Repeat cortisol levels at 30 and 60 min.

Patterns of response

- No response → continue steroid replacement therapy
- Flat response (increase of baseline less than 200 or total value less than 700 µg/mL) → continue steroid replacement
- Good response (↑ greater than 200 over baseline or total value over 700 µg/mL).

Administration of steroids should not be delayed pending results of the synacthen test. There is at present controversy regarding the use of fludrocortisone 50 mg orally daily, based not only on whether hydrocortisone has sufficient mineralocorticoid activity but also on its unpredictable absorption.

Recombinant activated protein C (rhAPC)

Coagulation abnormalities are common in the septic patient. Although DIC can occur this is not the most common abnormality found; the most common abnormality is in fact a hypercoaguable state with increased levels of D-dimers and decreased levels of protein C.

Although open to debate the PROWESS study showed that in septic patients with multiorgan failure and an APACHE II score > 25 the use of rhAPC significantly reduced mortality.

Because rhAPC increases the risk of bleeding it is contraindicated in:

- known allergy to it
- active internal bleeding
- patients with intracranial pathology; neoplasm or evidence of cerebral herniation
- concurrent heparin therapy > 15 iu/kg/h
- known bleeding diathesis other than related to sepsis

- chronic severe hepatic disease
- platelet count < 30 000.

  Caution should be taken in:

- administration < 3 days of thrombolytic therapy
- administration of oral anticoagulants within 7 days, including aspirin or other platelet inhibitors
- ischaemic stroke within 3 months
- any other circumstances where bleeding is likely, including recent surgery.

For procedures with an inherent bleeding risk, rhAPC must be stopped for 2 h prior to the procedures and may be restarted 12 h after major invasive procedures if adequate haemostasis has been achieved.

Blood product administration

Organ dysfunction in the septic patient is determined by inadequate oxygen delivery and or uptake, therefore low haemoglobin levels will significantly reduce oxygen delivery. The transfusion requirements in critical care (TRICC) trial suggests that target haemoglobin should be kept at 7.0–9.0 g/dL and that the transfusion threshold should be 7.0 g/dL as this is not associated with an increased mortality. In general, transfusion over this limit, although increasing oxygen delivery, does not usually increase oxygen uptake.

The results of this trial do not apply to the patient with significant coronary artery disease or the difficult-to-wean patient, where a higher haemoglobin may be beneficial.

The administration of fresh frozen plasma (FFP) to the patient with abnormal international normalized ratio (INR), other than to correct bleeding or facilitate surgical procedures, does not seem to have an impact on outcome, and hence routine use for these purposes is no longer recommended.

Patients in renal failure will not benefit from the administration of erythropoietin during an acute septic episode.

Tight glucose control

In the septic patient, high glucose levels are common. Recent evidence suggests that tight control of blood sugar (BM 4.4–6.1) in the septic patient with the use of insulin infusions improves outcome. This appears to be related to the actual glucose levels rather than the amount of insulin administered.

Tight control of blood sugar requires frequent sampling and monitoring as well as the establishment of nutrition, either enterally or parenterally.

Deep vein thrombosis (DVT) prophylaxis

As previously mentioned, septic patients tend to be hypercoaguable as well as less mobile. All these factors predispose the patient to DVT. Hence the administration of a low molecular weight heparin is recommended.

In patients where the administration of low molecular weight heparin is contraindicated, mechanical intermittent compression devices or graduated compression stockings are indicated. Contraindication to the use of these two devices is the presence of marked peripheral vascular disease.

Stress ulcer and aspiration prophylaxis

Alongside DVT prophylaxis, stress ulcer and aspiration prophylaxis comprise one of the critical care bundles. They are strategies that apply to most critical care patients and are proven to improve outcome. As such, they have no defined role for the treatment of ward patients, but serve as a reminder of the complications that result in increased mortality in these patients.

It has long been known that head elevation up to 45° decreases the risk of ventilator-acquired pneumonia and improves outcome; however this simple factor of care is often forgotten and ignored. Likewise respiratory function is improved for most patients in the sitting position. If the consciousness level is impaired, the patient should be nursed in the recovery position until the airway has been definitively secured.

Stress ulcer prophylaxis should be given to all patients with severe sepsis. H_2 receptor antagonists are more efficacious than sucralfate. Proton pump inhibitors are the currently preferred agent despite there being no evidence of their efficacy in improving overall mortality. They do, however, increase gastric pH to the same levels. Patients in whom full enteral nutrition is established do not require additional stress ulcer prophylaxis. Certain high-risk patients, however, such as spinally injured patients, may require stress ulcer prophylaxis for reasons independent of sepsis.

Mechanical ventilation

Should the septic patient require mechanical ventilation, standard critical care unit ventilatory care will be necessary. This entails the avoidance of high tidal volumes and high ventilatory pressures in order to avoid volu and barotrauma. Aim for tidal volumes of 6 mL/kg and peak pressures < 30 cmH$_2$O. Permissive hypercapnia and optimal PEEP are also recommended.

Induction of anaesthesia in the septic patient can be extremely challenging due not only to hypovolaemia but also to reduced cardiac contractility and increased oxygen demand. In general the patient will be difficult to pre-oxygenate and will be at high risk of aspiration, hence this should not be attempted by the novice or alone.

It is good practice to preload the patient with 500 mL of colloid or crystalloid prior to the use of the induction agent. This will minimize or prevent a drop in blood pressure after the administration of the induction agent. A rapid sequence induction will be indicated in most cases. Care must be taken with patients in renal failure as the use of suxamethonium may be contraindicated due to life-threatening hyperkalaemia.

If the patient requires surgery, preoptimization will improve outcome. The place to do it will depend on the urgency of surgery and space availability. If the patient is on a medical ward, preoptimization with oxygen, fluid and CVP monitoring should begin as soon as possible and not be delayed until surgical transfer.

Secondary assessment and continuous monitoring

Following initial assessment and resuscitation, the patient should have a secure airway, adequate ventilation, supplemental oxygen administration, and cardiovascular resuscitation should have commenced. These need to be reviewed regularly and every time a deterioration in the patient's condition is noted. The priorities during the next phase are:

- Accurate and complete history taking, including revision of medical notes
- Full physical examination
- Perform relevant investigations
- Communication with the other teams involved in the patient's management
- Continue resuscitation.

Once septic patients have been identified they should not be left unattended. Continuous monitoring will be necessary, not forgetting that the presence of trained staff is more important than any other bit of equipment.

Repeated observations of the patient's condition will allow determination of whether the patient is improving or deteriorating. Clear documentation aids the assessment of subtle changes in the patient's clinical state. Hourly observations will normally be required, including:

- body temperature
- pulse
- blood pressure
- CVP
- respiratory rate
- FiO_2
- SpO_2
- blood sugar
- urine output
- fluid balance
- level of consciousness.

Transfer to definitive care

Ideally all septic patients should be looked after in a high dependency area, however it cannot be emphasized enough that treatment should commence as soon as possible.

During transfer, adequately trained nursing and medical staff will be necessary as well as portable oxygen and monitoring equipment. Resuscitation equipment should also be available at all times.

A 65-year-old man with a background of alcohol abuse is admitted to the medical critical care unit with presumed alcoholic pancreatitis. Initial markers of severity are good and the patient makes a good recovery. Initial management consisted of humidified oxygen, NBM, TPN, and LMW heparin.

An abdominal CT scan showed no necrosis; he was, however, initially oliguric and a central line was inserted to assist fluid replacement and facilitate TPN.

He was discharged from the critical care unit on day five. On day 10 he developed an increased WCC and a swinging pyrexia. What are the possible causes and investigations?

Answers

The list in a case like this is endless. However, it was found that the patient had had his central line in for 11 days, the line having been inserted on admission, and line sepsis was found to be the cause.

The line was removed and after being given oxygen and fluids he continued to progress satisfactorily.

Line sepsis should be suspected in all patients with a CVP line, particularly if the line has been in for longer than 10 days, or there is doubt regarding the asepsis at the time of insertion, or the line has been heavily manipulated as in the case of an emergency abdominal aortic aneurysm. Infection rates are highest in femoral and internal jugular lines and lowest in subclavian lines. An episode of line-related sepsis has been shown to adversely affect outcome in critically ill patients.

Specific treatment will consist in its removal plus replacement if its use is still indicated. With current evidence there is no role for routine replacement of invasive lines on the basis of time but consider using antibiotic or silver coated lines and lines must always be removed as soon as they are no longer required, ideally by day 10. A list of manoeuvres to prevent catheter related sepsis have been published by the Department of Health.

CASE 6.2

A 55-year-old woman with a history of diabetes presented to hospital with a perforated duodenal ulcer for which she underwent an emergency laparotomy and oversewing. As, initially, she was shocked and oliguric, a central line was inserted to guide fluid management and she was nursed postoperatively in the high dependency area. Initially, she recovered very well and was discharged to a medical ward for ongoing diabetic management. However, on day 10 postoperatively, she developed respiratory failure, bronchopneumonia and sepsis, requiring admission to the medical critical care unit.

Again she initially recovered well and was discharged to the general ward, only to relapse with sepsis three days after antibiotics were stopped. Her CXR is shown in Figure 6.4.

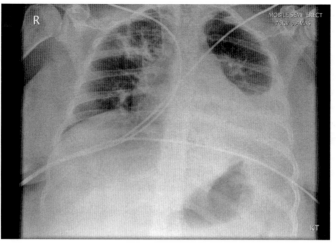

Figure 6.4 Chest X-ray.

**You are the physician on call. What does the CXR show?
What is the possible differential diagnosis?
What investigations would you organize?**

Answers
The CXR demonstrates elevated right and left hemidiaphragms with collapse/consolidation at both bases, which is particularly worse on the left. Owing to the suspicious CXR and repeated signs of infection, an abdominal CT was performed which demonstrated the existence of a left-sided subdiaphragmatic collection (Fig. 6.5). This was successfully drained percutaneously by the radiologist.

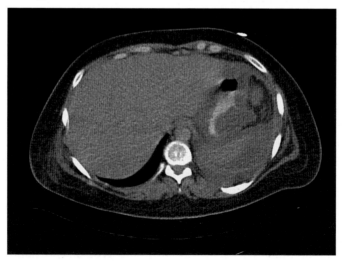

Figure 6.5 Abdominal CT scan.

After a slow recovery the patient was eventually discharged home.

Repeated bronchopneumonia can be due to pathology other than pulmonary pathology and the presence of a subdiaphragmatic collection is a good example of how consolidation is a symptom rather than the cause. Subdiaphragmatic abscesses are normally accumulations of purulent exudates beneath the diaphragm, also known as upper abdominal abscesses. They are usually associated with peritonitis or postoperative infections.

The usual cause is infected fluid ascending along the paracolic gutters from the pelvis. This movement is facilitated by the negative pressure caused by the movement of the right diaphragm. Left-sided subdiaphragmatic abscesses are less common and occur more frequently following splenectomy, perforation of high gastric ulcer, pancreatitis or left-sided colonic surgery.

Changes found in CXRs include changes in the level and configuration of the diaphragm, signs of pleural effusion, or basal lung opacities on the side of the suspected abscess.

On ultrasound a crescentic sonolucent area representing the fluid collection between the diaphragm and the dome of the liver is clearly displayed. On CT the abscess will be visible as an area of fluid or an entity of less than soft tissue attenuation with possibly an airfluid level situated outside the liver or spleen.

Symptoms may vary from very little to full blown sepsis and prognosis very much depends on timely surgical and radiological intervention as well as patient background and physiological reserve. Antibiotics and antifungals may be required.

FURTHER READING

Alderson P, Schierhout G, Roberts I et al 2000 Colloid versus crystalloid for fluid resuscitation in critically ill patients. Cochrane Database Systemic Review 2000(2):CD000567

Amato M B, Barbas C S, Medeiros D M et al 1998 Effect of protective-ventilation strategy on mortality in the acute respiratory distress syndrome. New England Journal of Medicine 338:347–354

American College of Chest Physicians/Society of Critical Care Medicine Consensus 1992 Conference: definitions for sepsis and organ failure and guidelines for the use of innovative therapies in sepsis. Critical Care Medicine 20:864–874

Cook D 2000 Ventilator-associated pneumonia: perspectives on the burden of illness. Intensive Care Medicine 26:S31–37

Dellinger R P, Carlet J M, Masur H et al 2004 Surviving sepsis campaign guidelines for management of severe sepsis and septic shock. Critical Care Medicine 32:858–873

Department of Health 2000 Comprehensive critical care: a review of adult critical care services. Department of Health

Department of Health 2001 EPIC guidelines. Journal of Hospital Infection 47:S5–9

Finfer S, Bellomo R, Boyce N et al 2004 A comparison of albumin and saline for fluid resuscitation in the intensive care unit. New England Journal of Medicine 350:2247–2256

Harvey S, Harrison D A, Singer M et al (on behalf of the PAC-Man study collaboration) 2005 Assessment of the clinical effectiveness of pulmonary artery catheters in management of patients in intensive care (PAC-Man): a randomised controlled trial. Lancet 366:472–477

Hebert P C, Wells G, Blajchman M A et al 1999 A multicenter, randomised controlled clinical trial of transfusion requirements in critical care. New England Journal of Medicine 340:409–417

Intensive Care Medicine. Supplement 2001; 27 Sepsis

Intensive Care Society 2002 Guidelines for transport of the critically ill adult. Intensive Care Society, UK

MacIntyre R C, Pulido E J, Bensard D D et al 2000 Thirty years of clinical trials in acute respiratory distress syndrome. Critical Care Medicine 28:3314–3331

McQuillan P, Pilkington S, Allan A et al 1998 Confidential inquiry into quality of care before admission to intensive care. BMJ 316:1853–1858

Rivers E, Nguyen B, Havstad S et al 2001 Early goal-directed therapy in the treatment of severe sepsis and septic shock. New England Journal of Medicine 345:1368–1377

Stenhouse C, Coates S, Tivey M et al 2000 Prospective evaluation of a modified Early Warning Score to aid earlier detection of patients developing critical illness on a general surgical ward. British Journal of Anaesthesia 84:663P

Surviving sepsis guidelines: http://www.survivingsepsis.org/

Van den Berghe G, Woulters P, Weekers F et al 2001 Intensive insulin therapy in critically ill patients. New England Journal of Medicine 345:1359–1367

Ware L B, Matthay M A 2000 The acute respiratory distress syndrome. New England Journal of Medicine 342:1334–1349

Webb A R, Shapiro M J, Singer M et al (eds) 1999 Oxford textbook of critical care. Oxford University Press, Oxford

Cardiac emergencies

Andrew Turley

7

OBJECTIVES

After reading this chapter you should have an understanding of:

● *Recognition and resuscitation of the acutely unwell cardiac patient*

● *Treatment of acute coronary syndromes*

● *Treatment of acute cardiac dysrhythmias*

● *Indications for temporary cardiac pacing*

ACUTE CORONARY SYNDROMES

The majority of patients seen with acute chest pain will not be having an acute myocardial infarction (AMI), however all cases of chest pain must be taken seriously and all patients assumed to have an acute cardiac problem until proven otherwise. The patient must be assessed in a critical care environment following the airway, breathing and circulation (ABC) approach described earlier.

The term 'acute coronary syndrome' (ACS) encompasses:

- unstable angina (UA)
- non ST elevation myocardial infarction (NSTEMI)
- ST elevation myocardial infarction (STEMI).

The ACSs share a common pathophysiology, namely, rupture or fissure of an atheromatous coronary plaque within an epicardial coronary artery. This leads to platelet activation and aggregation at the site of injury with associated local vessel vasoconstriction, thrombus formation and distal embolization. In STEMI, these usually result in complete occlusion of the vessel whereas in UA/NSTEMI the vessel is often only transiently or subtotally occluded.

CASE 7.1

A 47-year-old man is admitted directly to the coronary care unit with a three-hour history of central crushing chest pain. The pain radiates to the right arm and is associated with breathlessness. Onset was sudden whilst at work in an insurance office. The

89

patient smokes 30 cigarettes a day and is on treatment for hypertension.

On examination his pulse is 80 bpm and blood pressure (BP) 180/105 mmHg. Respiratory examination is unremarkable. (*To be continued.*)

> **KEY POINTS: IMMEDIATE MANAGEMENT OF ALL PATIENTS WITH AN ACS**
> **DO NOT DELAY**
> **Initial assessment:** ABCD
> **Oxygen:** high flow
> **IV access:** large bore cannula in a large calibre vein
> **Opiates:** diamorphine 5 mg IV slowly with 2.5 mg increments (as required)
> **Antiemetics:** metoclopramide 10 mg IV
> **Aspirin:** 300 mg chewed, unless the patient is allergic or has already been given aspirin
> **Monitor:** attach to cardiac monitor. Obtain a 12-lead electrocardiogram (ECG) if this has not already been taken
> **Beta-blockers:** metoprolol 5 mg IV (maximum dose 15 mg IV, in 3 × 5 mg aliquots) then continue orally, e.g. atenolol 50 mg od. If beta-blockers are contraindicated, consider calcium antagonists. Angiotensin converting enzyme (ACE)-inhibitors and statins should be prescribed for all patients in the absence of any absolute contraindication.

Risk stratification

Risk stratification aims to identify high- and low-risk patients and allows for the instigation of appropriate treatment. The initial assessment involves history taking and clinical examination, 12-lead electrocardiography and the measurement of markers of myocardial damage such as troponins T and I (TnT, TnI).

History

Ischaemic chest pain can present in many forms from jaw ache, to discomfort in the throat, shoulder, arm (right or left), precordium, back or epigastrium. Chest pain due to an aortic dissection is classically intrascapular and tearing in nature, although patients may have retrosternal pain. Chest pain of a pulmonary embolism is usually pleuritic in nature. Chest pain in an acute coronary syndrome is usually of recent onset, which is of increasing severity. Chest pain that occurs at rest or woke the patient must be taken seriously. Does the patient have any cardiac risk factors?

Examination

Does the patient look unwell? Check the vital signs and record the blood pressure manually in both arms; aortic dissection can present in many ways.

Clinical findings in ACS patients can be divided into three broad groups:

- **Autonomic upset**: sweating, pallor, tachycardia
- **Precipitating cause**: fever, hypertension, cyanosis, anaemia
- **Complications**: left ventricular failure, atrial fibrillation, hypotension.

Investigations

ECG: A 12-lead ECG on admission is mandatory. The ECG may be normal; do not discount the diagnosis of an ACS if the history is suggestive. Patients presenting with a normal ECG have a 94% chance of survival at 4 years. This compares to 53% in individuals with > 2 mm ST segment depression. The greater the ST segment depression, the worse the prognosis. T wave inversion alone is of less clinical significance with the exception of deep symmetrical T wave inversion across the anterior chest leads which is indicative of left anterior descending (LAD) coronary disease (Fig. 7.1).

Cardiac biomarkers: troponin T. Distinguishes UA from NSTEMI. Samples should be taken on admission and at 12 h. Troponin provides prognostic information.

Full blood count (FBC): excludes anaemia, thrombocytopenia and polycythaemia.

Urea and electrolytes (U&E): baseline renal function. Renal failure can complicate ACS. ACE-inhibitors can cause renal dysfunction.

Liver function tests (LFTs): statins can cause liver dysfunction.

Lipid profile: this is only of value if taken on admission.

Chest X-ray (CXR): is there any evidence of pulmonary oedema, cardiomegaly, aortic dissection?

EARLY MANAGEMENT OF THE PATIENT WITH UA/NSTEMI

General

In patients suffering UA/NSTEMI, buccal or intravenous nitrates can be administered if the patient still has chest pain. Antithrombotic strategies are a cornerstone of treatment. A combined approach is advocated, involving the use of dual antiplatelet therapy, aspirin 300 mg chewed, then 75 mg daily combined with clopidogrel 300 mg po stat, and 6 h later followed by 75 mg daily plus the use of low molecular weight heparin, e.g. dalteparin 120 U/kg bd (max. 10 000 units bd).

Cardiac catheterization

Urgent cardiac catheterization should be considered in patients with high-risk features, e.g. post-infarction angina, ECG features of severe or worsening ischaemia or elevated cardiac markers in the context of a typical ischaemic history. Troponin levels are an adjunct to clinical assessment and not a substitute. The decision to refer a patient for cardiac catheterization should only be taken after consultation with senior medical staff. The early invasive strategy, especially amongst the high-risk patient population, is superior to medical management alone. It is important that the patient and relatives are aware of the possible outcomes of cardiac catheterization, including cardiac revascularization.

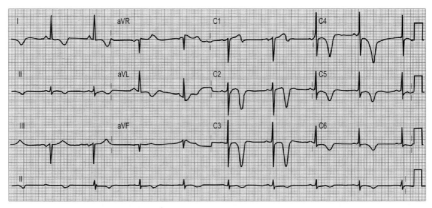

Figure 7.1   12-lead electrocardiogram showing T wave inversion in leads V1–V5 (LAD syndrome).

EARLY MANAGEMENT OF THE PATIENT WITH STEMI

The management of STEMI and patient survival depends on:

- restoration of antegrade coronary blood flow
- time taken to achieve reperfusion
- sustained patency of the infarct-related artery.

There are two approaches to re-open an occluded epicardial coronary artery: either pharmacological with a fibrinolytic agent or percutaneously (Fig. 7.2). Management will depend on the centre and on in-house protocol.

Indications for thrombolysis

- Typical ischaemic chest pain, onset within the last 12 h
- Plus ECG with either:
  - 1 mm ST elevation in two or more adjacent limb leads
  - new LBBB
  - posterior AMI
- ST depression in leads V1–4 with ST elevation > 1 mm in posterior leads V7–9
- Emergency 'cardiac enzymes' are not a prerequisite for thrombolysis.

Tip
Thrombolysis
Use of thrombolytic drugs should be reserved for patients presenting with an appropriate history of AMI and either ST segment elevation or new left bundle branch block (LBBB). Administration of a thrombolytic drug to other ACS patients results in a worse outcome (Figs 7.3, 7.4).

CARDIAC EMERGENCIES

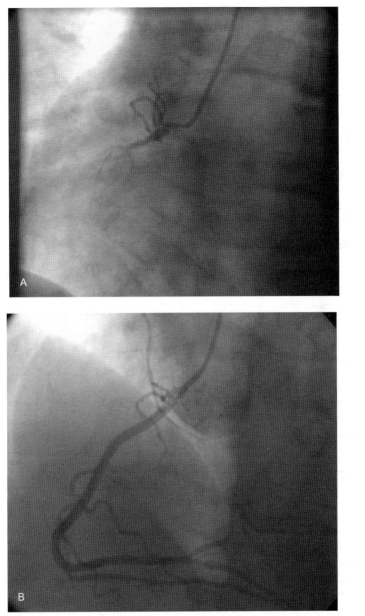

Figure 7.2 Primary percutaneous coronary intervention (PCI) (A) pre (B) post PCI to the RCA in a patient presenting with acute inferior STEMI.

Contraindications to thrombolysis

Absolute contraindications

- Absence of the inclusion criteria above
- More than 12 h from symptom onset

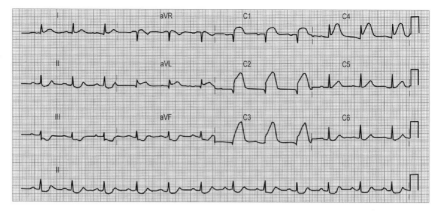

Figure 7.3   12-lead electrocardiogram showing anterior ST elevation.

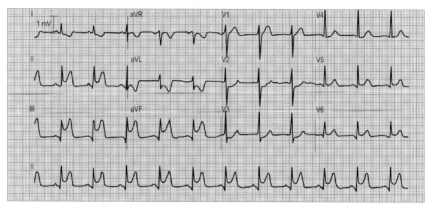

Figure 7.4   12-lead electrocardiogram showing an inferoposterior myocardial infarction.

- Previous cerebral haemorrhage or other cerebrovascular accident (CVA)/transcient ischaemic attack (TIA) within one year
- Intracranial lesion, oesophageal varices, pancreatitis
- Suspected aortic dissection
- Active bleeding or internal bleeding in the past four weeks.

Relative contraindications

- Surgery within 21 days
- Trauma including traumatic cardiopulmonary rescuscitation (CPR)
- Eye bleeding (vitreous)
- Peptic ulceration (active), pregnancy
- Bleeding tendency
- Warfarin, haemophilia, liver disease, thrombocytopenia
- Cardiogenic shock
- Severe hypertension (BP > 200/120 mmHg) despite diamorphine (risk of stroke is increased).

If in doubt, seek senior help.

Other cautions for the use of thrombolysis

Requirement for instrumentation, e.g. bradycardia requiring temporary pacing wire insertion. In this case, use the femoral venous access site where direct pressure can be applied if necessary. Proliferative retinopathy is not an absolute contraindication to thrombolysis.

Streptokinase and antistreplase are contraindicated if either has been given more than four days previously.

Problems with thrombolysis

If hypotension develops, the infusion should be stopped and the patient laid flat. Restart when BP normalizes. Recurrent or profound hypotension may require the use of an alternative agent, e.g. tPA. Always remember the possibility of occult gastrointestinal blood loss.

An allergic reaction to streptokinase can occur. Stop the infusion and administer IV chlorphenamine 10 mg and hydrocortisone 100 mg. Restart with tPA once the reaction has resolved.

Use of ACE-I post AMI

ACE-inhibitors reduce mortality after AMI. These agents should be given within 24 h of onset of AMI unless there is hypotension (BP < 100 mmHg), irrespective of left ventricular function.

Diabetic patients with AMI

Diabetic patients with AMI have higher morbidity (relative risk 1.5–2.2) and mortality rates than non-diabetics. The DIGAMI study showed that insulin/glucose infusion during the AMI followed by long-term insulin therapy was associated with an absolute mortality risk reduction of 11% over three years.

COMPLICATIONS OF ACUTE MYOCARDIAL INFARCTION

CASE 7.1 (continued)

A 47-year-old man is admitted directly to the coronary care unit with a three-hour history of central crushing chest pain. The pain radiates to the right arm and is associated with breathlessness. Onset was sudden whilst at work in an insurance office. The patient smokes 30 cigarettes per day and is on treatment for hypertension.
On examination his pulse is 80 bpm and BP is 180/105 mmHg. Respiratory examination is unremarkable.

The admission 12-lead ECG shows 6 mm inferior ST elevation. The patient is given aspirin and thrombolysis is commenced after checking for contraindications. Two hours later the patient is still in pain and the ECG changes have not altered.

Failed thrombolysis

Failed thrombolysis reflects failure of the infarct-related artery to reperfuse. Clinical markers are ongoing ischaemic symptoms and failure of ST segment resolution.

- Identify the lead with the highest degree of ST elevation.
- Reperfusion has occurred if the ST segment elevation has resolved by at least 50%, 120 min after the commencement of thrombolysis.

If a patient has failed to reperfuse then advice should be sought immediately from the regional cardiac centre.

Reinfarction

This will manifest as new ST elevation or ST re-elevation and requires IV nitrates and IV heparin; consider beta-blockade if not already given and discuss urgently with the regional cardiac centre. Never readminister thrombolysis.

Pericarditis

A bruised feeling is common after an AMI. The pain of pericarditis is typically pleuritic in nature and positional, and is worse when lying flat. A pericardial rub may be heard on auscultation. Treat with paracetamol or a non-steroidal anti-inflammatory drug (NSAID). Pericarditis can cause ST elevation and should not be confused with reinfarction.

Recurrent ischaemia/post-infarct angina

This will manifest as ongoing ischaemic chest pain and ST segment depression. The patient requires buccal or IV nitrates in addition to beta-blockers, heparin and dual antiplatelet therapy. Such patients may require emergency cardiac catheterization and revascularization. Advice should be sought immediately from the regional cardiac centre.

Left ventricular failure

Cardiogenic shock is the most serious haemodynamic complication. Prompt recognition and treatment is essential. Even with prompt and effective treatment mortality remains high.

Acute mitral regurgitation: this can occur due to papillary muscle ischaemia or rupture, or due to left ventricular dilatation. Papillary muscle rupture can be sudden and catastrophic. All patients should be auscultated daily and new murmurs investigated promptly.

Ventricular septal defect (VSD): always consider this in a patient who decompensates after AMI. It produces a harsh pansystolic murmur.

Cardiac tamponade: see below.

Arrhythmias

Management of arrhythmias post AMI differs from most other situations. The arrhythmia is usually a manifestation of ischaemia or reperfusion and does not necessarily require intervention.

Sinus tachycardia

Sinus tachycardia can reflect increased sympathetic drive. In the absence of ventricular failure, patients need to be beta-blocked, aiming for a target heart rate of 60 bpm, hence reducing myocardial oxygen demand.

Sinus bradycardia/junctional bradycardia

This is common after an inferior AMI. Treat if the patient is haemodynamically compromised (atropine 0.5 mg IV).

Atrial fibrillation/flutter (Fig. 7.5)

Both rhythms can aggravate cardiac failure, worsen ischaemia and cause haemodynamic compromise. If the patient is haemodynamically compromised then synchronized DC cardioversion is required. Treatment is as in other settings with the aim of ventricular rate control. If rapid control is needed, IV beta-blockade, e.g. metoprolol 5 mg, is useful.

Atrial or ventricular ectopic beats

No treatment is required.

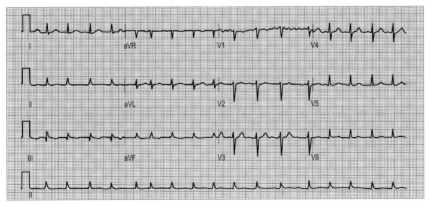

Figure 7.5   12-lead electrocardiogram showing atrial fibrillation.

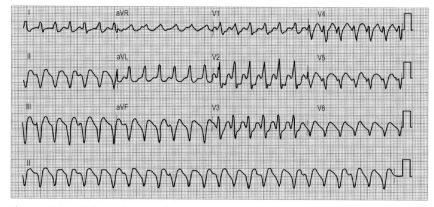

Figure 7.6 12-lead electrocardiogram showing ventricular tachycardia.

Accelerated idioventricular rhythm

This is often a sign of reperfusion. It is a broad complex automatic ventricular rhythm < 120 bpm. No treatment is needed.

Ventricular tachycardia (VT) (Fig. 7.6)

VT is common in the first 48 h post AMI. Non-sustained episodes < 30 s require no treatment if there is no haemodynamic compromise. For sustained VT without haemodynamic compromise, treat as in other situations.

If there is hypotension then the patient requires urgent synchronised DC cardioversion. Recurrent or incessant VT may reflect ongoing ischaemia and is an indication for cardiac catheterization. If VT occurs late, i.e. > 48 h, then the risk of fatal arrhythmia is high; seek help.

Atrioventricular (AV) block

First-degree AV block

First-degree AV block requires no treatment.

Second-degree AV block

Wenkebach phenomenon
Wenkebach phenomenon requires no treatment.

Anterior myocardial infarction (MI) with Mobitz type II AV block
This is an indication for temporary cardiac pacing (Fig. 7.7). There is a high chance of complete heart block (CHB) (Fig. 7.8).

Complete heart block
In anterior MI, CHB almost always requires permanent pacemaker insertion.

In the setting of an inferior AMI this will usually resolve. It may take several days or weeks. Temporary pacing will be required meanwhile.

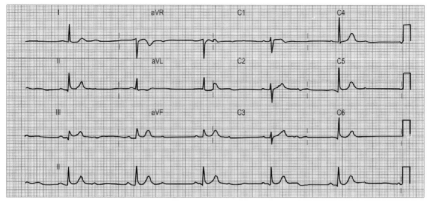

Figure 7.7 12-lead electrocardiogram showing Mobitz II.

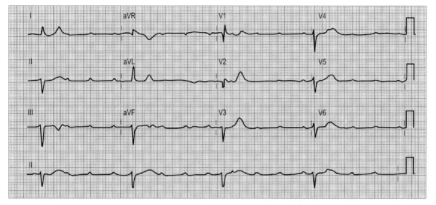

Figure 7.8 12-lead electrocardiogram showing complete heart block.

Bifascicular block

Bifascicular block is seen more commonly with anterior AMIs than inferior AMIs. There is a risk of progression to CHB and so this is an indication for temporary pacemaker insertion.

Trifascicular block

This requires pacing. Alternating left bundle branch block (LBBB) and right bundle branch block (RBBB) always requires a temporary pacemaker.

ACUTE LEFT VENTRICULAR FAILURE

Cardiac output = stroke volume × heart rate

Stroke volume, the amount of blood pumped out of the ventricle with each beat, is determined by preload (venous filling pressure), afterload (the resistance against which the ventricle ejects blood) and myocardial contractility. In the majority of patients, cardiac failure is due to reduced left ventricular systolic function and stroke volume, leading to a reduction in cardiac output. This causes a reduction in oxygen delivery at the cellular level resulting in cellular hypoxia and metabolic acidosis. In diastolic dysfunction (failure of relaxation of the ventricle), reduced ventricular compliance limits diastolic filling, increases left and right atrial pressures and can limit cardiac output, e.g. after a large myocardial infarction, in cardiomyopathies or mitral stenosis. Cardiac failure can occur in the context of a high output state, e.g. sepsis, or a low output state, e.g. hypothyroidism.

Pulmonary oedema ≠ acute left ventricular failure

Pulmonary oedema may occur in the absence of cardiac disease if loading conditions are altered, e.g. acute renal failure. Acute left ventricular failure can occur de novo, or in the background of chronic heart failure. A common mistake is to not look for the cause.

CASE 7.2

A 68-year-old man was admitted at 2 a.m. with acute shortness of breath. The patient had recently been discharged following an acute anterior myocardial infarction complicated by pulmonary oedema. Over the previous week he had noticed a decrease in exercise tolerance and had woken several times in the preceding two nights with acute breathlessness.

On examination the patient was agitated and confused; he was pale and sweating and peripherally cool. His heart rate was 136 beats per min irregularly irregular, and BP 145/90 mmHg. Inspiratory crepitations were heard on auscultation throughout the lung fields.

Management

Patients should receive treatment prior to completion of all investigations. The key to treatment is rapid venodilation to remove fluid from the thorax. All patients should be managed in a critical care environment.

Immediate management

Initial assessment: ABCD.

Oxygen: Sit the patient upright to reduce venous return and give high flow oxygen via a re-breathe bag.

IV access: A large bore cannula is inserted in a large calibre vein.

IV opiates: Reduce preload and help to reduce sympathetic drive. Opiates also act as anxiolytics. Consider an antiemetic at the same time.

IV loop diuretics: The initial effect is due to venodilation (reducing preload) followed by diuresis. Insert a urinary catheter; this will help fluid balance monitoring.

IV nitrates: The main problem in left ventricular failure is misdistribution of fluid. Nitrates redistribute fluid into capacitance vessels and also acutely reduce left atrial pressure. The nitrate dose is titrated upward every 10 min until clinical improvement is seen or systolic blood pressure is < 100 mmHg.

Digoxin: This is of use in patients with atrial fibrillation with a fast ventricular response.

History

Patients present with rapidly worsening fatigue and extreme breathlessness. A history of dyspnoea, effort tolerance, orthopnoea and paroxysmal nocturnal dyspnoea may be present. The precipitating cause may be suggested by symptoms such as chest pain or palpitations.

The condition is an acute medical emergency and usually occurs in the nocturnal hours.

Examination

General: Patients are classically distressed/agitated. They are usually tachypnoeic although they can have a reduced respiratory rate secondary to exhaustion or opiates. A reduced respiratory rate is often a pre-arrest sign: **act immediately**. The patient can be hypotensive (cardiogenic shock) or hypertensive. In cases of cardiac tamponade, pulsus paradoxus could be present. The JVP is usually elevated. The apex beat may be dyskinetic in anterior MI and is often displaced in chronic heart failure. A gallop rhythm is invariably present. Inspiratory crepitations will be heard on auscultation of the lung fields.

Autonomic upset: Sympathetic activation results in pallor, sweating, cool peripheries and peripheral cyanosis. The pulse is tachycardic in an attempt to maintain cardiac output and some patients will have atrial fibrillation. Bradycardia worsens ventricular filling and is an ominous sign.

Precipitating cause: The patient may exhibit signs of non-cardiac illness including anaemia, fever and signs of thyroid dysfunction or endocarditis. The presence of a systolic murmur may indicate valve pathology, e.g. aortic stenosis or acute VSD.

Impaired tissue perfusion: An impaired consciousness level can represent tissue hypoxia and is an ominous sign.

Investigations

U&E: Acute renal failure may result in fluid retention. Hypo/ hyperkalaemia may precipitate arrhythmias.

FBC: To exclude anaemia. A rise in the white cell count is common and does not necessarily imply sepsis.

Others: TFTs, viral titres and blood cultures are useful.

ABGs: To assess acidosis (usually metabolic: impaired tissue perfusion).

ECG: To look for evidence of myocardial infarction (recent or old), ischaemia, rhythm disturbance, e.g. atrial fibrillation/ventricular tachy-cardia or left ventricular hypertrophy (LVH), e.g. hypertension/aortic stenosis.

CXR: Pulmonary oedema or pleural effusions may be present in patients with acute or chronic heart failure. Other factors to look for are fluid in the horizontal fissure, and cardiomegaly – if this is globular, it is suggestive of pericardial effusion. Pulmonary pathology can also be excluded.

Echocardiogram: To assess left ventricular function as well as providing structural information, e.g. LVH, valve pathology, pericardial effusions and acute VSDs. This is indicated acutely for patients in cardiogenic shock.

Advanced management steps

Renal failure

Patients resistant to diuretic therapy may require extracorporeal haemo-filtration.

Respiratory failure

Consider mechanical ventilation if respiratory compromise persists. Ominous signs are bradypnoea, persistent arterial hypoxia, worsening acidosis and hypercapnia.

Non-invasive ventilation/continuous positive airway pressure (CPAP)
CPAP may avoid the need for formal ventilation. It is simple to use and delivers nearly 100% oxygen. It can be applied in most high dependency areas. In simple terms it pushes fluid back into the circulation from the alveoli by applying continuous positive airway pressure.

Invasive ventilation/intermittent positive pressure ventilation (IPPV)
IPPV reduces respiratory effort and metabolic demand, increases alveolar pressure which clears alveolar oedema, improves oxygenation and acidosis, and relieves hypercapnia. Like CPAP, cardiac output may be reduced owing to increased intrathoracic pressure. IPPV is not without risks and senior help should be enlisted to decide the appropriateness of critical care unit admission in chronic heart failure.

CARDIOGENIC SHOCK

Cardiogenic shock, a state of progressive reduction in tissue perfusion and hypotension despite adequate preload and heart rate, remains the commonest cause of death in patients admitted to hospital with AMI. The incidence in the setting of STEMI is over 7% with mortality rates exceeding 70%. It is usually secondary to left ventricular dysfunction and can be defined clinically or haemodynamically. The fall in cardiac output leads to increased sympathetic tone. The non-ischaemic portions of myocardium become hyperdynamic and hence oxygen consumption increases. A vicious cycle is set in motion leading to progressive hypotension and worsening myocardial ischaemia.

Definitions of cardiogenic shock

Clinical: decreased cardiac output and evidence of tissue hypoxia in the presence of adequate intravascular volume.

Haemodynamic: sustained hypotension, systolic BP < 90 mmHg for at least 30 min and a reduced cardiac index < 2.2 L/min per m² in the presence of elevated pulmonary capillary occlusion pressure > 15 mmHg.

CASE 7.3

A 58-year-old man presents with an 8-hour history of central crushing chest pain. The pain radiates to the neck and is associated with marked breathlessness. The patient is a known diabetic and ex-smoker.

On examination the patient is peripherally cool, with a pulse of 110 beats per min and BP 70/54 mmHg. On auscultation a systolic murmur is heard at the lower left sternal edge. Respiratory rate is 40 bpm. Breath sounds are very quiet. 12-lead ECG shows 8 mm anterior ST elevation.

History

- Has there been a recent MI?
  - Territory is very important. Has thrombolysis been given? Which and when?
  - If the timing of presentation is 2–3 h post MI suspect myocardial rupture.
  - Is there sudden haemodynamic collapse? If so, suspect a rupture, VSD or acute myocardial rupture (or regurgitation?).
- Has there been previous heart failure? Valve disease? Fluid balance?
- Are drugs involved? Are there any negative inotropes? Is there known cardiomyopathy?

Examination

Examination relates to either low output state or impaired ventricular function:

Blood pressure	Hypotension. Systolic BP < 90 mmHg
Pulse	Sinus tachycardia (note effect of beta-blockade)
Peripheral circulation	Cool, low volume pulse, peripheral cyanosis
Reduced organ perfusion	Anuria/oliguria, urine output < 0.5 ml/kg/h. Confusion/impaired consciousness level
Lactic acidosis	If tissue perfusion is poor.

Investigations

Investigation is as for acute left ventricular failure.

Echocardiography: This will usually reveal the cause (Fig. 7.9). If left ventricular function is not badly impaired, consider other causes.

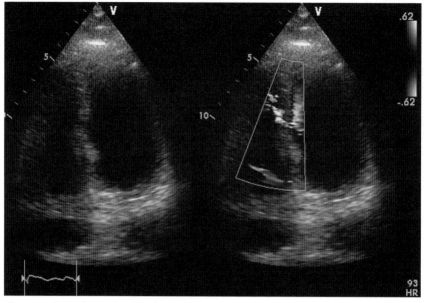

Figure 7.9 Echocardiogram demonstrating a ventricular septal defect.

Left ventricle (LV) function: There are usually extensive regional wall motion abnormalities in infarct territory.

Right ventricle (RV) function: There is a hypokinetic free wall in RV infarct and dilated, poor function with a massive pulmonary embolus (PE). It is compressed in cardiac tamponade.

Ventricles: There is a visible VSD, and a ventricular aneurysm.

Valves: There is flail, a prolapsing mitral valve, and acute aortic regurgitation in type A aortic dissection.

Aortic root: This is dilated in type A aortic dissections and a visible dissection flap may be seen.

CXR: Look for evidence of coexisting pulmonary oedema/lower respiratory tract infection, and aortic root and mediastinal contour. Identify position of CVP/pulmonary artery catheters. Identify iatrogenic pneumothorax.

Management

Management requires consultant input involving critical care services and cardiologists. Prompt recognition of symptoms and instigation of treatment is vital. It should be remembered that mortality is high despite maximal medical intervention. Escalation of care to intensive care may not always be in the patient's best interest

Treatment is aimed at improving myocardial perfusion by following several basic principles:

- The patient's left ventricular filling volume should be optimized.
- Gas exchange needs to be maintained and the appropriateness of non-invasive and invasive ventilation needs to be addressed early in the treatment course.
- The patient requires systemic blood pressure support and reperfusion therapies. Blood pressure can be supported with inotropes to maintain adequate organ perfusion but mechanical methods, such as intra-aortic balloon counterpulsation (IABP) may be of benefit if combined with reperfusion therapy.

Oxygenation
High-flow oxygen is mandatory; consider CPAP/IPPV. Patients are peripherally shut down so peripheral pulse oximetry may be misleading.

Effective monitoring is vital:

- Continuous ECG
- Blood pressure monitored invasively via arterial line
- Urinary catheter to monitor fluid output
- CVP line or pulmonary artery catheter to assess fluid input and to optimize filling pressure. Optimum filling pressure is the highest filling pressure that can be achieved without inducing pulmonary oedema. Low pulmonary capillary wedge pressure (PCWP) often accompanies right ventricular infarction or reduced intravascular volume.

Haemodynamic management
Hypotensive patients in acute left ventricular failure may benefit from inotropes. However, the gain from cardiac output is offset by an increase in cardiac workload and the risk of arrhythmias. Inotropes should be used in conjunction with measures to optimize ventricular filling.

Preload
Optimize ventricular filling.

If filling pressures are high start a venodilator, e.g. IV nitrates.

Contractility: inotropic support
Dobutamine: 5–20 µg/kg/min. Dobutamine is an inodilator causing peripheral vasodilatation and positive inotropy. It is the inotrope of choice in cardiac failure.

Adrenaline (epinephrine): 1–12 µg/kg/min. More arrhythmogenic than dobutamine. Vasoconstriction may worsen cardiac ischema by increasing cardiac work.

Noradrenaline (norepinephrine): Ionoconstrictor 1–12 µg/kg/min. Mainly used in septic shock and of little use in carcinogenic shock.

Afterload

Intra-aortic balloon pumping (IABP): Availability is limited outside cardiac centres and is best used as a bridge to definitive treatment such as cardiac revascularization. A helium-filled balloon is inserted via the femoral artery under fluoroscopic guidance. The balloon fills during diastole augmenting coronary perfusion pressure and distal aortic flow. Rapid deflation during systole causes a reduction in afterload.

Definitive therapy

Treat reversible myocardial ischaemia. All patients who present with or develop cardiogenic shock in the context of an ACS should be discussed urgently with a cardiologist. Thrombolysis is ineffective in patients with cardiogenic shock. In the under 75 years age group the preferred treatment is haemodynamic support and percutaneous coronary intervention to the infarct-related artery with concomitant use of glycoprotein IIb/IIIa antagonists. In patients with severe three-vessel coronary disease or left main stem stenosis, coronary artery bypass grafting (CABG) is the treatment of choice.

Treat other reversible causes. Surgical repair of VSD and flail mitral leaflet carries a high operative mortality, but is the only option if cardiogenic shock ensues. IABP can help stabilize such patients preoperatively.

Arrhythmias should be corrected to optimize cardiac output. IV amiodarone 5 mg/kg over 30 min limits heart rate rapidly and may restore sinus rhythm. It is also the treatment of choice for ventricular arrhythmias.

RIGHT VENTRICULAR INFARCTION

This is a variant of AMI in which there is extensive RV involvement, usually associated with an inferior of inferoposterior AMI. Always check leads in all patients presenting with inferior AMI. RV infarction is associated with a significant increase in all peri-infarct complications (Fig. 7.10).

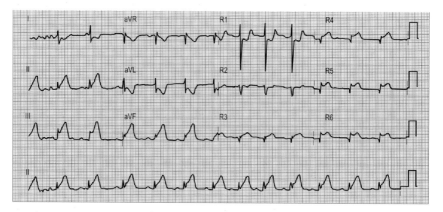

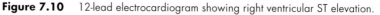

Figure 7.10   12-lead electrocardiogram showing right ventricular ST elevation.

Characteristics of RV infarction

- Inferior or inferoposterior AMI on ECG
- Impaired RV function
- Hypotension due to decreased left heart filling
- Increased RA pressure
- Low/low-normal PCWP
- Markedly raised JVP, low blood pressure, dry lung fields
- Cardiac enzymes elevated disproportionately to degree of LV dysfunction.

Investigations

Patients present with a history of cardiac ischaemia and classical ECG changes. Clinically they display signs of shock and right-sided heart failure.

ECG: To show inferior MI pattern plus tall R waves in V1–V3, indicating posterior involvement. Right ventricular involvement is implied by ST elevation in V4R–V6R (V4R lies in the mid-clavicular line 5th intercostal space on the right. Greater than 1 mm ST elevation implies RV infarction).

Echocardiography: To demonstrate a dilated RV with reduced RV free wall movement. There will be variable LV involvement. Echocardiography also excludes cardiac tamponade.

CXR: To exclude pulmonary oedema.

Pulmonary artery catheterization: To show typically elevated RA pressure and RV end-diastolic pressure with normal or reduced RV and PA systolic pressure. The PCWP is low or low-normal.

Management

Management is as for STEMI.

In addition, patients need volume expansion to increase RV preload and output. Aliquots of fluid (250 ml) should be given and the patient examined frequently (every 30 min) for signs of cardiac failure. Several litres of fluid may be needed to drive the RV output sufficiently to increase LV filling and reverse hypotension. Consider pulmonary artery catheterization if response to fluids is poor. Patients with RV infarction should not be treated with diuretics or nitrates as this can cause a dangerous fall in blood pressure.

RV infarction with LV failure

This is a severe condition with mortality > 80%. Treat as for cardiogenic shock.

AV block and RV infarction

Atrial transport is critical for RV filling in RV infarction. High-grade second degree AV block and complete heart block should be treated with temporary dual chamber cardiac pacing to maintain AV synchrony. Discuss with a cardiologist.

Right ventricular infarction

CARDIAC TAMPONADE

A pericardial effusion is the accumulation of fluid in the pericardial space. Cardiac tamponade occurs when a pericardial effusion causes haemo-dynamically significant cardiac compression. Adequate diastolic filling is prevented.

CASE 7.4

A 50-year-old man presented with increasing shortness of breath (SOB) and haemoptysis after returning from holiday in the Balearics. He was an ex-smoker. CXR revealed consolidation in the right mid-zone and he was treated with intravenous antibiotics. In spite of treatment and multiple investigations he remained unwell and hypoxic. A 12-lead ECG showed electrical alternans (see Fig. 7.11).

Presentation

Many of the findings in cardiac tamponade are non-specific. Presentation relates to speed of fluid accumulation. Very rapid accumulation may lead to cardiac arrest (PEA) or shock. In the sub-acute setting, patients are unwell but not necessarily in *extremis*.

Causes of cardiac tamponade

Acute
- Myocardial rupture post acute myocardial infarction
- Type A aortic dissection
- Iatrogenic:
  - post cardiac surgery
  - post cardiac procedure, e.g. cardiac catheterization, temporary/permanent pacemaker insertion
  - anticoagulation-spontaneous bleed
  - erosion of CVP line through right atrial wall
- Thoracic trauma.

Sub-acute

- Malignancy
- Hypothyroidism
- Uraemia
- Pericarditis
- Infection (viral, bacterial, fungal)
- Radiation (rare).

Examination

When fluid accumulation is rapid, e.g. acute aortic dissection, patients are often in a shocked state with cool peripheries and evidence of organ dysfunction.

The majority of patients are tachycardic (heart rate > 90 beats per min), however patients who are uraemic, hypothyroid or on beta-blockade may be bradycardic. Cardiac tamponade is suggested by pulsus paradoxus, which is characteristically:

- An inspiratory fall in systolic arterial pressure of > 10 mmHg during normal breathing. If this is marked, the pulse and Korsakoff sounds may be completely absent during inspiration. This sign can be difficult to demonstrate with a low cardiac output.

Venous distension is common, involving not only the jugular veins but also those of the forehead, scalp and ocular fundi.

- Characteristically the JVP is elevated and may paradoxically rise on inspiration (Kussmauls sign). This is not a specific sign of cardiac tamponade.

> **KEY POINT**
> - Falling BP, rising JVP and muffled heart sounds (due to the insulating effects of the pericardial fluid) on auscultation constitute Becks triad.

Other clinical signs that may be present relate to compression of adjacent structures and include hoarseness, dyspnoea and dysphagia.

Investigations

The diagnosis of cardiac tamponade is a clinical one.

ECG: Electrical alternans, variation in the QRS amplitude from cycle-to-cycle, is almost pathognomonic of cardiac tamponade, occurring in one-third of cases. It results from periodic swinging of the heart within the pericardial fluid, usually at a frequency equal to half that of the heart rate (2:1) whilst the surface ECG electrodes remain static (Fig. 7.11).

Echocardiography: This is used principally as a non-invasive investigative tool. It demonstrates the presence of fluid collection (usually circumferential) and compressed cardiac chambers.

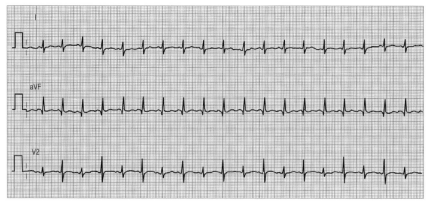

Figure 7.11 Electrocardiogram rhythm strip showing electrical alternans.

The most characteristic finding is diastolic chamber collapse, usually of the right atrium and ventricle. During early diastole the right ventricular free wall is compressed, and at end diastole the right atrial wall is compressed. Right atrial collapse can be seen in patients with hypovolaemia without cardiac tamponade. A highly specific feature of cardiac tamponade is left atrial collapse, which occurs in 25% of patients (Fig. 7.12).

Management

The immediate management of cardiac tamponade following initial assessment is drainage of the pericardial contents by needle paracentesis guided by cardiac ultrasound or fluoroscopy. Two approaches are used: the subxiphoid or apical approaches.

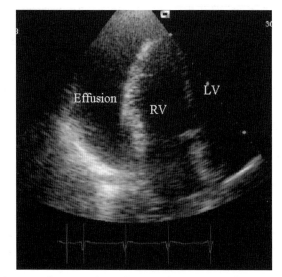

Figure 7.12 Transthoracic echocardiogram showing a significant pericardial effusion.

For prolonged drainage a pigtail catheter can be inserted and sutured in place. Echocardiography can monitor the residual pericardial volume. Any pericardial fluid aspirated should be sent for cytology, microscopy, culture and biochemical analysis.

Pericardiocentesis is not without risk and complications include:

- laceration of ventricle or coronary artery
- aspiration of ventricular blood
- arrhythmias
- pneumothorax
- puncture of peritoneum, oesophagus or aorta.

Once cardiac tamponade has been relieved, the underlying cause must be sought and this ultimately governs long-term prognosis.

ACUTE THORACIC AORTIC DISSECTION

Acute thoracic aortic dissection is usually due to an intimal tear, which is propagated along the media of the aorta and its main branches. Rupture outward results in catastrophic haemorrhage and sudden death. Tears in the branches result in many of the complications of aortic dissection. Less commonly, rupture of the vasa vasorum within the media occurs with development of a intramural haematoma.

The most clinically useful classification system for thoracic aortic dissections is the Stanford classification:

Type A: all aortic dissections involving the ascending thoracic aorta
Type B: all aortic dissections not involving the ascending thoracic aorta.

CASE 7.5

A 62-year-old man with a 7-year history of hypertension is admitted acutely unwell with severe chest pain. It had a sudden onset, was retrosternal and occurred whilst eating. There is no radiation. It is associated with shortness of breath. The patient then develops intrascapular pain although there is a history of osteoarthritis. He also complains of bloody diarrhoea and abdominal pain.

On examination his pulse rate is 106 bpm and manual BP is 185/105 mmHg in both arms. There are no audible murmurs.

12-lead ECG shows inferior and anterior ST elevation. CXR is normal.

History

Patients classically present with sudden onset, severe, tearing and intrascapular back pain, which may migrate along the path of the dissection. The pain of acute aortic dissection can be difficult to differentiate from AMI and should always be considered in the differential diagnosis of any patient presenting with chest pain.

Type A: usually anterior chest pain radiating to the face.
Type B: usually back pain.

Factors associated with aortic dissection

- hypertension (80% cases)
- aortic atherosclerosis
- bicuspid aortic valve
- congenital abnormalities:
  - coarctation of aorta, Turner or Noonan syndromes
- connective tissue diseases:
  - Ehlers–Danlos syndrome, Marfan's syndrome (cystic medial necrosis)
- advanced age
- pregnancy (usually 3rd trimester)
- trauma
- iatrogenic:
  - cardiac catheterization/IABP insertion/cocaine use.

Examination

The patient is usually distressed in severe haemodynamic compromise.

Check ABCD: Look for signs of poor peripheral perfusion and low cardiac output.

Pulse: The pulse will be low volume and tachycardic. Peripheral pulses may be absent because of subclavian or iliac artery dissection. Check for arterial bruits.

Blood pressure: This may be high or low; check for pulsus paradoxus (cardiac tamponade). Blood pressure must be manually recorded in both upper limbs. Unequal upper limb systolic BP > 20 mmHg may indicate subclavian artery involvement.

Cardiac auscultation: The patient may have an early diastolic murmur consistent with acute aortic regurgitation. This is an ominous sign, suggesting aortic root dilatation, a flail valve or distortion of the aortic root by haematoma.

Other: Respiratory examination may reveal signs of a pleural effusion, either reactive or secondary to an aortic leak. The patient may be in acute pulmonary oedema.

Examine the abdomen for signs of an abdominal aortic aneurysm. Are there any signs of mesenteric ischaemia? Neurological examination may reveal evidence of hypertensive retinopathy or focal neurological signs.

Rarely, dissection compromises one of the coronary ostia and causes acute MI. Thrombolytic therapy in this setting is likely to be fatal as it will cause massive bleeding. Always consider acute aortic dissection in a patient with chest pain and ST elevation in an unusual combination of leads, e.g. anterior and inferior.

Patients may present with symptoms and signs of occlusion of one of the branches of the aorta/aortic valve:

Coronary artery	Myocardial infarction, typically inferior MI
Aortic valve	Acute aortic regurgitation, pulmonary oedema
Head and neck vessels	Stroke
Renal arteries	Acute renal failure, anuria, haematuria
Spinal arteries	Paraplegia
Mesenteric arteries	Acute abdominal pain
Iliac arteries	Acute ischaemic limb

Investigations

ECG: To provide evidence of myocardial infarction/ischaemia, heart block or hypertension, e.g. LVH.

CXR: To show widened mediastinum and pleural effusion.

Echocardiography: To provide evidence of a visible dissection flap, dilated aorta, pericardial effusion, cardiac tamponade and regional wall motion abnormalities. Transoesophageal echocardiography (TOE) is particularly good at imaging the aortic valve and ascending aorta (Fig. 7.13).

Contrast enhanced CT of the thorax: This is used if TOE is not available.

Cardiac catheterization and aortography: This is not a routine investigation.

Management

Untreated acute aortic dissections have a high mortality rate with 70% of patients dying within 1 week of presentation. Mortality is significantly greater with type A dissections.

Initial assessment and stabilization

All patients require aggressive medical therapy to limit the extent of the medial tear. Particular attention should be paid to blood pressure control and

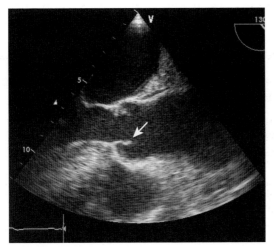

Figure 7.13 Transoesophageal echocardiogram demonstrating aortic dissection (intimal flap arrowed).

urine output. The main medical management is analgesia and anti-hypertensive therapy with target systolic BP of 100–120 mmHg. Patients should have invasive haemodynamic monitoring, e.g. arterial and central venous pressure line insertion, and be managed in a critical care environment.

Anti-hypertensive therapy

The extent of propagation of the dissection is determined by:

- shear stress
- rate of pressure rise in the aorta
- heart rate.

Negatively inotropic and negatively chronotropic agents minimize these effects and are preferable to vasodilators. Continuous intravenous infusion of labetalol 1–2 mg/min is useful as a negatively inotropic, negatively chronotropic agent with additional α-antagonist effects. If beta blockade is contraindicated consider a rate-limiting calcium channel blocker, e.g. verapamil.

If blood pressure remains elevated, commence a vasodilator, e.g. sodium nitroprusside.

Surgical management

Type A dissections: emergency surgical repair is indicated because of the risk of retrograde dissection into the pericardium and fatal tamponade. Aortic root replacement, reimplantation of the coronary arteries and valve replacement/resuspension may be necessary.

Surgical repair is considered for type B dissections complicated by:

- rupture
- saccular aneurysm formation
- limb ischaemia
- vital organ ischaemia or persistent pain
- dissections associated with Marfan's syndrome.

Otherwise acute type B dissections are managed medically with aggressive antihypertensive medication.

INFECTIVE ENDOCARDITIS

Infective endocarditic refers to infection of the endothelial surface of the heart, and is usually bacterial. Symptoms are often non-specific and mortality rates remain high.

Native valve endocarditis usually affects abnormal or diseased heart valves. In intravenous drug abusers (IVDAs) the tricuspid valve is a common site of infection. Endocarditis also occurs at sites of vascular or cardiac anomalies, e.g. VSD or patent ductus arteriosus.

Presentation

Typically, non-specific symptoms prevail including fever, malaise, myalgia, arthralgia, anorexia and sweating. In 75% of patients a history of cardiac or valvular abnormalities is present. Symptoms and signs may date back over several months or can present as an acute fulminant infection. The speed of presentation relates to the infective organism. Patients will present in one of three ways:

- Symptoms and signs of the infection
- Complications of the infection
- Symptoms and signs of immune complex deposition.

History

In any patient where infective endocarditis is suspected a detailed history needs to be taken including:

- history of recent invasive procedures/dental history
- history of IVDA
- history of rheumatic fever
- history of congenital heart disease.

Examination

A detailed examination is essential. Fever, murmur and haematuria are the commonest features. In a minority, neurological abnormalities and embolic signs will be present. A new cardiac murmur or change of an existing murmur may indicate valve damage and must be treated as a significant finding. Patients may present in overt septic shock.

Investigations

Blood cultures: key diagnostic investigation: These should be taken before antibiotics are administered. At least three sets (i.e. six bottles) from three separate sites are required. Sampling during pyrexia does not improve sensitivity. Avoid antibiotic administration until the organism is identified and ensure good aseptic technique to minimize the risk of sample contamination.

FBC: To provide evidence of anaemia of chronic disease (usually normochromic) and a neutrophilia. Thrombocytopenia may indicate disseminated intravascular coagulation.

CRP/ESR: Acute phase reactant. They provide an indication of activity and help monitor response to treatment.

U&E/LFT: Renal and hepatic involvement is common secondary to septic microemboli. Renal function can be impaired due to immune complex glomerulonephritis or from aminogylcoside antibiotics.

Urine dipstix/microscopy: Haematuria is an early sign. Formal microscopy is also needed to look for casts (glomerulonephritis)

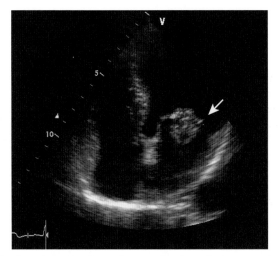

Figure 7.14 Transthoracic echocardiogram showing a large vegetation (arrow).

Microbiology: Culture any suspicious site, e.g. intravenous cannulae.

ECG: This should be done at least twice weekly. New PR prolongation suggests aortic root abscess formation and urgent cardiology review is needed.

CXR: Lung abscesses may be present if there is right-sided involvement. There may be evidence of pulmonary oedema.

Echocardiography: This is not a diagnostic test although it is helpful to identify the site and size of vegetation (Fig. 7.14). Transthoracic echocardiography cannot exclude endocarditis. TOE is required to exclude aortic root abscess formation.

Criteria for diagnosis

There are two groups of criteria: major and minor. Diagnosis can be based on:

- two major criteria   **or**
- one major and three minor   **or**
- five minor criteria.

Major criteria

- Positive blood culture:
  - typical organism from two blood cultures
- Endocardial involvement:
  - positive echocardiographic findings (vegetation/abscess)
  - new valvular regurgitation
  - dehiscence of a prosthesis.

Minor criteria

- Predisposing valvular or cardiac abnormality
- Fever > 38°C
- Intravenous drug abuser
- Embolic phenomenon
- Vasculitic phenomenon
- Blood cultures suggestive of endocarditis but not with a typical organism
- Echocardiographic features suggestive of endocarditis but not with major criteria.

Management

Management is two-fold:

- Treat infection
- Treat/prevent complications.

The choice of antibiotic regimen and duration of therapy should be decided on only after discussion with the microbiology staff and local cardiology team. Any failure to respond to medical treatment requires careful management.

Once blood culture results are known, therapy tailored to the specific causative organism can be started. If the patient is critically ill, and either haemodynamically compromised or overtly septic, IV antibiotics can be started after all blood cultures have been taken. Initial treatment should include flucloxacillin and fusidic acid to cover *Staphyloccocus aureus*.

Infection resides within the vegetation and, as such, high-dose antibiotics are required and usually given in synergistic combinations lasting up to 6 weeks. A tunnelled central line is often required to reduce infection risk.

Complications

Complications are classified into three groups:

- Locally destructive effects
  - paravalvular abscess formation, valvular incompetence leading to pulmonary oedema
- Embolic phenomenon
  - mycotic aneurysms
- Immune mediated
  - glomerulonephritis, encephalopathy, arthralgia.

Surgery

Surgery is indicated for:

- high degree AV block
- paravalvar infection, e.g. aortic root abscess
- cardiac failure due to valve incompetence

- uncontrolled infection despite appropriate medical therapy
- relapse after optimal medical therapy
- threatened or actual systemic embolization on treatment
- sinus of valsalva aneurysm
- valve obstruction.

PROSTHETIC VALVE ENDOCARDITIS

This affects up to 1% of patients after their valve replacement. It is most common in the early (< 2 months) postoperative period. Mortality is high (50%) partly because *Staphylococcus* is a common cause. The condition usually affects valves but can also affect vascular grafts or pacing leads.

The most important aspect of management is to have a high index of suspicion for the condition in the prosthetic valve patient with pyrexia. Presentation and diagnosis are the same as for native valve endocarditis, but complications are more serious. The majority of prosthetic valve patients with endocarditis will require further surgery. Endocarditis affecting pacing systems requires removal of the system, and if the patient is pacemaker dependent, temporary cardiac pacing may be required.

> **Tip**
> Infective endocarditis should always be considered in any patient with a heart murmur and fever.

DISORDERS OF CARDIAC RHYTHM: TACHYARRYTHMIAS

Narrow complex tachycardia (NCT)

An NCT is any cardiac rhythm > 100 bpm with a QRS duration of < 120 ms. Electrophysiologically the majority of these rhythms are supraventricular due to an automatic focus or a re-entry circuit with an atrial and/or atrio-ventricular (AV) nodal component.

Broad complex tachycardia (BCT)

Clinically a BCT is any cardiac rhythm > 100 bpm with a QRS duration of > 120 ms. Most of these arrhythmias are ventricular in origin involving an automatic focus or re-entry circuit within the ventricles.

Assessment of the patient with tachyarrhythmia

The initial assessment of a patient with a tachyarrhythmia is identical to that for a narrow or broad complex tachyarrythmia.
Initial assessment: ABCD.

Oxygen: Provide high-flow oxygen. Consider ventilation: CPAP or IPPV.

IV access: Insert a large bore venflon in a large calibre vein and start IV fluids.

Cardiac monitor: Attach an ECG monitor and obtain 12-lead ECG plus rhythm strip.

If the patient is haemodynamically compromised (systolic BP < 90 mmHg or in acute cardiac failure) and arrhythmia is continuous, consider immediate DC cardioversion:

- Perform under general anaesthetic
- Use synchronized DC shock.

If there is no response, consider the possibility that the diagnosis is sinus tachycardia with systemic compromise.

If sinus rhythm is only temporarily restored then further attempts at DC cardioversion are unlikely to be successful; treat pharmacologically or with temporary pacemaker insertion.

Factors to look for in the history

Check cardiac history for: ischaemic heart disease, valve disease, hypertension, long QT syndrome, LV impairment. Check current drug history for: proarrhythmic prescribed drugs or illicit drugs. Look for acute triggers including AMI, hypo/hyperkalaemia, hypoxaemia, cardiac failure and drug toxicity, e.g. tricyclic antidepressants.

Examination

Examination should be brief and focused. Look for signs of haemodynamic compromise and possible causes. Listen for carotid bruits.

Investigations

12-lead ECG plus rhythm strip: Examine 12-lead ECG in sinus rhythm (if possible) and during arrhythmia. Are there any atrial ectopics that can initiate SVT? Check the PR interval. Is there any evidence of pre-excitation (i.e. short PR interval and delta waves)?

CXR: Are there any signs of pulmonary oedema or cardiomegaly?

Bloods: To check electrolytes (particularly magnesium and potassium).

Echocardiogram: This is not essential in the immediate management but will provide information regarding cardiomyopathies, valvular disease and chamber dimensions.

Management of NCT

NCTs can be regular or irregular.

For all NCTs, AV nodal blocking manoeuvres should be considered. These may terminate an AV nodal or re-entry tachycardia, whilst slowing atrial fibrillation/flutter to allow the diagnosis to be made. They therefore have diagnostic and therapeutic actions.

AV nodal blocking manoeuvres

Always record a continuous ECG during AV nodal blocking manoeuvres.

Carotid sinus massage (CSM)

Check for carotid bruits and if present do not perform CSM. Apply firm pressure over the carotid artery for at least 10 s. Try both sides but not at the same time. CSM increases vagal tone and so prolongs AV node conduction time.

Valsalva manoeuvre

Ask the patient to exhale forcefully for at least 15 s, with the mouth and nose sealed.

Adenosine

Adenosine is a purine nucleoside with a half-life of 10 s. It acts via K^+ channels to cause temporary AV nodal block.

Check the patient has no contraindications and reassure the patient that side effects are transient. Insert a large bore cannula into a large vein, e.g. antecubital vein. Run a continuous rhythm strip (lead II usually shows clearest P wave morphology). Give each dose rapidly followed by a rapid saline flush.

Start with 3 mg and if there is no response increase incrementally to 6 mg, 12 mg and 18 mg. Allow up to 30 s between doses to look for AV block. Do not go beyond the effective dose.

Side effects of adenosine

- Flushing
- Chest pain/tightness
- Bronchospasm.

Contraindications to adenosine

Concomitant treatment with:

- dipyridamole: adenosine effect potentiated (reduce dose to 0.5–1 mg)
- aminophylline: unpredictable dose response
- sick sinus syndrome
- second or third degree AV block
- asthma.

> **Tip**
> If a contraindication to adenosine exists, IV verapamil 5 mg over 2 min should be considered. Verapamil should never be used in patients on beta-blockers or in broad complex tachycardia.

Irregular NCT

Atrial fibrillation

Atrial fibrillation is a common arrhythmia, especially in critically ill patients, and is due to multiple micro re-entry circuits within the atria. This results in a chaotic ventricular rhythm with absent P waves. AV nodal blocking manoeuvres will temporarily slow, but not terminate, the tachycardia. The rhythm is irregularly irregular. The severity of symptoms relates to ventricular response rate.

Atrial flutter

Atrial flutter is due to a rapid intra-atrial circuit resulting in an atrial rate of between 250–300 bpm. The AV node rarely conducts all atrial impulses and there can be a fixed relation between the atrial and ventricular rate, e.g. 2:1 block (i.e. atrial rate 300 bpm and ventricular rate 150 bpm). Cardioversion can be achieved electrically (synchronised DC cardioversion) or pharmaco-logically with the use of amiodarone, sotalol or flecainide. Control of ventricular rate can be achieved with beta-blockers or verapamil with or without digoxin. Cardioversion is less likely to be achieved with long-standing atrial fibrillation.

Regular NCT

Sinus tachycardia

Sinus tachycardia is due to autonomic imbalance or sinus node re-entry. The P wave axis is the same as in sinus rhythm. Inappropriate or pathological sinus tachycardia can occur with many non-cardiac situations, e.g. thyrotoxicosis, pain, sepsis. Administration of adenosine may cause sinus bradycardia or at higher dose, AV block, but does not terminate the tachycardia. Treatment is aimed at correcting the underlying cause.

Atrial flutter with regular AV block

This is easily identifiable by the underlying flutter waves.

Junctional tachycardia/supraventricular tachycardia (SVT)

This may be due to:

- AV nodal re-entrant tachycardia (AVNRT)
- accessory pathway (atrioventricular) re-entry tachycardia.

AV nodal re-entrant tachycardia (AVNRT)

AVNRT is due to dual AV node conduction via a fast and slow pathway. In 'typical' AVNRT, antegrade conduction goes down a slow pathway in the AV node; the retrograde conduction is via the fast pathway at the same time the ventricles are activated. This causes a short R–P, long P–R tachycardia with rates of 130–250 bpm. The QRS complexes often mask the P waves. In 'atypical' AVNRT antegrade conduction is via the fast pathway giving rise to long R–P, short P–R tachycardia. The tachycardia is usually of sudden onset and offset. Intravenous adenosine will often terminate the tachycardia.

Accessory pathway (atrioventricular) re-entry tachycardia

This is due to an abnormal anatomical connection between atrium and ventricle known as an accessory pathway, which is usually rapidly conducting, and inserts into ventricular myocardium, e.g. the bundle of Kent in Wolff-Parkinson White syndrome (WPW).

In sinus rhythm there is often (but not always) a short PR interval. In WPW a delta wave may be present. During the tachycardia, antegrade conduction is via the AV node (orthodromic tachycardia) and retrograde conduction is via the accessory pathway; the delta wave is absent and the heart rate is usually 170–220 bpm. P waves may be visible occurring within or shortly after the QRS complex. The less common antidromic tachycardia is caused by antegrade accessory pathway conduction and retrograde AV nodal conduction, and delta waves are present during tachycardia. Intravenous adenosine will often terminate the tachycardia.

Management of BCT

Ventricular tachycardia (VT): there are three or more consecutive ventricular beats occurring at a rate > 120 bpm. It is usually associated with ischaemic heart disease (see Fig. 7.6).

The main differential diagnosis of VT is SVT with aberrant conduction. If in doubt all BCTs must be treated as VT as this is life threatening and requires prompt treatment.

Initial assessment: ABCD.

Cardiac monitor: Attach ECG monitor and obtain 12-lead ECG plus rhythm strip. Check the QT interval in sinus rhythm if the tachycardia is intermittent.

Discontinue all pro-arrhythmic medication.

If the patient is haemodynamically stable and the diagnosis is unclear give adenosine IV.

Correct electrolyte disturbances, particularly hypokalaemia and hypomagnesaemia.

If LV is not known to be impaired: give lidocaine 100 mg IV slowly over 2 min followed by an infusion of 4 mg/min over 30 min, 2 mg/min over 2 h and then 1 mg/min maintenance. Beware of toxicity with abnormal neurological signs, fits, perioral numbness and blurred vision.

If LV is impaired or the patient has evidence of pulmonary oedema: give IV amiodarone administered via a long line (in ante-cubital fossa) or preferably via a central line.

If above options fail consider:

- synchronized DC cardioversion
- second line drug, e.g. procainamide
- overdrive pacing
- contact cardiology as pacing regimen is complex.

Tip

Tachyarrhythmias

- Treat urgently any arrhythmia causing symptoms or haemodynamic compromise.
- Electrical DC cardioversion is the treatment of choice if there is haemodynamic compromise.
- 12-lead ECG is essential in sinus rhythm and during the arrhythmia.
- A rhythm strip is very useful.
- Always correct electrolyte imbalances.
- Anti-arrhythmic drugs have pro-arrhythmic properties.
- Avoid the use of multiple anti-arrhythmic drugs.
- Never use verapamil in BCT.
- Differentiating between VT and SVT can be difficult.
- BCT is VT until proved otherwise.

Torsade de Pointes

Torsade de Pointes (Fig. 7.15), or polymorphic VT, occurs when cardiac repolarization is delayed. During the arrhythmia the ECG shows an irregular rhythm, which twists about the isoelectric line. During sinus rhythm the QT interval is prolonged. The arrhythmia is classically non-sustained and repetitive, although it can degenerate into ventricular fibrillation.

QT interval

The QT interval represents the time taken for ventricular depolarization and repolarization and is measured from the start of the QRS complex to the end of the T wave. The QT interval is rate dependent; it will shorten as heart rate increases and widen as heart rate slows. To standardize recordings a corrected QT interval (QTc) is often quoted, correcting for heart rate. The QTc interval should be < 0.44 ms.

Management of Torsade de Pointes

Torsade de Pointes is different from VT and is treated differently. Enlist senior help early. Treatment is aimed at identifying and removing causative factors.

Initial assessment: ABCD.

Cardiac monitor: Attach ECG monitor and obtain 12-lead ECG plus rhythm strip.

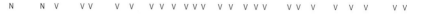

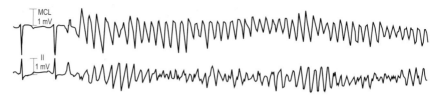

16/03/05 18:28:35 *** V-FIB/TACH 25.0 mm/s Strip

Figure 7.15   Electrocardiogram rhythm strip showing Torsade de Pointes.

Discontinue all pro-arrhythmic medication.

Correct electrolyte disturbances.

In acquired long QT syndrome Torsade de Pointes is often triggered by bradycardia:

- IV isoprenaline 0.5–10 μg/min, may prevent bradycardia.
- Overdrive atrial pacing, or if AV block, ventricular pacing at 100 bpm will usually suppress Torsade de Pointes. Contact the cardiology department for advice.

Other drug options for Torsade de Pointes should be discussed with the local cardiologist. **DO NOT USE ANTIARRYTHMIC DRUGS INCLUDING AMIODARONE** as they lengthen the QT interval, exacerbating the situation.

DISORDERS OF CARDIAC RHYTHM: BRADYARRYTHMIAS

Bradyarrhythmias are due to:

- failure of impulse formation, e.g. sinus node disease
- failure of impulse propagation via AV node.

Clinical definition: any heart rate that causes haemodynamic compromise, or places the patient at risk of cardiac arrest.

Examination

Check the patient's blood pressure, temperature and consciousness level. Is there evidence of cardiac failure? Does the patient have signs of aortic valve disease, jaundice, raised intracranial pressure or hypothyroidism?

Causes of bradycardia

- Physiological:
  - athletes, young adults
- Parasympathetic response:
  - vasovagal faint
  - vagal response, e.g. vomiting, acute MI
  - carotid sinus hypersensitivity

- Drugs
  - beta-blockers, calcium channel blockers, digoxin, antiarrhythmic agents
- Cardiac
  - sinus node disease, especially in the elderly
  - AV node disease
  - myocardial ischaemia or infarction
- Other
  - raised intracranial pressure
  - hypothyroidism
  - hypothermia
  - cholestatic jaundice.

Investigations

ECG: Examine the ECG during the bradycardia. Are any P waves visible? When do the P waves occur and what is the relation of the P waves to the QRS complex? If P waves are absent is the QRS complex broad or narrow? Broad complex escape rhythms are more likely to degenerate to asystole, as they usually originate from a ventricular origin with no back up if the focus should fail.

CXR: Check for cardiac enlargement and pulmonary oedema.

Bloods: To check FBC, U&Es, TFTs, digoxin levels, cardiac enzymes, Ca^{2+}, Mg^{2+}.

Echocardiogram: Look for regional wall motion defects (suggesting ischaemic heart disease), aortic valve disease and vegetations.

Tip

AV dissociation ≠ complete heart block.

In AV dissociation the atria and ventricles act independently. This can occur in CHB, but can also occur when:

- the intrinsic ventricular rate speeds up above sinus (accelerated idioventricular rhythm, ventricular tachycardia)
- the sinus rate slows below the intrinsic juntional or ventricular rate, e.g. extreme sinus bradycardia with ventricular/junctional escape.

Differentiating the two conditions is important because:

- CHB can lead to asystole
- AV dissociation is benign.

Management of bradycardia

Initial assessment: ABCD.

Cardiac monitor: Attach an ECG monitor and obtain a 12-lead ECG plus rhythm strip.

If the patient is haemodynamically compromised (systolic BP < 90 mmHg or in acute cardiac failure) and arrhythmia is continuous, follow the peri-arrest guidelines of the UK Resuscitation Council:

- If the patient is compromised, give atropine, and if this is unsuccessful consider isoprenaline or temporary pacemaker insertion.
- If the patient is uncompromised then monitor.

Definitive treatment relates to the actual bradyarrythmia. Treat acutely if the patient is at risk of asystole or has adverse signs.

Risk of asystole

- History of asystole
- 2nd degree AV block
- Pauses > 3 s
- Complete heart block with broad QRS complex.

Adverse signs

- Low cardiac output
- Hypotension (systolic BP < 90 mmHg)
- Heart failure
- Heart rate < 40 bpm
- Ventricular arrhythmias.

Atropine

Give 0.5–1.0 mg atropine IV. The maximum dose is 3 mg in 24 h. Side effects include tachycardia, blurred vision, hallucinations and urinary retention.

Isoprenaline

This is indicated for symptomatic bradycardia unresponsive to atropine. It is given by continuous IV infusion titrated up to 10 µg/min. It is also used as a temporary measure whilst awaiting transvenous temporary pacing wire insertion. Isoprenaline leads to increased oxygen consumption and can cause myocardial irritability.

TEMPORARY CARDIAC PACING

Pacemakers deliver electrical stimuli via pacing leads to the heart, and can be used on a temporary or permanent basis. Wherever possible a permanent system should be inserted (if facilities allow).

Indications for temporary cardiac pacing wire (TPW) insertion

AMI

Inferior AMI commonly causes CHB as the right coronary artery supplies the AV nodal artery. This rarely requires a TPW. Any sign of haemodynamic compromise, e.g. hypotension, poor urine output, the patient becoming cerebrally obtunded, would necessitate IV atropine. If there is no response, consider TPW insertion.

Anterior AMI complicated by second or third degree AV block carries a poor prognosis. The infarct is large and involves the bundle branches. The risk of ventricular asystole is high and a TPW is indicated.

Indications for TPW post anterior AMI

- Asystole
- Second or third degree AV block
- Bifascicular block (RBBB plus LAD)
- Trifascicular block (RBBB plus LAD plus first degree AV block or LBBB plus first degree AV block)
- Alternating LBBB and RBBB
- Sinus/junctional bradycardia with inadequate response to atropine
- Recurrent ventricular tachycardia (overdrive pacing).

Other indications

- Heart failure or haemodynamic compromise associated with inappropriate bradycardia unresponsive to atropine
- Profound bradycardia associated with drug overdose complicated by haemodynamic compromise unresponsive to atropine/isoprenaline
- Asystole or ventricular standstill
- Aortic valve or root endocarditis with evidence of AV block
- Overdrive suppression of bradycardia-mediated ventricular tachycardia, e.g. Torsade de Pointes.
- Overdrive termination of recurrent or persistent tachyarrhythmias, e.g. recurrent ventricular tachycardia.

Methods of temporary cardiac pacing

Emergency temporary cardiac pacing can be performed in one of two ways: transcutaneous ventricular pacing or transvenous pacing.

Transcutaneous ventricular pacing

This is an emergency measure reserved for the treatment of severe bradycardia or asystole, usually in the setting of a cardiac arrest or peri-arrest situation. The pacing system is usually incorporated into a defibrillator unit.

Temporary cardiac pacing

It allows time until more definitive transvenous temporary pacing can be organized. Two large pads are attached to the chest wall, one at the V3 lead position, the other posteriorly under the left scapula. The patient may require sedation.

Transvenous pacing

The most commonly used pacing mode for the treatment of bradyarrythmias is ventricular demand pacing. This is achieved with a single bipolar temporary pacing wire inserted in the right ventricle. When it is important to maintain cardiac synchrony, e.g. critically ill patients with impaired LV function, dual chamber pacing (atrioventricular sequential pacing) is the preferred method as it can improve cardiac output by up to 20%.

Placement of a TPW is difficult and must not be attempted by an unsupervised, inexperienced operator. Most coronary care units will have a fully equipped temporary pacing room. At least one other assistant and a radiographer need to be present.

Venous access

Dictated by the clinical setting. If recent thrombolysis has been administered the internal jugular or femoral vein is the route of choice as direct compression can be applied if a haematoma or excessive bleeding occurs. Venous access is secured by the Seldinger technique. A sheath is inserted through which a bipolar pacing electrode (wire) can be introduced.

Technique

All TPW manipulation must be performed under fluoroscopic guidance. Ventricular temporary leads either have a straight or angulated tip. Once the lead is in the right atrium it is positioned so the tip points towards the cardiac apex (pointing towards the left hip). Transient ventricular arrhythmias, as the TPW passes through the tricuspid valve, are normal. The tip should point downwards in the RV apex.

Checking function

Once positioned, connect the TPW to the external pacemaker box, switch to demand pacing, with at least 3 volts output and a rate at least 20 bpm greater than the patient's intrinsic rate. If pacing is successful the heart rate will increase and an LBBB appearance should occur. Slowly turn the output down until pacing capture is lost, i.e. the patient's intrinsic rhythm returns. This point is known as the 'ventricular threshold' and should be less than 1 volt. If this is not achieved, further attempts to reposition the TPW should be made.

Check wire sensing by turning the pacing rate below the patient's intrinsic rate (this is not always possible in the acute setting). If the wire is sensing correctly, pacing should not occur. Poor sensing requires TPW re-position.

Initiating pacing

The pacing rate (demand rate) should be set as per clinical need. A low pacing rate is adequate for prophylaxis against bradycardia; a higher rate is needed if the bradycardia is inappropriate, e.g. Torsade de Pointes. The output should be three times the ventricular threshold and checked at least twice daily to avoid inadvertent loss of capture. The ventricular threshold will rise after TPW insertion. As the ventricular threshold climbs, the output should be reset, always keeping the output three times the ventricular threshold. If the ventricular threshold exceeds 5 volts lead replacement is indicated.

High or rising ventricular threshold

- Check lead connections
- Check pacing box function and settings
- Consider lead displacement or perforation through RV wall.

Other considerations

As for any central venous line insertion the TPW needs to be secured in place at the point of venous access.

A CXR must be performed after TPW insertion to exclude a pneumothorax, and to check wire position once the patient has returned to the critical care area.

Further reading

FURTHER READING

Erbel R, Alfonso F, Boileau C et al; Task Force on Aortic Dissection, European Society of Cardiology 2001 Diagnosis and management of aortic dissection. European Heart Journal 22:1642–1681

Fox K F 2005 Investigation and management of chest pain. Heart 91: 105–110

French J K, White H D 2004 Clinical implications of the new definition of myocardial infarction. Heart 90:99–106

Hochman J S, Sleeper L A, Webb J G et al 1999 Early revascularization in acute myocardial infarction complicated by cardiogenic shock. Shock Investigators. New England Journal of Medicine 341:625–634

Markides V, Schilling R J 2003 Atrial fibrillation: classification, pathophysiology, mechanisms and drug treatment. Heart 89:939–943

Mylonakis E, Calderwood S B 2001 Medical progress: infective endocarditis in adults. New England Journal of Medicine 345:1318–1330

Silber S, Albertsson P, Avilés F F et al; Task Force for Percutaneous Coronary Interventions of the European Society of Cardiology 2005 Guidelines for percutaneous coronary interventions. European Heart Journal 26:804–847

Spector P S 2005 Diagnosis and management of sudden cardiac death. Heart 91:408–413

Spodick D H 2003 Current concepts: acute cardiac tamponade. New England Journal of Medicine 349:684–690

Turley A J, de Belder M A 2004 Management of acute coronary syndromes: an update. CPD Anaesthesia 6(3):105–115

7

Van de Werf F, Ardissino D, Betriu A et al 2003 Management of acute myocardial infarction in patients presenting with ST-segment elevation. Task Force on the Management of Acute Myocardial Infarction of the European Society of Cardiology. European Heart Journal 24:28–66

Wellens H J J 2001 Electrophysiology: ventricular tachycardia: diagnosis of broad QRS complex tachycardia. Heart 86:579–585

Yusuf S, Zhao F, Mehta SR et al; Clopidogrel in Unstable Angina to Prevent Recurrent Events Trial Investigators 2001 Effects of clopidogrel in addition to aspirin in patients with acute coronary syndromes without ST-segment elevation. New England Journal of Medicine 345:494–502

Respiratory emergencies 8

Sean Parker, Richard Harrison, Andrew Fisher

OBJECTIVES

After reading this chapter you will:

◗ *Understand the concept of respiratory failure and its treatment with oxygen and non-invasive ventilation*

◗ *Have a greater understanding of the treatment of the following respiratory emergencies:*
  - *Acute severe asthma*
  - *Severe pneumonia*
  - *Acute pulmonary embolism*
  - *Pneumothorax*
  - *Exacerbation of chronic obstructive airways disease*
  - *Acute upper airways obstruction*

RESPIRATORY FAILURE

Respiratory failure occurs when the lungs fail to maintain effective gas exchange and results in hypoxaemia ($PaO_2 < 8$ kPa), hypercapnea ($PaCO_2 > 6$ kPa) or both. A PaO_2 of 8 kPa is close to the steep part of the oxygen dissociation curve where rapid desaturation occurs, resulting in significantly impaired oxygen delivery. Respiratory failure can be classified into two main groups: type 1 and type 2. Although both types frequently coexist in the same patient, the classification can be useful when considering the cause of respiratory failure and in guiding management.

Type 1 'hypoxaemic respiratory failure'

PaO_2 is low and $PaCO_2$ low or normal. The main mechanism is ventilation perfusion (VQ) mismatch. As the condition progresses a combination of fatigue, hypoxia and acidosis causes respiratory muscle weakness and ventilatory failure that will complicate the picture. This is reflected in a blood gas picture similar to type 2 respiratory failure. It is important to recognize that type 2 respiratory failure which has progressed from type 1 failure is a bad prognostic sign, implying the possibility of imminent respiratory arrest.

Type 2 'ventilatory failure'

PaO_2 is low and $PaCO_2$ is high. $PaCO_2$ is determined by alveolar ventilation (V_A) and is normally tightly controlled; any reduction in V_A will cause hypoxia and hypercapnea. Hypoxia associated with ventilatory failure is usually readily correctible by an increase in the inspired oxygen concentration (FIO_2). In structurally abnormal lungs (e.g. chronic obstructive pulmonary disorder (COPD)) VQ mismatch also contributes. Chronic ventilatory failure results in a persistently elevated $PaCO_2$ and renal compensation with an elevation of serum bicarbonate normalizes arterial pH. Any superimposed acute ventilatory failure in these patients will cause a further rise in $PaCO_2$ and a consequent fall in arterial pH. The arterial pH is the best marker of acute ventilatory failure in these patients rather than absolute values of $PaCO_2$ which can be misleading.

Assessment of the patient with respiratory failure

The differential diagnosis is wide but can be narrowed significantly through clinical assessment and some simple investigations. Causes of respiratory failure are shown in Figure 8.1. Respiratory failure is potentially life-threatening and assessment should be rapid and follow the ABC method below.

Airway: Is the airway patent? Is there noisy breathing with gurgling or stridor suggesting upper airway obstruction?

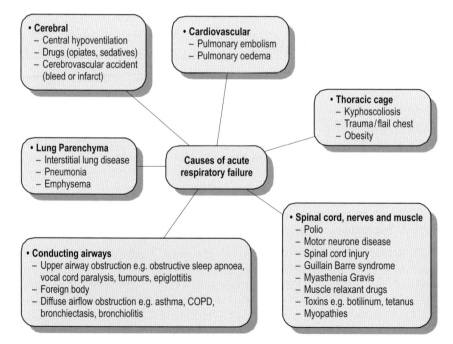

Figure 8.1 Causes of acute respiratory failure.

Breathing: Check for chest wall movement, cyanosis, respiratory rate and SpO_2; if the patient is hypoxaemic, give high-flow oxygen and aim for SpO_2 > 92% (unless there is significant COPD, in which case, start with controlled 24–28% O_2 and aim for an SpO_2 of 93% at most), and check arterial blood gases. Listen to the chest.

Circulation: Check the pulse, blood pressure and capillary refill. Listen to heart sounds and assess the JVP.

- History, physical examination and routine investigations: chest X-ray (CXR), arterial blood gases (ABGs), electrocardiogram (ECG), full blood count (FBC), urea and electrolytes (U&E), C-reactive protein (CRP), glucose. If a neuromuscular cause is suspected, perform spirometry to assess FEV1 and, more importantly, vital capacity if possible. These should point to the likely cause.
- If the patient has impaired consciousness, pinpoint pupils and respiratory effort is poor, consider an empirical trial of naloxone 400 µg IV in the case of opiate overdose, or flumazenil 200 µg IV then 100 µg/min up to a maximum of 1 mg to reverse benzodiazepine toxicity (caution, there is a risk of inducing seizures).
- Consider intensive care if it is not possible to maintain PaO_2 > 8 kPa despite maximum oxygen, worsening hypercapnea/acidosis, exhaustion and deteriorating respiratory effort, comatose/drowsy, shock or other organ dysfunction.

Specific treatment depends on the cause, e.g. bronchodilators in asthma, and diuretics and nitrates in pulmonary oedema. There are some specific methods of respiratory support that can be used in most patients to treat respiratory failure.

Oxygen (see also Chapter 2)

Hypoxaemia compromises vital organ metabolic functions and can result in death if not treated. Rapid correction of hypoxaemia by administration of supplementary oxygen can be life-saving. Other indications for supplemental oxygen include: myocardial infarction, pneumothorax, carbon monoxide poisoning, acute anaemia and shock. Oxygen can be delivered by a number of different methods (Fig. 8.2):

- A high concentration mask such as a 'Hudson' or 'reservoir' mask allows an FIO_2 of about 60–80% to be delivered to the patient. The main problem is that excessive oxygen can be inadvertently delivered to patients with chronic type 2 respiratory failure who are sensitive to the effects of oxygen, and this causes worsening hypercapnea.
- Fixed performance masks work on the venturi principle and deliver a fixed FIO_2 that can be varied according to the mask used and the oxygen flow rate. Masks available include: 24, 28, 35, 40 and 60%.
- Nasal cannulae are comfortable and well tolerated but the FIO_2 delivered is variable and depends on minute ventilation. They should not be used in unstable patients, or those with a tendency to retain CO_2.

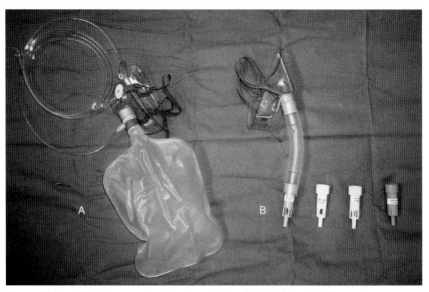

Figure 8.2 (A) Hudson mask with rebreathe bag for delivering high-flow oxygen.
(B) Venturi mask with various attachments for delivering oxygen at fixed concentrations; 24,
28, 35 and 40%.

Oxygen and patients with chronic respiratory failure

In patients with chronic type 2 respiratory failure ('CO_2 retainers', most
commonly seen in COPD), the persistently elevated CO_2 levels lead to
adaptation and a loss of drive from the CO_2 sensing central chemoreceptors.
Ventilatory drive in these patients depends largely on stimulation of hypoxia
sensing peripheral chemoreceptors. If excessive oxygen is administered,
PaO_2 rises to a level where there is a loss of hypoxic chemoreceptor
stimulation and a consequent reduction in ventilatory drive. This can result
in alveolar hypoventilation, worsening hypercapnea, acidosis and ultimately
respiratory arrest. These patients must be given sufficient oxygen to correct
hypoxia but not so much as to cause ventilatory depression and retention
of carbon dioxide. Concern about administering excessive oxygen should not
prevent correction of life threatening hypoxaemia rapidly; remember:
'hypoxia kills quickly, hypercapnea kills slowly'. Additionally, most patients
do not depend on a hypoxic drive and these patients will be harmed if they
do not have their hypoxaemia corrected rapidly. Patients who depend on a
hypoxic drive are usually the COPD patients with severe exercise limitation.
  A simple approach in these chronic COPD patients would be:

* If the patient is hypoxic ($SpO_2 < 92\%$) administer oxygen at a fixed
  concentration via a venturi mask, usually 24–28%, sufficient to correct
  hypoxaemia. Aim for an SpO_2 of around 93% at most; if it is higher than
  this then the patient is being given too much O_2. Check arterial blood gas
  after 30 min. During this period further medical treatment such as
  nebulizers can be given.

- Acute type 2 respiratory failure (pH < 7.35, high $PaCO_2$) and a high PaO_2 (> 10) after the administration of oxygen in a patient with severe COPD may suggest loss of hypoxic ventilatory drive. Consider reducing FIO_2 and recheck after 30 min, do not remove the oxygen as this, combined with hypoventilation, can result in dangerous hypoxia. Aim for a PaO_2 of around 8 kPa; if the acidosis persists despite these measures then non-invasive ventilation (NIV) may be indicated.
- If there is no evidence of acute CO_2 retention (pH normal) and the patient is still hypoxic (PaO_2 < 8 kPA), increase FIO_2 and recheck after 30 min.
- If there is acute type 2 respiratory failure (pH < 7.35) and PaO_2 is not high, NIV or invasive ventilation may be indicated. Most patients will correct the abnormality after administration of medical treatment such as bronchodilators; the arterial blood gases should be rechecked after 1 h and if the acidosis is not correcting or is worsening then consider NIV/invasive ventilation.
- Nebulizers should be driven by oxygen at 5 L/min for a maximum of 5 min and then replaced with controlled oxygen so as to minimize the possibility of delivering excess oxygen.
- Nasal cannulae can be used only in patients who are stable with no evidence of acute type 2 respiratory failure; arterial blood gases should be checked after 1 h.

Respiratory stimulants

Analeptic drugs act to stimulate neural output to respiratory muscles and therefore increase ventilation. They are only useful if there is capacity in the respiratory muscles to do more work and they should not be used in exhausted patients. NIV has largely rendered these drugs obsolete but they are useful if NIV is not available, not tolerated or is unsuccessful in a patient in whom invasive mechanical ventilation is inappropriate. Senior advice should be sought before using respiratory stimulants. The drug most often used is doxapram which acts on peripheral chemoreceptors to cause an increase in both the rate and depth of ventilation. Its use is limited by significant side effects that include nausea, cough, agitation and in some cases convulsions.

Non-invasive ventilation

NIV allows the delivery of positive pressure ventilatory support via the upper airway to patients in respiratory failure. NIV avoids some of the risks associated with intubation and mechanical ventilation but is not a substitute for invasive ventilation in patients where this is appropriate. NIV can be used as:

- a holding measure in patients who are not yet sick enough to require invasive ventilation
- a trial, with invasive ventilation used if NIV fails
- a 'ceiling of treatment' in those patients where invasive ventilation is not appropriate.

Prior to commencing treatment a decision needs to be made by a senior clinician as to whether or not invasive ventilation is appropriate if NIV fails. Issues to consider here include premorbid condition, the potential to recover to an acceptable quality of life and the wishes of the patient and family. NIV should only be administered by experienced practitioners who have received appropriate training.

Absolute contraindications to NIV include: facial injury, recent facial or upper airway surgery, vomiting, fixed upper airway obstruction and an undrained pneumothorax. Relative contraindications include upper gastro-intestinal surgery, excessive secretions, confusion and bowel obstruction; NIV can be attempted with caution in these patients.

NIV machines deliver a positive airway pressure that varies between inspiration (IPAP) and expiration (EPAP). The main indication for NIV is acute type 2 respiratory failure (pH < 7.35, $PaCO_2$ > 6 kPa) that persists

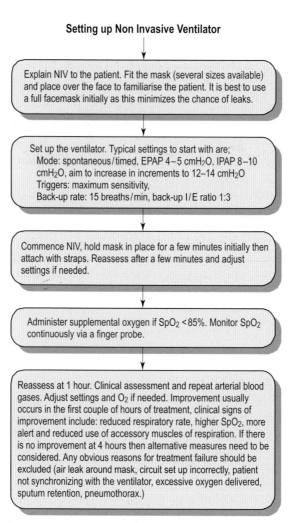

Setting up Non Invasive Ventilator

Explain NIV to the patient. Fit the mask (several sizes available) and place over the face to familiarise the patient. It is best to use a full facemask initially as this minimizes the chance of leaks.

Set up the ventilator. Typical settings to start with are;
Mode: spontaneous/timed, EPAP 4–5 cmH₂O, IPAP 8–10 cmH₂O, aim to increase in increments to 12–14 cmH₂O
Triggers: maximum sensitivity,
Back-up rate: 15 breaths/min, back-up I/E ratio 1:3

Commence NIV, hold mask in place for a few minutes initially then attach with straps. Reassess after a few minutes and adjust settings if needed.

Administer supplemental oxygen if SpO₂ <85%. Monitor SpO₂ continuously via a finger probe.

Reassess at 1 hour. Clinical assessment and repeat arterial blood gases. Adjust settings and O₂ if needed. Improvement usually occurs in the first couple of hours of treatment, clinical signs of improvement include: reduced respiratory rate, higher SpO₂, more alert and reduced use of accessory muscles of respiration. If there is no improvement at 4 hours then alternative measures need to be considered. Any obvious reasons for treatment failure should be excluded (air leak around mask, circuit set up incorrectly, patient not synchronizing with the ventilator, excessive oxygen delivered, sputum retention, pneumothorax.)

Figure 8.3 Setting up non-invasive ventilation.

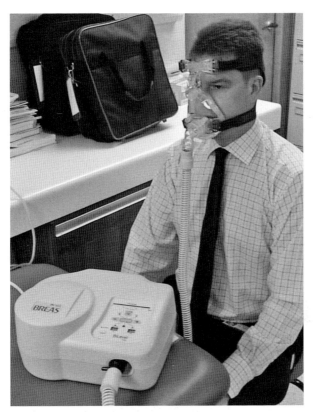

Figure 8.4   NIV mask set up on a normal subject.

despite initial medical therapy. NIV should not be attempted in patients with asthma or pneumonia; as invasive ventilation is usually more appropriate. Patients with a more severe acidosis (pH < 7.25) are less likely to succeed with NIV and should be managed in a critical care unit if progression to invasive ventilation is thought to be appropriate (Figs 8.3, 8.4).

Patients in whom NIV should be attempted include those with:

- acute exacerbation of COPD (evidence is best for this)
- acute type 2 failure associated with chest wall deformity, neuromuscular disease and obstructive sleep apnoea
- acute cardiogenic pulmonary oedema where CPAP has failed
- acute exacerbation of bronchiectasis.

Weaning from NIV: during the first 24 h the time spent on the ventilator should be maximized but breaks for food and nebulizers are acceptable. If the patient's clinical condition stabilizes (RR < 24 breaths/min, pulse < 110, pH > 7.35, SpO_2 > 90% on 4L/min O_2) then the time spent on the ventilator can be gradually reduced and should be guided by frequent clinical assessment. Care must be taken in allowing relief of pressure from the face, particularly the bridge of the nose where pressure necrosis may occur.

KEY POINT
• During weaning from NIV, nocturnal ventilation should be withdrawn last.

Continuous positive airway pressure (CPAP)

CPAP is considered to be a form of ventilatory support rather than non-invasive ventilation. A facemask delivers a continuous positive airway pressure throughout the respiratory cycle; this allows delivery of a high FIO_2 and improves gas exchange by recruitment of underventilated lung and reduction in the work of breathing. It should only be used in a critical care environment. Indications for acute use include:
• Acute cardiogenic pulmonary oedema with hypoxaemia that is not responding to medical therapy (this is the only situation where there is any good evidence for CPAP)
• Chest wall trauma and hypoxia despite high flow oxygen and regional anaesthesia
• Pneumonia and type 1 respiratory failure
• Weaning from mechanical ventilation.

Invasive mechanical ventilation

Invasive mechanical ventilation may be required in some patients with severely impaired and deteriorating respiratory function. If a patient is unable to maintain a PaO_2 of 8 kPa with high-flow oxygen then invasive mechanical ventilation is likely to be necessary if indicated. Patients are often very ill with coexisting cardiovascular compromise as a result of sepsis. The details of invasive mechanical ventilation are beyond the remit of this chapter.

ACUTE SEVERE ASTHMA

CASE 8.1

A 43-year-old smoker was admitted to accident and emergency (A&E) with a 2-day history of worsening breathlessness, wheeze and a cough productive of yellow sputum. She normally used 'blue and brown' inhalers and had been hospitalized with asthma in the past. She was unwell and unable to speak more than a few words at a time; her pulse was 110 bpm, blood pressure 130/60 mmHg, SpO_2 92% on room air, respiratory rate 30 breaths/min. Her chest was wheezy with poor air entry throughout and she could only manage a peak expiratory flow measurement of 200 L/min (best 450). Arterial blood gases showed pH 7.48, PCO_2 3.4, PO_2 8.6, HCO_3^- 24 on room air. She was

diagnosed with acute severe asthma (see Fig. 8 6) and given high flow oxygen, nebulized bronchodilators and 40 mg oral prednisolone. Despite the administration of several nebulizers, she failed to improve and remained wheezy and breathless after 30 min of treatment. What treatment would you consider next?

Answer
Administration of 2 g intravenous magnesium sulphate resulted in a marked improvement and she was admitted to a medical ward to continue treatment. Magnesium acts as a smooth muscle dilator and magnesium levels are low in asthma. There is increasing evidence of its efficacy in asthma. Repeated doses should not be given in a short time-frame without checking serum levels first as at high dose it can act as a muscle relaxant.

Asthma is a common problem and is defined as a 'chronic inflammatory disorder of the airways associated with reversible airflow obstruction and an exaggerated airway response to a variety of stimuli'. The diagnosis is clinical and is based on symptoms (typically wheeze, shortness of breath and cough) that tend to be variable, worse at night and frequently made worse by specific triggers such as exercise and common allergens (e.g. dust mite, pollen). Objective measures of airflow obstruction such as spirometry and peak expiratory flow rate (PEFR) measurements may support the diagnosis.

The majority of deaths from asthma are preventable; they occur outside the hospital in chronically severe asthmatics who deteriorate over days or weeks. Only a minority (8.5–14%) deteriorate suddenly over hours or minutes from a background of only mild or moderately severe disease.

There should be a low threshold for admitting patients to hospital; if there is any doubt, err on the side of caution. Admit anyone with near fatal or life-threatening asthma and those with any features of acute severe asthma that do not settle with treatment (see Fig. 8.6).

Investigations

Investigations are required in all patients and include:

- Chest radiograph to exclude a pneumothorax or pneumonia
- Peak expiratory flow rate to assess the degree of airway narrowing (expressed as a percentage of predicted best). This measurement is not as

KEY POINT
- Evidence suggests that medical staff frequently underestimate the severity of asthma and as a consequence do not provide adequate treatment. An objective assessment of the severity of acute severe asthma (Fig. 8.5) made on the basis of symptoms, signs and measurements is essential to guide treatment and identify patients needing intensive care at an early stage.

Management of acute severe asthma in adults in A&E

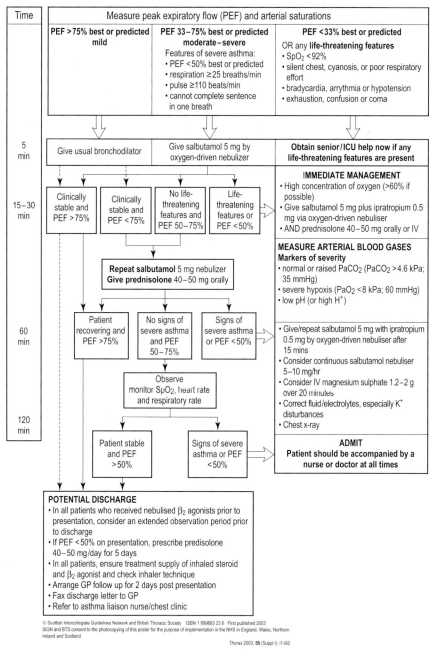

Thorax 2003; **58** (Suppl I): i1-i92

Figure 8.5   Management of acute severe asthma in adults in A&E.

useful in those with a degree of chronic fixed airflow obstruction, such as severe chronic asthmatics and smokers with coexistent COPD

- Pulse oximetry should be measured continuously and arterial blood gases taken if SpO$_2$ is < 92% or there are signs of a life-threatening attack

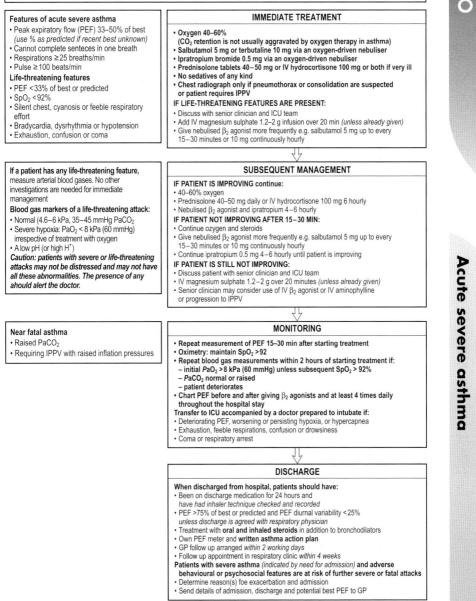

Management of acute severe asthma in adults in hospital

Features of acute severe asthma
- Peak expiratory flow (PEF) 33–50% of best
  (use % as predicted if recent best unknown)
- Cannot complete sentences in one breath
- Respirations ≥ 25 breaths/min
- Pulse ≥ 100 beats/min

Life-threatening features
- PEF <33% of best or predicted
- SpO_2 <92%
- Silent chest, cyanosis or feeble respiratory effort
- Bradycardia, dysrhythmia or hypotension
- Exhaustion, confusion or coma

IMMEDIATE TREATMENT
- **Oxygen 40–60%**
  (CO_2 retention is not usually aggravated by oxygen therapy in asthma)
- **Salbutamol 5 mg or terbutaline 10 mg via an oxygen-driven nebuliser**
- **Ipratropium bromide 0.5 mg via an oxygen-driven nebuliser**
- **Prednisolone tablets 40–50 mg or IV hydrocortisone 100 mg or both if very ill**
- **No sedatives of any kind**
- **Chest radiograph only if pneumothorax or consolidation are suspected or patient requires IPPV**

IF LIFE-THREATENING FEATURES ARE PRESENT:
- Discuss with senior clinician and ICU team
- Add IV magnesium sulphate 1.2–2 g infusion over 20 min *(unless already given)*
- Give nebulised β_2 agonist more frequently e.g. salbutamol 5 mg up to every 15–30 minutes or 10 mg continuously hourly

If a patient has any life-threatening feature, measure arterial blood gases. No other investigations are needed for immediate management

Blood gas markers of a life-threatening attack:
- Normal (4.6–6 kPa, 35–45 mmHg $PaCO_2$
- Severe hypoxia: PaO_2 < 8 kPa (60 mmHg) irrespective of treatment with oxygen
- A low pH (or high H^+)
Caution: patients with severe or life-threatening attacks may not be distressed and may not have all these abnormalities. The presence of any ahould alert the doctor.

SUBSEQUENT MANAGEMENT

IF PATIENT IS IMPROVING continue:
- 40–60% oxygen
- Prednisolone 40–50 mg daily or IV hydrocortisone 100 mg 6 hourly
- Nebulised β_2 agonist and ipratropium 4–6 hourly

IF PATIENT NOT IMPROVING AFTER 15–30 MIN:
- Continue ozygen and steroids
- Give nebulised β_2 agonist more frequently e.g. salbutamol 5 mg up to every 15–30 minutes or 10 mg continuously hourly
- Continue ipratropium 0.5 mg 4–6 hourly until patient is improving

IF PATIENT IS STILL NOT IMPROVING:
- Discuss patient with senior clinician and ICU team
- IV magnesium sulphate 1.2–2 g over 20 minutes *(unless already given)*
- Senior clinician may consider use of IV β_2 agonist or IV aminophylline or progression to IPPV

Near fatal asthma
- Raised $PaCO_2$
- Requiring IPPV with raised inflation pressures

MONITORING
- **Repeat measurement of PEF 15–30 min after starting treatment**
- **Oximetry: maintain SpO_2 > 92**
- **Repeat blood gas measurements within 2 hours of starting treatment if:**
  – initial PaO_2 > 8 kPa (60 mmHg) unless subsequent SpO_2 > 92%
  – $PaCO_2$ normal or raised
  – patient deteriorates
- **Chart PEF before and after giving β_2 agonists and at least 4 times daily throughout the hospital stay**

Transfer to ICU accompanied by a doctor prepared to intubate if:
- Deteriorating PEF, worsening or persisting hypoxia, or hypercapnea
- Exhaustion, feeble respirations, confusion or drowsiness
- Coma or respiratory arrest

DISCHARGE

When discharged from hospital, patients should have:
- Been on discharge medication for 24 hours and
  have had inhaler technique checked and recorded
- PEF >75% of best or predicted and PEF diurnal variability <25%
  unless discharge is agreed with respiratory physician
- Treatment with **oral and inhaled steroids** in addition to bronchodilators
- Own PEF meter and **written asthma action plan**
- GP follow up arranged *within 2 working days*
- Follow up appointment in respiratory clinic *within 4 weeks*
- Patients with **severe asthma** *(indicated by need for admission)* **and adverse behavioural or psychosocial features** are at risk of further severe or fatal attacks
- Determine reason(s) foe exacerbation and admission
- Send details of admission, discharge and potential best PEF to GP

© Scottish Intercollegiate Guidelines Network and British Thoracic Society ISBN 1 899893 23 8 First published 2003
SIGN and BTS consent to the photocopying of this poster for the purpose of implementation in the NHS in England, Wales, Northern Ireland and Scotland

Thorax 2003; **58** (Suppl I): i1-i92

Figure 8.6 (A) Management of acute severe asthma in adults in hospital.

Normal or raised values of $PaCO_2$ are a very worrying sign that suggest a serious state of hypoventilation that could deteriorate rapidly. A lactic acidosis may also be seen

- FBC and U&E to look for evidence of infection. Hypokalaemia may be due to steroids and beta-agonists.

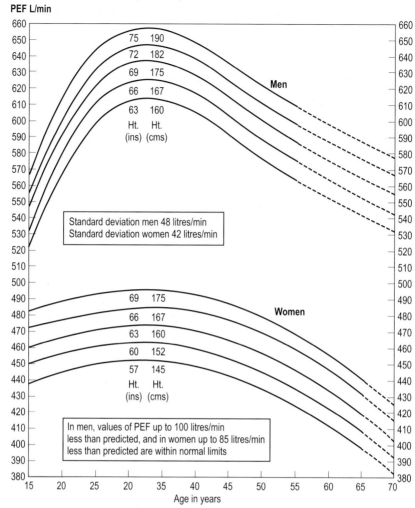

Peak expiratory flow in normal adults

PEF L/min

Men

75	190
72	182
69	175
66	167
63	160
Ht.	Ht.
(ins)	(cms)

Standard deviation men 48 litres/min
Standard deviation women 42 litres/min

Women

69	175
66	167
63	160
60	152
57	145
Ht.	Ht.
(ins)	(cms)

In men, values of PEF up to 100 litres/min
less than predicted, and in women up to 85 litres/min
less than predicted are within normal limits

Age in years

Nunn A.J., Gregg I. New regression equations for predicting peak expiratory flow in adults.
BMJ 1989; 298: 1068-70

Figure 8.6   (B) Peak expiratory flow in normal adults.

General management

General management of acute severe asthma is outlined in Figures 8.5 and 8.6. Severity should be assessed and the intensive care department should be contacted, if necessary, without delay as asthmatic patients can deteriorate rapidly (Fig. 8.7). Treatment should be commenced immediately and includes the following.

Oxygen: Hypoxaemia should be corrected as early as possible using high-flow oxygen via a Hudson mask (and humidified whenever possible). Hypoventilation due to loss of hypoxic respiratory drive that is seen in some patients with COPD is not a problem in acute asthma.

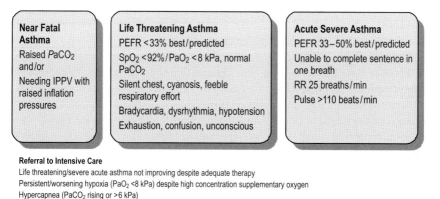

Asthma Severity assessment

Near Fatal Asthma

Raised $PaCO_2$ and/or

Needing IPPV with raised inflation pressures

Life Threatening Asthma

PEFR <33% best/predicted

SpO_2 <92%/PaO_2 <8 kPa, normal $PaCO_2$

Silent chest, cyanosis, feeble respiratory effort

Bradycardia, dysrhythmia, hypotension

Exhaustion, confusion, unconscious

Acute Severe Asthma

PEFR 33–50% best/predicted

Unable to complete sentence in one breath

RR 25 breaths/min

Pulse >110 beats/min

Referral to Intensive Care

Life threatening/severe acute asthma not improving despite adequate therapy

Persistent/worsening hypoxia (PaO_2 <8 kPa) despite high concentration supplementary oxygen

Hypercapnea ($PaCO_2$ rising or >6 kPa)

Exhausted, feeble respiration, drowsy or unconscious

Respiratory arrest

Figure 8.7 Asthma severity assessment.

Bronchodilators: A combination of nebulized beta-agonist (salbutamol 5 mg or terbutaline 10 mg) and anticholinergic (ipratropium bromide 0.5 mg) via an oxygen-driven nebulizer is most effective. The beta-agonist can be repeated in boluses every 10–15 min or given continuously if the initial response is inadequate. Intravenous bronchodilators do not normally offer any advantage over inhaled therapy and should be reserved for patients who are unable to take inhaled therapy, such as very serious cases where the degree of bronchoconstriction and sputum plugging prevents adequate drug delivery for ventilated patients.

Steroids: Oral prednisolone at a dose of 40–50 mg od should be given to all patients. Intravenous steroids (e.g. hydrocortisone 200 mg immediately then 100 mg qds) usually offer no advantage over the oral route and should be reserved for those who are very seriously ill with hypercapnea and where there may be a problem with swallowing and absorption. Steroids will need to be continued until the patient's symptoms have stabilized; usually at least 5 days are required and some patients will need a more prolonged course.

Magnesium sulphate: 1.2–2.0 g IV over 20 min is an effective treatment in those with acute severe asthma not responding to therapy and life-threatening or near fatal asthma. It should be given as a single dose and only repeated after levels of magnesium checked as hypermagnesaemia may cause muscle weakness that could exacerbate respiratory failure.

Aminophylline: This is not likely to be of additional benefit in most patients presenting with acute severe asthma. It should be used on an individual basis in patients with near fatal or life-threatening asthma who are not responding to other treatment. A loading dose of 5 mg/kg should be given over 20 min followed by an infusion of 0.5 mg/kg/h. The loading dose should be withheld if the patient is on oral aminophylline/theophylline and the dose halved if cirrhosis, CCF or taking erythromycin, cimetidine or ciprofloxacin. Toxicity can be a problem and side effects include palpitations, arrhythmias and vomiting. Blood levels should be monitored daily whenever intravenous aminophylline is continued for more than 24 h.

Antibiotics: These should only be given if there is objective evidence of infection; they should not be given routinely.

Intravenous fluids: These may need to be given if the patient is dehydrated. Hypokalaemia as a result of beta-agonist therapy will need to be corrected.

Non-invasive ventilation (NIV): This may be of value in treating some patients with hypercapneic respiratory failure due to asthma. Hypercapnea is a sign of very severe asthma and these patients can deteriorate rapidly and require urgent intubation. NIV for acute asthma should therefore only be considered in an intensive care unit. More studies are required before the routine use of NIV can be recommended.

Intermittent positive pressure ventilation (IPPV): This may be used to correct hypoxaemia when other methods have failed. IPPV is a useful treatment in some patients but is not without risk and should only be attempted by someone with appropriate expertise.

Further management

Patients' symptoms may improve rapidly with treatment despite still having severe underlying airflow obstruction. Continued objective monitoring is required to assess progress:

- The PEFR should be repeated 15–30 min after starting treatment to assess response and four times a day pre- and post-nebulizer thereafter. If the patient is improving then nebulized bronchodilators should be continued 4–6 hourly and as required. If the patient is not making satisfactory progress then beta-agonist nebulizers can be given more frequently, every 15 min or continuously.
- Oxygen should be continued at an appropriate concentration to keep $SpO_2 > 92\%$. Arterial blood gas measurement will need repeating within 2 h if: initial $PO_2 < 8$ kPa, initial PCO_2 is normal or raised or if the patient's condition is deteriorating.
- Heart rate, blood pressure and respiratory rate should be monitored.
- Serum potassium, glucose and, if appropriate, aminophylline levels should be monitored daily.

If the patient makes satisfactory progress then treatment can be weaned. Oxygen can be stopped once the patient is able to maintain $SpO_2 > 92\%$ on room air; nebulized bronchodilators should be substituted for inhalers (salbutamol 100 µg as required and long-acting beta-agonist if previously taking or thought appropriate, e.g. salmeterol 50 µg bd). An adequate dose of inhaled corticosteroid should be commenced (e.g. beclometasone 1 g inhaled bd) and intravenous steroids should be switched to the oral route. The patient should be switched to these medications at least 48 h prior to discharge.

Patient education is essential and should include inhaler technique, PEFR record keeping and a written symptom-based action plan. The patient can be discharged once stable with a PEFR > 75% predicted and no nocturnal symptoms. Large (> 25%) diurnal dips in PEFR suggest that the patient needs further observation and more prolonged high intensity treatment.

CASE 8.2

A 67-year-old woman with a history of hypertension and a 40-year history of smoking 20 cigarettes per day presented with 6-day history of cough and green sputum. Over the previous 2 days the patient's general condition had deteriorated markedly with the development of left-sided pleuritic chest pain, breathlessness and rigors. A 5-day course of amoxicillin prescribed by the GP had had no effect. On arrival at the medical admissions unit the patient was pyrexial (38.5°C), warm and sweaty. Clinical observations showed: pulse 72 bpm, blood pressure 100/60, respiratory rate 30 breaths/min. Auscultation of the chest revealed coarse crepitations at the left base and oxygen saturations were 85% on room air. Her chest radiograph and CT scan are shown (Figs 8.8, 8.9). Blood tests showed: Na 132, K 4.1, urea 10.1, creatinine 102, Hb 14.5, WCC 19.6 (neutrophils 18.1), Plt 130. Arterial blood gas analysis on 4 L/min of oxygen showed pH 7.33, PO_2 8.1, PCO_2 6.2, HCO_3^- 20, BXS 4.5.

The CXR reveals left basal shadowing, but the CT scan confirms the severity of the left-sided pneumonic changes with extensive areas of consolidation, which is not as visible on the CXR. The patient was diagnosed with a severe community-acquired pneumonia, fulfilling all the CURB-65 severity criteria (Fig. 8.10). Initial management included administration of high-flow oxygen via a Hudson rebreathe mask,

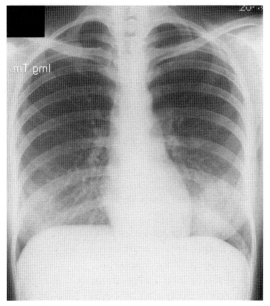

Figure 8.8 Chest X-ray.

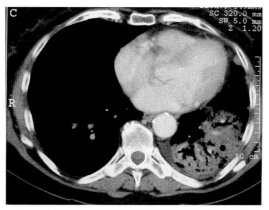

Figure 8.9 CT scan of thorax.

intravenous fluids, paracetamol and NSAIDs for the pleuritic pain and intravenous antibiotics, cefuroxime and clarithromycin, were chosen in accordance with guidelines to cover most pathogens that cause severe community-acquired pneumonia. Mycoplasma was subsequently confirmed on sputum culture.

The high severity score blood gases showing type 2 respiratory failure suggested the patient was seriously ill and a critical care opinion was sought. Because of the need for regular blood gases, an arterial line was inserted and she was transferred to the medical high-dependency unit where she gradually improved over the following week.

Pneumonia is defined as inflammation and consolidation of lung tissue due to an infectious agent. It is important to distinguish between 'community-acquired pneumonia' (CAP) that develops outside hospital and 'nosocomial' or 'hospital-acquired pneumonia' (HAP) that develops more than 48 h after admission (this definition includes nursing homes and similar institutions), as the pathogens responsible may be quite different.

The classical presentation of pneumonia is of productive cough, shortness of breath, pleuritic chest pain, fever and physical and radiographic signs of consolidation. Pneumonia frequently presents with non-specific features, particularly in the elderly. Radiographic evidence of consolidation is required to reliably diagnose pneumonia.

Investigations

Investigations required include:
- Chest radiograph: this should show evidence of consolidation.
- Blood tests: FBC, U&E, LFTs, CRP.
- Pulse oximetry and arterial blood gases if $SpO_2 < 92\%$.
- Blood cultures (preferably before antibiotics).
- Sputum culture (and Gram stain if severe).
- Paired serological tests for 'atypical' pathogens if: severe, unresponsive to beta lactam antibiotics or during an outbreak. Take on admission and 7–10 days later.

- Thoracocentesis if there is pleural fluid; samples should be sent for culture, Gram stain, pH, protein and glucose.
- If the patient is seriously ill, immunosuppressed or the diagnosis is uncertain, consider invasive investigation such as bronchoscopy and lavage, and occasionally lung biopsy.

Severity assessment

Severity assessment is the key to management of the patient with pneumonia. The overall average hospital mortality is 5.7–12% and mortality rates can be as high as 50% in those admitted to intensive care for ventilatory support. It is essential that those patients who are at increased risk of death are identified at the earliest opportunity as this influences where (critical care unit or ward) and how (antibiotic choice and route) the patient is treated. A validated and simple to remember bedside guide to assessing pneumonia severity is the CURB-65 score (see Fig. 8.10). It should be remembered that this score is not absolute and it may be inaccurate in the elderly and those with comorbidity.

Management

Management of severe pneumonia includes:

1. Oxygen: aim to keep PaO_2 > 8 kPa/SpO_2 > 92% and much higher in patients with sepsis and without COPD (> 12 kPa). High-flow O_2 should be used initially in uncomplicated pneumonia. More care is required if

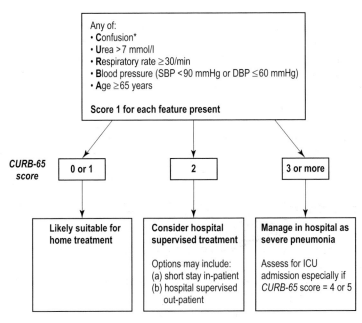

*Defined as a Mental Test Score of 8 or less, or new disorientation in person, place or time

Figure 8.10 Management of community acquired pneumonia in adults. Adapted from British Thoracic Society Guideline Update 2004.

the patient also has documented chronic type 2 respiratory failure as the patient may rely solely on hypoxic drive to stimulate ventilation; these concerns should not, however, prevent the patient receiving adequate oxygen therapy. Arterial blood gases should be used to guide therapy; an elevated CO_2 in a patient with no underlying lung disease suggests exhaustion and mechanical ventilation is likely to be imminently required.

2. Fluid balance: patients may be dehydrated and hypotensive and require intravenous fluids. Raising blood pressure may significantly improve oxygenation by reducing shunt.
3. Analgesia if pleuritic pain: an NSAID is usually sufficient but opiates may be required if severe.
4. Nebulized bronchodilators if there is evidence of airflow obstruction. Treat any other underlying respiratory disease.
5. Monitoring of temperature, respiratory rate, heart rate, blood pressure, mental status and pulse oximetry at least twice daily and more frequently if severe.
6. Chest physiotherapy for patients who have bronchiectasis or patients who have difficulty with sputum expectoration.
7. Antibiotics: it is not possible to predict the likely pathogen responsible on the basis of clinical or radiographic features alone. Most prescribing is therefore empirical and should be started without delay after blood cultures have been sent. Factors influencing the choice of antibiotic include: severity, comorbidity, whether the infection was hospital- or community-acquired, and age. Many hospitals have local prescribing guidelines and these should be followed. These will take into account the local incidence of acquired resistance to antibiotics.

   - **Non-severe community-acquired pneumonia** can usually be treated with oral antibiotics. Most infections are caused by *Streptococcus pneumoniae* but 'atypical' pathogens including *Mycoplasma*, *Chlamydia* and *Legionella* account for approximately 20% of cases. A combination of a beta-lactam and macrolide is recommended to cover most pathogens, e.g. amoxicillin 500 mg tds and clarithromycin 500 mg bd. If the patient is at high risk of *Clostridium difficile* diarrhoea (age > 70 years, repeated antibiotics or on a ward with a high rate of *C. difficile* infection) or has a history of penicillin hypersensitivity, a fluoroquinolone with activity against *S. pneumoniae* such as moxifloxacin 400 mg od, may be used.
   - **Severe community-acquired pneumonia** should be treated with broad-spectrum parenteral antibiotics to cover all likely pathogens. *S. pneumoniae* is again the commonest pathogen but infections caused by *Staphylococcus aureus*, Gram-negative enteric bacilli and *Legionella* species carry a high mortality so it is essential that the initial antibiotic regimen adequately covers these. A combination of a beta-lactamase stable antibiotic (e.g. co-amoxiclav or 2nd or 3rd generation cefalosporin) and a macrolide is recommended, e.g. cefuroxime 1.5 g tds IV and clarithromycin 500 mg bd IV. If the pneumonia occurs during an outbreak of influenza, additional antistaphylococcal cover with flucloxacillin should be considered and rifampicin may be added if *Legionella* is a real possibility.

- **Hospital-acquired pneumonia (HAP)** tends to occur in patients with impaired defences as a result of illness and medical intervention (such as ventilation). The commonest organisms are Gram-negative enteric bacilli, anaerobes, *S. aureus* and *Pseudomonas*. Non-severe HAP should be treated with a single agent such as a 2nd or 3rd generation cefalosporin, e.g. cefuroxime 1.5 g tds IV. Severe cases should be treated with a combination of an aminoglycoside plus an antipseudomonal beta-lactamase stable antibiotic, e.g. gentamicin IV and meropenem 1 g tds IV. It is advisable to discuss the case with a microbiologist if the case is complex, previous antibiotics have been used or if methicillin-resistant *Staphyloccus aureus* (MRSA) is a possibility.

If the patient fails to show signs of improvement by 48–72 h then the case should be reviewed by a respiratory specialist and further investigations should include a repeated chest radiograph, blood tests including CRP; white cell count and cultures should be repeated. Failure to improve or deterioration can be due to a number of factors (Fig. 8.11).

The commonest complication of pneumonia is the development of a parapneumonic effusion, seen in 36–57% of those admitted to hospital. Most

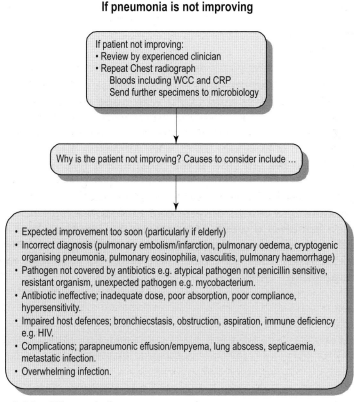

If pneumonia is not improving

If patient not improving:
- Review by experienced clinician
- Repeat Chest radiograph
  Bloods including WCC and CRP
  Send further specimens to microbiology

Why is the patient not improving? Causes to consider include ...

- Expected improvement too soon (particularly if elderly)
- Incorrect diagnosis (pulmonary embolism/infarction, pulmonary oedema, cryptogenic organising pneumonia, pulmonary eosinophilia, vasculitis, pulmonary haemorrhage)
- Pathogen not covered by antibiotics e.g. atypical pathogen not penicillin sensitive, resistant organism, unexpected pathogen e.g. mycobacterium.
- Antibiotic ineffective; inadequate dose, poor absorption, poor compliance, hypersensitivity.
- Impaired host defences; bronchiecstasis, obstruction, aspiration, immune deficiency e.g. HIV.
- Complications; parapneumonic effusion/empyema, lung abscess, septicaemia, metastatic infection.
- Overwhelming infection.

Figure 8.11 What to do if pneumonia is not improving.

KEY POINTS
- Pneumonia is treated with oxygen, fluids and antibiotics.
- Always consider TB in a patient not improving with pneumonia.

of these effusions resolve after antibiotics, but a small proportion of these develop into an empyema. Any pleural effusion should be sampled by needle thoracocentesis at the earliest opportunity and the fluid drained if there is frank pus, organisms found on Gram stain or culture, or the fluid is pH < 7.2.

Indications for referral to intensive care

Pneumonia is associated with high mortality and often results in multi-organ failure. This cannot be managed adequately in the ward situation and consideration should be given to transfer to a higher level of care if there is a high chance of death after assessing severity or the patient exhibits one of the following poor prognostic markers:

- Failure to achieve adequate oxygenation despite high-flow oxygen
- Exhaustion or rising $PaCO_2$
- Co-existing other organ system failure, such as hypotension, renal failure or coagulopathy.

CASE 8.3

A 74-year-old man presents with shortness of breath. He is an ex-miner and has mild COPD with good exercise tolerance, although he has had increasing shortness of breath over recent weeks. He has green sputum at presentation, is pyrexial 38°C, with extensive bronchial breathing on the left side of his chest and is hypoxic, saturating at 88% on 40% oxygen. His CXR is shown (Fig. 8.12). He initially improves after treatment with cefuroxime and clarithromycin and humidified high-flow oxygen but after a week of treatment he remains short of breath with discoloured sputum and a niggling intermittent pyrexia. What does his CXR show? What do you think may be happening? Outline a plan of treatment.

Answer
His CXR shows extensive left-sided pneumonic changes with an overlying pleural effusion. Despite an initial improvement his lack of improvement is likely to be due to an underlying abnormality. This is likely to be infective or neoplastic. He requires an infection screen, necessitating blood cultures, sputum culture, bronchoscopy with bronchoalveolar lavage (BAL) samples for culture. If negative, particularly for a hospital-acquired superadded

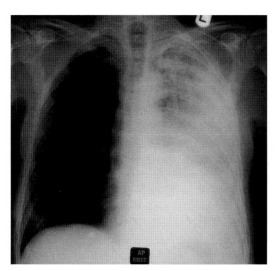

Figure 8.12 Chest X-ray.

infection, a sample of pleural fluid should be sent for culture. A CT chest scan may also be required to look for neoplastic lesions. In fact his pleural fluid revealed acid-fast bacilli on ZN staining. He was treated with antituberculous drugs and was discharged home after 2 months in hospital.

ACUTE PULMONARY EMBOLISM

The commonest form of pulmonary embolism (PE) is related to venous thromboembolism (VTE), usually from a distal site such as a leg deep vein thrombosis (DVT). Other sources of pulmonary embolism include bone marrow, amniotic fluid, air and fat. PE is a common problem (incidence 60–70/100 000) that carries a significant mortality depending on the severity at presentation and is often associated with serious underlying disease such as malignancy.

Acute minor PE

Acute minor PE occurs when less than 50% of the pulmonary circulation is occluded and it may be asymptomatic. The commonest symptoms are exertional breathlessness, pleuritic chest pain and haemoptysis. Physical signs tend to be the result of pulmonary infarction: breathlessness, tachycardia, chest pain, fever, pleural rub, consolidation and sometimes pleural effusion. Pulmonary artery pressure is not significantly elevated so there is no right ventricular impairment or cardiovascular collapse; heart sounds and jugular venous pressure are therefore usually normal. Hypoxaemia, if present, will only be modest.

Acute massive PE

Acute massive PE results from significant obstruction (> 50%) of the pulmonary vasculature and an elevated pulmonary artery pressure that causes right ventricular dilatation and dysfunction, consequent reduction in left ventricular filling and a reduction in cardiac output. Hypoxaemia occurs as a result of ventilation/perfusion mismatch and the severity correlates approximately with the size of the blood clot. In the presence of underlying cardiopulmonary disease the patient may be more severely affected. The clinical presentation is of acute breathlessness and low cardiac output and there may be symptoms and signs associated with a preceding minor embolism. The patient will be breathless and peripherally and centrally cyanosed; acute right ventricular strain results in elevated venous pressure, right ventricular gallop and widely split second heart sound. Reduced cardiac output causes circulatory shock with hypotension, tachycardia and cool peripheries. Mortality is high and massive PE may present as a pulseless electrical activity (PEA) arrest; poor prognosis is particularly associated with hypotension, hypoxia and ECG changes.

Diagnosis of PE

Diagnosis of PE is difficult and is impossible to make on clinical grounds alone; PE is notorious for being both under and over diagnosed, even by experienced clinicians. The most powerful method of diagnosing PE is through a combination of clinical assessment, D-Dimer and more definitive tests such as isotope ventilation–perfusion (VQ) scanning and CT pulmonary angiogram. A simple and robust method for assessing clinical probability of pulmonary embolism is outlined in Figure 8.13. Such a method should be

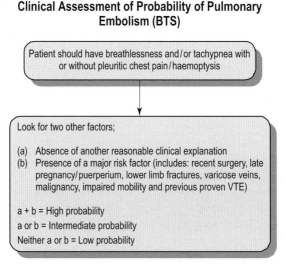

Clinical Assessment of Probability of Pulmonary Embolism (BTS)

Patient should have breathlessness and/or tachypnea with or without pleuritic chest pain/haemoptysis

Look for two other factors;

(a) Absence of another reasonable clinical explanation
(b) Presence of a major risk factor (includes: recent surgery, late pregnancy/puerperium, lower limb fractures, varicose veins, malignancy, impaired mobility and previous proven VTE)

a + b = High probability
a or b = Intermediate probability
Neither a or b = Low probability

Thorax 2003; 58 (suppl II) ii1–ii59.

Figure 8.13 Clinical assessment of probability of pulmonary embolism.

used in all patients with suspected PE. The importance of this cannot be overemphasized; it is a useful tool that stratifies patients into groups of low, medium and high probability of PE. This allows sensible decisions to be made regarding subsequent choice and interpretation of investigations and management.

Investigations

Investigations that should be performed in all patients include:

Chest radiograph: A normal film in a breathless and hypoxaemic patient should alert the clinician to the possibility of PE. Often there are no signs and the chest radiograph is useful to exclude other conditions such as pulmonary oedema. Subtle and non-specific signs include atelectasis, reduced lung volume and a small effusion. Hyperluscency due to oligaemia in affected parts of the lung (Westermark's sign) may sometimes be present but is often difficult to see.

ECG: Changes are often non-specific and in acute minor PE, tachycardia is the only abnormality seen. In massive PE the classic signs associated with right heart strain may be seen: right axis deviation, right bundle branch block, T wave inversion in V1–3, S1Q3T3 and enlarged P waves (Fig. 8.14). Other conditions such as myocardial infarction can be excluded.

Arterial blood gases: These may be normal. With minor PE the PaO_2 may be normal or only slightly reduced; with larger clots the degree of hypoxaemia increases. The alveolar–arterial (A–a) gradient is increased. $PaCO_2$ tends to be low as a result of hyperventilation. A metabolic acidosis may be seen if the patient is shocked.

D-Dimers: These are degradation products of fibrinolysis and are sensitive but non-specific markers of intravascular thrombosis. D-Dimers may be elevated in conditions other than PE/DVT such as malignancy, disseminated intravascular coagulation (DIC), trauma, infection and other

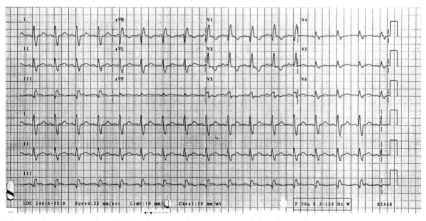

Figure 8.14 12-lead ECG showing deep S wave in lead I, with Q wave and inverted T wave in lead III and RSR pattern in the anterior leads. This is a classic ECG pattern of PE representing acute right-sided strain; however, most ECGs of patients with acute PE only show a mild tachycardia.

inflammatory states. The D-Dimer should only be interpreted in the context of clinical probability. A normal D-Dimer can reliably exclude PE where the clinical probability of PE is low or intermediate. In patients with a high clinical probability of PE there is a significant chance of a false negative and the test is not useful.

Leg ultrasound: Leg DVT is seen in 70% of patients with proven PE. A leg ultrasound demonstrating DVT is sufficient to confirm the diagnosis of venous thromboembolism without the need for lung imaging. A negative scan in a patient with appropriate clinical signs is not sufficient to exclude the diagnosis and should be followed up by further imaging.

Ventilation/perfusion (V/Q) scan: This is performed following injection and inhalation of radioisotopes (injected technetium 99 albumin micro-aggregates for perfusion and inhaled Xenon 133 for ventilation). Underlying lung disease such as COPD makes interpretation impossible and a V/Q scan should only be done in patients with a normal chest radiograph and no evidence of underlying cardiopulmonary disease. The scan should be interpreted in the context of clinical probability and standardized reporting criteria should be used. The scan is reported as showing a high, intermediate or low probability of PE (Fig. 8.15). A normal scan reliably excludes a PE. A high probability scan is associated with a significant rate of false positives and should be interpreted in association with the clinical probability; a high probability scan and high clinical probability is associated with a 96% rate of PE – this falls to 88% if the clinical probability is intermediate and 56% if low (Table 8.1). Any high probability scan with low or intermediate clinical probability should be regarded as indeterminate. Most scans fall into the 'indeterminate' category and all these should be followed with further imaging such as CTPA.

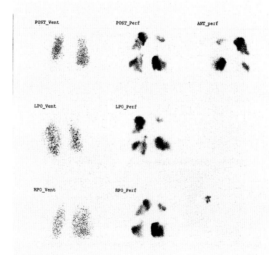

Figure 8.15   V/Q scan showing near normal ventilation but multiple perfusion defects consistent with a high probability of PE.

Table 8.1 Probability of PE (%) after clinical assessment of probability and V/Q scanning (from PIOPED study)

Clinical likelihood	V/Q scan probability			
	Normal/very low	Low	Intermediate	High
Low	2	4	16	56
Intermediate	6	16	28	88
High	0	40	66	96

CT pulmonary angiography (CTPA): This has established itself as a reliable method of looking for PE and can be used in patients with underlying cardio-pulmonary disease in whom V/Q scanning is unreliable (Fig. 8.16). CTPA should be the first investigation of choice when imaging PE although a lack of ready availability means that V/Q continues to be used. The false negative rate is low and a patient with a negative CTPA usually does not need further investigation or treatment for PE, unless there is a high clinical probability of PE in which case specialist advice should be sought regarding further imaging, e.g. conventional pulmonary angiography.

Echocardiography: This is useful in the diagnosis of massive life-threatening PE where a dilated pulmonary artery and right ventricle may be seen; clot may occasionally be directly visualized in the pulmonary artery. Echo is less reliable for diagnosing other types of PE.

Management

A scheme for management is outlined in Figures 8.17 and 8.18. The patient should have a rapid clinical assessment using the ABCD method. If PE is thought likely the clinical probability should be assessed. High-flow oxygen should be administered to correct hypoxaemia and IV access should be obtained. Some patients require analgesia for pleuritic pain; NSAIDs may be

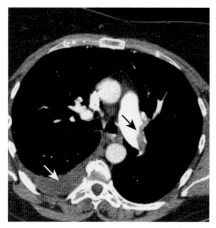

Figure 8.16 A CT pulmonary angiogram showing a large filling defect in the left pulmonary artery (black arrow) consistent with pulmonary thromboembolism. Note also right-sided pleural effusion (white arrow). Image courtesy of Dr L Michell.

adequate, opiates should only be used cautiously as they may lower blood pressure and respiratory drive. Subsequent management depends on the haemodynamic state of the patient.

If the patient is *haemodynamically stable* and PE is likely (intermediate/high probability) then anticoagulation should be given immediately and prior to more definitive investigations. An initial bolus of fast-acting unfractionated heparin, e.g. 80 units/kg IV should be given along with a low molecular weight heparin, e.g. tinzaparin 175 u/kg od. If rapid reversal of anticoagulation might be required then an intravenous infusion of unfractionated heparin should be used. Warfarin should be commenced only when the PE is confirmed by further imaging such as a V/Q scan or CTPA; the target INR is 2–3 in most cases. Warfarin has procoagulant effects when first given and it is essential that heparin anticoagulation is continued for the first 5 days of anticoagulation and until the INR is therapeutic. The duration of anticoagulation depends on the cause of the PE: 4–6 weeks if a temporary risk factor (surgery), 3 months for the first idiopathic embolism and at least 6 months for other cases. If PEs are recurrent and there are ongoing risk factors then long-term anticoagulation may be required.

Haemodynamic instability implies an acute massive embolism. Intravenous fluids should be given and, unless the patient is rapidly deteriorating, a single dose of unfractionated heparin should be given and an urgent CTPA or echo obtained to confirm the diagnosis. If a PE is seen then senior advice should be sought and thrombolysis considered if there is haemodynamic instability or acute right ventricular dysfunction. If there

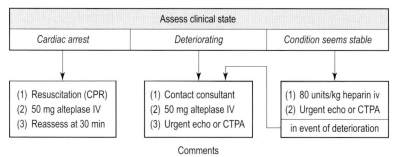

Comments

1. Massive PE is highly likely if:
   - collapse/hypotension, and
   - unexplained hypoxia, and
   - engorged neck veins, and
   - right ventricular gallop (often)

2. In stable patients where massive PE has been confirmed, IV dose of alteplase is 100 mg in 90 min (i.e. accelerated myocardial infarction regimen).

3. Thrombolysis is followed by unfractionated heparin after 3 h, preferably weight adjusted.

4. A few units have facilities for clot fragmentation via pulmonary artery catheter. Elsewhere, contraindications to thrombolysis should be ignored in life threatening PE.

5. 'Blue light' patients with out-of-hospital cardiac arrest due to PE rarely recover.

Figure 8.17 A scheme for management of pulmonary embolism. Reproduced with permission of the BMJ publishing group.

A

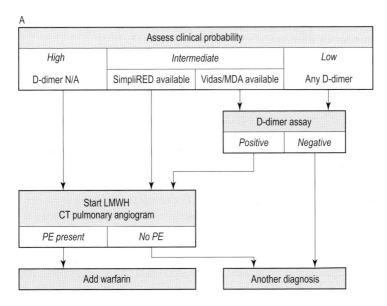

B

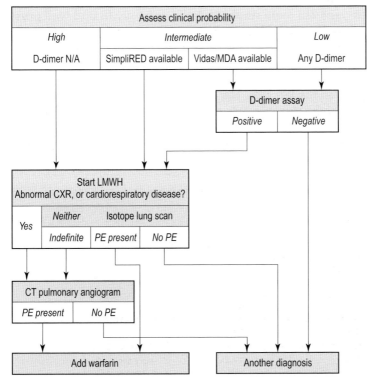

Figure 8.18 Management of suspected non-massive pulmonary embolism (A) with isotope lung scanning off site only and (B) with isotope lung scanning available on site. Reproduced with permission of the BMJ publishing group.

are no contraindications to thrombolysis, RtPA should be given at a dose of 100 mg over 2 h. If the patient is rapidly deteriorating and in danger of imminent cardiorespiratory arrest then thrombolysis should be administered before echo or CTPA are performed. If a patient presents with a PEA arrest that is thought to be related to a PE, RtPA 50 mg IV, preferably via a central catheter, should be given during resuscitation and the patient reassessed if cardiac output returns, or 30 min after rescuscitation; few patients survive. In the event of continued deterioration despite thrombolysis, specialist advice should be sought; the patient may require mechanical ventilation and inotropic support. Pulmonary embolectomy should be considered if there is continued deterioration or thrombolysis is contraindicated and this can be performed percutaneously using a catheter or surgically with the patient on cardiopulmonary bypass; it carries a high mortality rate (30%) and is only readily available in specialist centres.

PNEUMOTHORAX

CASE 8.4

A 26-year-old male smoker who is normally fit and well presented to A&E with a 2-h history of breathlessness and sharp left-sided chest pain that was worse on inspiration. On examination he looked comfortable, SpO$_2$ was 95% on room air, pulse 90 regular, BP 130/80; auscultation of the chest revealed reduced breath sounds on the left side. His CXR shows a pneumothorax on the left side with the distance between the lung and chest wall more than 2 cm. How would you manage this?

A distance greater than 2 cm indicates a 'large' pneumothorax. Because of the breathlessness and the size of the pneumothorax, aspiration was performed using a large bore venflon and a chest aspiration system. The procedure removed 1.4 L air and was stopped when no more air was able to be aspirated, the patient's symptoms settled after the procedure and a repeat CXR showed only a small residual pneumothorax (< 1 cm) at the apex. The patient was well after the procedure and was discharged home with instructions to return if symptoms recurred; a review appointment was made for 1 week in the chest clinic.

Pneumothorax is defined as air in the pleural space.

- Primary spontaneous pneumothorax usually occurs in healthy people without underlying lung disease. It is more frequent in males, tall people and smokers and is generally a benign condition with a very low mortality rate.
- Secondary spontaneous pneumothorax is associated with underlying lung disease, most frequently emphysema, interstitial lung disease and cystic fibrosis. It is a potentially serious problem with an overall mortality of about 10%.

KEY POINT

- The presence of severe cardiorespiratory compromise suggests a tension pneumothorax that will require immediate treatment. Signs include: hypotension/shock, tachycardia, raised JVP, midline shift away from the affected side, hyper-expanded and hardly moving hemithorax on the affected side and severe respiratory distress.

- Iatrogenic pneumothorax is commonly seen in hospitals and the severity of presentation depends on the degree of comorbidity. Procedures that cause pneumothorax include: needle aspiration of a lung mass, subclavian venepuncture, thoracocentesis, pleural biopsy and mechanical ventilation.

The commonest symptoms are of sudden onset breathlessness and pleuritic chest pain. The patient may present non-specifically with an acute exacerbation of underlying lung disease. The severity of symptoms at presentation varies: a patient with a primary spontaneous pneumothorax may have very mild or absent symptoms and many patients delay presentation for several days. A secondary spontaneous pneumothorax places additional strain on an already compromised respiratory system so symptoms tend to be more severe. Examination of the chest reveals hyper-resonance to percussion and reduced chest expansion and air entry on the affected side.

Investigations

Investigations required include:

- Assessment of the patient's cardiorespiratory status. Pulse rate, blood pressure and oxygen saturations should be checked.
- Arterial blood gases should be checked if $SpO_2 < 92\%$, the patient is very breathless or there is known underlying lung disease. Blood gas measurements are frequently abnormal and relate to the severity of underlying lung disease as well as to the size of the pneumothorax.
- A standard posteroanterior (PA) chest radiograph is usually sufficient to confirm the diagnosis; a routine expiratory film is not necessary. The lung edge should be seen detached from the chest wall and the area of hemithorax that is not occupied by lung will be hyperlucent and absent of lung markings. If a pneumothorax is suspected but the findings on the standard PA radiograph are unclear then a lateral decubitus radiograph should be performed. Difficulty in the interpretation of chest radiographs arises particularly in the presence of small or mediastinal pneumothoraces, anterior pneumothorax (best seen on a lateral radiograph or CT scan (Fig. 8.19)), consolidated lung, superimposed chest wall artefact, intrapulmonary cavities that cause air-fluid levels, subcutaneous emphysema and most importantly emphysematous bullae. Insertion of a chest tube into a bulla mistakenly thought to be a pneumothorax can be disastrous. The 'edge sign' helps differentiate the

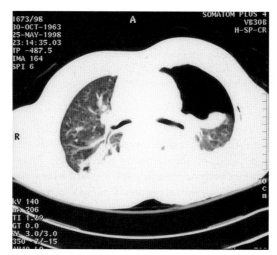

Figure 8.19 CT scan revealing left-sided anterior pneumothorax not visible on the CXR.

two; a pneumothorax will usually form a convex line in relation to the chest wall whereas a bulla forms a concave line. Where there is uncertainty about the diagnosis a CT scan should be performed (Figs 8.20a, b, c). A reliable estimation of the size of a pneumothorax is essential to guide management but exact measurement is complicated. A common error is to underestimate the size of the pneumothorax by basing any estimation on the two-dimensional area occupied by the pneumothorax on a standard PA radiograph. A practical and easy to remember method is to divide pneumothorax size into two groups on the basis of the distance between the lung edge and chest wall. A 'small' pneumothorax is less than 2 cm and a 'large' pneumothorax > 2 cm.

Algorithms for the management of pneumothorax are outlined in Figures 8.21 and 8.22. Treatment options are outlined in more detail below.

Tension pneumothorax (Fig. 8.23)

This is a medical emergency requiring prompt action; the patient may deteriorate rapidly and should not be left unattended. High-flow oxygen should be administered and a large cannula (green venflon or larger) inserted into the chest wall of the affected side at the second intercostal space in the mid-clavicular line. If a tension pneumothorax is present then air should hiss out via the cannula as the tension decompresses. A chest drain should be inserted as soon as possible, and the cannula removed only when it is confirmed that the chest drain is working.

Observation

• If the patient is breathless then conservative management is not an option and some intervention will be required.

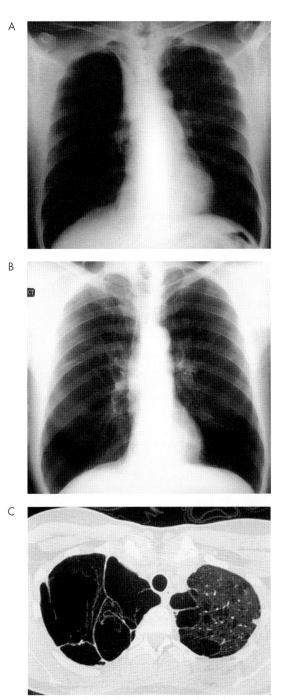

A

B

C

Figure 8.20   CXR in (A) may initially be mistaken for right-sided pneumothorax. However comparison with the patient's normal CXR reveals a large right-sided bulla (B) and this is confirmed on CT scan (C). (A) actually reveals a tension bulla. This may still require a small chest drain, but the risks of producing a bronchopleural fistula are significant and such cases must be managed with advice from experienced respiratory physicians and cardiothoracic surgeons. Fortunately such cases are rare and must not prevent you from treating pneumothoraces urgently. Compare with tension pneumothorax in Figure 8.23.

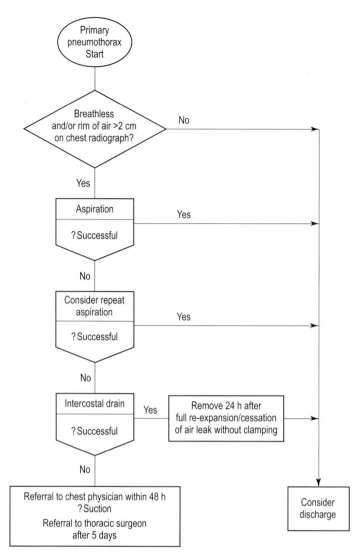

Figure 8.21   Recommended algorithm for the treatment of primary pneumothorax.

- Most patients with small primary pneumothoraces not associated with breathlessness can be considered for discharge home with advice to return if symptoms deteriorate. Follow-up should be in outpatients with a repeat chest radiograph at 14 days.
- Small, asymptomatic iatrogenic pneumothoraces can usually be observed (unless on positive pressure ventilation or significant underlying lung disease).
- Secondary pneumothoraces can only be observed if very small (less than 1 cm or an isolated apical pneumothorax) and the patient is not breathless. These patients have the potential to deteriorate and should be admitted. Oxygen should be administered as this speeds reabsorbtion of

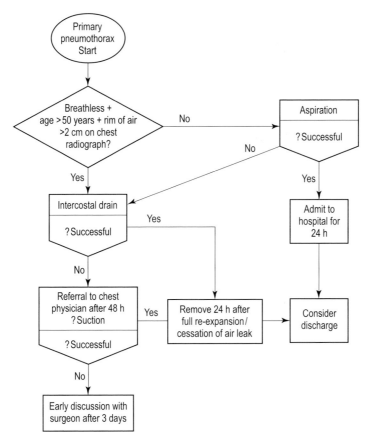

Figure 8.22   Recommended algorithm for the treatment of secondary pneumothorax.

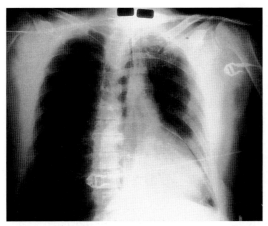

Figure 8.23   Right-sided tension pneumothorax.

the pneumothorax. High-flow oxygen is best (10 L/min) but care needs to be taken in patients with COPD who may be sensitive to high concentrations of oxygen.

Simple aspiration

This is a relatively straightforward procedure that is quicker and more comfortable than conventional intercostal pleural drains. Aspiration can only be used in certain patients:

- Aspiration should be the first line treatment for all patients with primary spontaneous pneumothorax and iatrogenic pneumothorax needing intervention. It should be repeated if the first attempt is unsuccessful, unless the pneumothorax is very large or > 2.5 L of air was aspirated at the first attempt. If a repeat chest radiograph shows the aspiration was successful and the patient is clinically stable with no breathlessness then they can be considered for discharge home. If repeat aspiration is unsuccessful then an intercostal pleural drain may be required.
- Aspiration is less likely to work in secondary spontaneous pneumothorax and most patients will need a chest drain; only patients who are < 50 years with minimal symptoms and with a small pneumothorax should be considered. Aspiration should not be repeated if the first attempt failed. Following successful aspiration, patients should be given high-flow oxygen and observed in hospital for at least 24 h prior to discharge.

Intercostal pleural drainage (see Ch. 13 for more detail on insertion of intercostal drains)

This is a very effective treatment but unfortunately it carries a significant risk of complications including: scars, pain, infection, visceral trauma and surgical emphysema. It is therefore important that, where appropriate, less invasive strategies are attempted. There is no evidence to suggest that, in most situations, the size of the drain matters. A small (10–14F) drain should be the first choice as these are less traumatic to the patient. Drains that employ the Seldinger technique are particularly simple to use and are recommended for use in these situations. A larger drain may be needed later if higher flow rates are required to deal with an air leak or the drain becomes blocked. It is important that the patient is given adequate analgesia during insertion and whilst the drain is in place.

A chest drain should be used:

- in patients with primary pneumothorax not adequately treated after aspiration
- in most cases of secondary pneumothorax, except where the pneumothorax is very small, and the patient is < 50 years and has no symptoms
- where there is associated pleural fluid
- in ventilated patients.

Most pneumothoraces resolve rapidly with insertion of a chest tube but drainage time varies widely between individuals. It is important that chest drains are not removed prematurely (Table 8.2). Once the lung has re-expanded and the drain has stopped bubbling the patient should be left for a further 24 h and a chest radiograph repeated. If the lung remains expanded then the drain can be removed. It is important that the drain is never

Table 8.2 Managing an intercostal pleural drain

Bubbling	Swinging	Action
Yes	Yes	In pleural space, leak is still present
No	Yes	In pleural space, leak is stopped
		Repeat CXR
		Remove if the lung is fully expanded
No	No	Blocked or not in pleural space
		Reposition/unblock
		Remove if the lung is fully expanded

Do not clamp or drain except under expert supervision!

clamped, except under expert supervision. Persistent bubbling of the chest drain indicates an air leak (bronchopleural fistula). If the drain is not working and the lung has not expanded, blockage of the drain is a possibility and the drain should be flushed with saline to ensure its patency. If after 48 h of drainage the lung has not expanded or the drain is still bubbling, the advice of a respiratory physician should be sought. High volume, low pressure suction can be applied (2–5 kPa). Suction should not be used routinely as rapid lung re-expansion can result in re-expansion pulmonary oedema. This occurs due to excessive lung capillary permeability made worse by mechanical stress as the lung expands. Patients typically develop a cough and may become breathless; a chest radiograph will show pulmonary oedema that is usually unilateral. Although most patients are not compromised, it can occasionally be fatal. If respiratory failure develops the only effective treatment is invasive ventilation.

Surgical treatment

It is not clear when is the most appropriate time for surgical intervention in cases of a persistent air leak or failure of lung expansion. Most spontaneous pneumothoraces with persistent air leaks (100% primary, 79% secondary) will settle within 14 days. However, leaving a chest drain in situ for 14 days is not without significant infection risk, therefore it is recommended that patients be referred for a surgical opinion early (3–5 days). Other indications for surgical intervention are: recurrent spontaneous pneumothorax, bilateral pneumothoraces, spontaneous haemothorax and where there are professional implications, e.g. divers, pilots. The 'gold standard' procedure is an open thoracotomy and pleurectomy but, more recently, minimally invasive video-assisted thoracoscopy (VATS) and talc pleurodesis have been used.

Follow-up

Follow-up should be in outpatients with a repeat chest radiograph two weeks after discharge. The patient should not fly until six weeks after a chest radiograph has shown resolution of the pneumothorax. Diving should be avoided for life unless a definitive surgical procedure has been performed.

EXACERBATION OF CHRONIC OBSTRUCTIVE PULMONARY DISEASE (COPD)

An exacerbation of COPD is said to occur when there is acute and sustained worsening of symptoms beyond the usual day-to day-variation. Commonly reported symptoms include increased breathlessness, cough, increased sputum volume, wheeze and chest tightness and ankle swelling. On examination the patient may be tachypnoeic at rest, cyanosed, using accessory muscles and purse lip breathing. Sputum purulence suggests infection that is most frequently viral. Other precipitants include allergens and airborne pollutants. It is important to exclude other conditions that can mimic an exacerbation in patients with established COPD such as pneumonia, pneumothorax, pulmonary oedema, pulmonary embolism, lung cancer, pleural effusion and upper respiratory tract obstruction.

Investigations

Investigations should include: chest radiograph, arterial blood gases, ECG, bloods including FBC and U&E, sputum culture if purulent, blood culture if pyrexial, theophylline level if the patient is taking oral theophylline.

Management

Most patients, including those with markedly abnormal blood gases on presentation, will improve rapidly with nebulized bronchodilators and controlled oxygen. Unless the patient is in extremis it is best to repeat the arterial blood gases after one hour of medical therapy before considering NIV or invasive mechanical ventilation.

Oxygen therapy: This should be given at a fixed concentration via a venturi mask (24–28% initially) and titrated to an SpO_2 88–93%. (See 'Respiratory Failure' section earlier in the chapter).

Bronchodilators: Nebulized salbutamol 2.5 mg and ipratropium 0.5 mg should be given via an oxygen-driven nebulizer (5 L/min, maximum 5 min). Salbutamol can be repeated in boluses every 15 min. Intravenous aminophylline may be considered where the patient is unable to tolerate nebulized therapy or in occasional cases where there is inadequate response to nebulized treatment. However, care must be taken to minimize the chance of toxicity (see 'Acute Severe Asthma' earlier in the chapter).

Systemic steroids: These should be given to all patients, the earlier the better. Prednisolone 30 mg od for 5 days is preferred.

Antibiotics: These are not routinely indicated and should be reserved for cases where there are good objective signs of infection such as increased sputum purulence, pyrexia and elevated inflammatory markers. Sputum should be sent for culture. Treatment with a single agent is usually sufficient, e.g. amoxicillin, a macrolide or doxycycline.

If acute type 2 respiratory failure persists (pH < 7.35, $PaCO_2$ > 6 kPa) despite the above measures, some form of ventilatory support may be necessary and this has been described fully in the section on respiratory failure.

Non invasive ventilation: This is the first line treatment and can usually be performed on a general medical ward with appropriately trained staff. **Invasive mechanical ventilation** is an effective treatment for respiratory failure and should be considered in patients who do not respond to NIV, have complex multi-organ failure or impaired consciousness. Careful thought is needed when considering if invasive mechanical ventilation is appropriate and should take into account a number of factors, not just age and FEV1. Issues to consider include: patient wishes, functional status (being housebound is a poor prognostic marker), BMI, comorbidities, long-term oxygen therapy use, and previous episodes of artificial ventilation.

ACUTE UPPER AIRWAY OBSTRUCTION

KEY POINT
- Upper airway obstruction is a surgical and anaesthetic emergency. Call for senior help early and **do not** attempt to instrument the airway if signs of significant obstruction are present.

Upper airway obstruction only manifests clinically when there is significant (> 80%) obstruction by which time even a small worsening in the degree of obstruction can lead to a marked clinical deterioration. Acute causes include: inhaled foreign bodies, oedema (anaphylaxis, angioneurotic oedema and smoke inhalation), infection and subcutaneous emphysema. Subacute processes may present slowly over a prolonged period or can be rapid in onset and severe. Causes include: vocal cord paralysis/dysfunction, tumours (intrinsic or extrinsic causing compression), trauma, sarcoid, Wegener's, and tracheal cartilage abnormalities such as tracheobronchomalacia.

Clinical presentation

Stridor is a noise caused by collapse of the upper airway on inspiration and is characteristic; expiratory noise may occur in more severe cases. Stridor can easily be confused with the wheeze found in COPD or asthma and the diagnosis missed. Breathlessness is common and often associated with distress. Other symptoms include: cough, dysphagia, dysphonia and drooling. The patient may be cyanosed and show signs of respiratory distress that may progress to exhaustion and respiratory arrest.

Investigations

These should not delay treatment of a severely ill patient. Standard tests include FBC, U&E, CRP, arterial blood gases (which may be normal even with severe obstruction), chest radiograph and peak expiratory flow. CT scanning is useful and will usually identify the cause. Visualization of the airway either by nasopharyngoscopy or bronchoscopy is the best diagnostic method and rigid bronchoscopy allows intervention. If the patient is stable enough then spirometry and flow volume loops will show characteristic changes. Examination of the airway may precipitate complete obstruction in patients with acute epiglottitis; an anaesthetist and ENT surgeon should be present in case urgent intubation or tracheostomy is required.

Management

The priority is to secure the airway to allow adequate ventilation and gas exchange; once this is achieved further investigation and more definitive treatment can be undertaken.

Critical airway narrowing is suggested by: respiratory distress at rest, respiratory failure, drooling as a result of inability to swallow secretions, confusion, drowsiness and collapse. Administer high-flow oxygen or Heliox. An anaesthetist should be called immediately and an ENT surgeon if possible as the patient may need urgent endotracheal intubation or a surgical airway, e.g. tracheostomy. If obstruction is severe this may be performed under local anaesthesia with the patient sitting up.

If the patient has symptoms but is not severely unwell then basic medical treatment can be given and the patient observed. ENT advice should be sought at the earliest opportunity and more definitive treatment such as surgery or stenting performed after appropriate investigations. Measures include:

- Sit the patient up.
- High-flow oxygen should preferably be humidified.
- Nebulized adrenaline (epinephrine) may 'buy time' whilst other treatments take effect.
- Heliox is a mix of oxygen and helium (21:79) that is low density and will reduce airflow resistance and the work of breathing. Heliox will give symptomatic relief and can 'buy some time' prior to more definitive treatment.
- Corticosteroids may be of benefit if there is soft tissue oedema, e.g. hydrocortisone 200 mg IV.
- Antibiotics should be given if infection is suspected. The commonest infective cause in adults is *Haemophilus influenzae*-associated epiglottitis that should be treated with intravenous cefotaxime or chloramphenicol.

FURTHER READING

British Thoracic Society/ Scottish Intercollegiate Guidelines Network 2003 British guideline on the management of asthma. Thorax 58 (suppl 1):i1–i94

British Thoracic Society standards of care committee 2001 British Thoracic Society guidelines for the management of community acquired pneumonia in adults. Thorax 56 (suppl IV):IV1–IV64

British Thoracic Society standards of care committee 2002 Non invasive ventilation in acute respiratory failure. Thorax 59:192–211

British Thoracic Society standards of care committee 2003 British Thoracic Society guidelines for the management of pleural disease. Thorax 58 (suppl II) II1–II59

British Thoracic Society standards of care committee pulmonary embolism guidelines development group 2003 British Thoracic Society guidelines for the management of suspected acute pulmonary embolism. Thorax 58:470–484

Gibson G J, Geddes D M, Costabel U et al 2003 Respiratory medicine, 3rd edn. Saunders (Elsevier Science), London

McFarlane J T, Boldy D 2004 Update of BTS pneumonia guidelines: what's new? Thorax 59:364–366

National Collaborating Centre for Chronic Diseases 2004 Chronic obstructive pulmonary disease. National clinical guideline on management of chronic obstructive pulmonary disease in adults in primary and secondary care. Thorax 59 (suppl 1):1–232

Ramrakhan P S, Moore K P 2004 Respiratory emergencies. In: Ramrakhan P S, Moore K P (eds) Oxford handbook of acute medicine. Oxford University Press, Oxford

Sprigings D C, Chambers J B 2001 Acute medicine: a practical guide to the management of acute medical emergencies. Blackwell Science, Oxford

8

Further reading

Neurological emergencies 9

Richard Parris

OBJECTIVES

After reading this chapter you should be able to:

● *Understand the aetiology and management of common neurological emergencies, including coma*

● *Understand how to stablize these patients and monitor clinical progress*

● *Recognize the need for intubation or critical care managment*

INTRODUCTION

The involvement of critical care teams in the management of patients with a neurological emergency may be necessary for a variety of reasons. Primarily, critical care physicians should be involved in a patient's initial resuscitation to ensure early and correct management of the ABC method. This may not only be life saving but also may prevent deterioration, removing the need for invasive ventilation on the critical care unit. Critical care specialists may also offer facilities, advice or therapy either for management of non-specific conditions such as raised intracranial pressure or more specific therapies such as thrombolysis of patients with stroke. Whatever the reason for a critical care involvement, it must be recognized that early senior expertise improves the outcome for a patient with a neurological emergency.

ABC

Compromise of a patient's airway, breathing and circulation (ABC) may alter neurological function; conversely, altered neurological function may compromise the ABC. Strict attention to management of the ABC is therefore necessary and may significantly alter a patient's prognosis.

Airway

It is accepted practice that if a patient has a Glasgow Coma Score (GCS) of 8 or less, i.e. the patient is comatose, or if an oropharyngeal airway can be tolerated, then the patient is unable to maintain and protect the airway which should be secured and protected with an endotracheal tube. In addition, a lower threshold for intubation should be considered for any patient who is to be transferred to another hospital, one who is vomiting with a reduced consciousness level or one with a falling GCS. The gag reflex is unhelpful in assessing the need for intubation and may only serve to promote vomiting and pulmonary aspiration. If the patient is not intubated and has a lowered GCS, they should be nursed in the recovery position to maintain airway patency and prevent aspiration.

Breathing and circulation

It has been consistently shown that even a brief period of hypoxia or hypotension may cause a marked increase in morbidity and mortality in patients with brain injury. Whilst excellent management of the ABC may not reverse the underlying *primary* brain injury, it will prevent the development of *secondary* brain injury and this may make the difference between a dependent and independent existence post illness.

Controlled oxygen therapy should be provided to all patients with a neurological emergency to maintain saturations or the partial pressure of oxygen. Similarly, if the patient is intubated, the PCO_2 should be maintained within normal limits.

Cerebral autoregulation of blood flow is lost in brain-injured patients. Perfusion of the brain becomes dependent therefore on maintaining an adequate mean arterial blood pressure and controlling or reducing intracranial pressure.

The mean arterial blood pressure may be controlled through the use of invasive monitoring, fluids and vasopressors. Intracranial pressure (ICP) may be controlled by the insertion of an ICP monitor, sedation, mannitol and more simple measures including, if possible, nursing the patient in a head up position and ensuring that there are no constraints around the neck such as endotracheal tube (ET) ties and cervical collars.

The decision to transfer the patient to a critical care area is affected by several considerations including the likely underlying diagnosis and prognosis, the clinical state of the patient and the presence of any severe comorbidity, as well as taking into account the views of the patients themselves, many of whom may have been living with chronic and progressively worsening neurological disease for many years and who will be very aware of the likely progression of the disease.

D for disability

Initial assessment

The clinical condition of the patient may preclude a detailed neurological examination. A more rapid neurological assessment should initially include an assessment of a patient's level of consciousness, the presence or absence of pupillary and eye signs, localizing neurological signs and the presence or absence of meningism.

The purpose of this assessment is to determine the severity of the underlying illness, including possible requirement for critical care, to establish a baseline to monitor changes in neurological assessment and to detect signs that help in the diagnosis of the patient's illness.

Level of consciousness

A brief gross assessment of a patient's level of consciousness may be made using the AVPU scale.

A – **alert**
V – the patient responds to your **voice**
P – the patient responds to a **painful** stimulus
U – the patient is **unresponsive** to any stimulus

A more prolonged detailed assessment and the internationally standardized method of assessing a patient's consciousness level is by use of the GCS (Table 9.1).

A GCS of 8 corresponds approximately to P on the AVPU scale. The GCS should be described both as a total and by its individual components, e.g. GCS = 9, (E3, V2, M4). It should be noted that certain aspects of the GCS can be subjective and that serial trends are more important than a single initial measurement.

Table 9.1 Glasgow Coma Score

	Response	Score
Eye opening	Spontaneously	4
	To speech	3
	To pain	2
	None	1
Verbal response	Orientated	5
	Confused	4
	Inappropriate words	3
	Incomprehensible sounds	2
	None	1
Motor response	Obeys commands	6
	Localizes to pain	5
	Normal flexion/withdrawal	4
	Abnormal flexion*	3
	Extension*	2
	None	1
	Maximum total	15

*Flexion of the upper limb with extension of the lower limb is known as a decorticate posture whereas extension of the upper and lower limbs is known as a decerebrate posture. A decerebrate posture suggests a more serious insult and poorer prognosis. In his original paper Teasdale actually scored the total GCS out of 14, owing to the motor scale only being a 5 point scale (Teasdale and Jennett 1974)

ABC

Coma is accepted to be a GCS less than or equal to 8, e.g. with a patient failing to open their eyes in response to voice (E ≤ 2), vocalizing with incomprehensible sounds (V ≤ 2) and flexing/withdrawing to a painful stimulus (M ≤ 4).

Circumstances may, however, make it difficult to accurately record the GCS, e.g. facial trauma may make it extremely difficult to assess eye opening accurately, a high spinal cord injury will make motor assessment difficult and the patient may have a tracheostomy in situ making it impossible to speak. Recording each numerical value for the GCS will help to clarify this.

> **Tip**
> If there is asymmetry in assessing the motor response, the **best** motor response should be recorded.

CASE 9.1

A 25-year-old man is found at home with an empty bottle of amitriptyline beside him. There is no response when you talk to him but on pressing firmly on his sternum, you find that he tries to push away your hand and at the same time opens his eyes and shouts words that you are unable to understand. How would you record his GCS?

Answer
His GCS is: E = 2 (eyes opening to pain), V = 2 (incomprehensible sounds), M = 5 (localizes to pain). Total GCS = 9.

CASE 9.2

A 40-year-old woman alcoholic is found collapsed at the bottom of the stairs. She has a suspected spinal injury and is immobilized on a spinal board with head blocks and a cervical collar in situ. What problems might you encounter in assessing this woman's GCS?

Answer
Assessment might be complicated by both intoxication and spinal injury. For a patient with a spinal cord injury, it would be appropriate to assess motor movements of the cranial nerves, such as asking a patient to follow your finger with their eyes or assessing a painful stimulus by pressing on the supra-orbital nerve. In this case the woman had a high spinal cord injury at C5 making it difficult to assess a painful stimulus on the sternum (T3, T4 level) and for her to move her arms. She was able to move her eyes and smile on command (M = 6), was orientated (V = 5) and spontaneously opened her eyes (E = 4).

Eye position and eye movements

Observation of the resting position of the eyes, and any spontaneous movements may give some clues when assessing patients with an altered consciousness level (Table 9.2).

Pupillary signs

Careful examination of the pupillary size and response may give valuable information about the cause and site of the brain injury as well as possible information about likely outcome (Table 9.3).

Care must be taken to remember other possible causes of pupillary abnormalities, including normal asymmetry, previous cataract operations, traumatic mydriasis and the use of therapeutic or recreational drugs.

Table 9.2 Eye position and movement

Eye position and movement	Site of lesion
Lateral conjugate deviation of eyes	Ipsilateral frontal lesion
Lateral conjugate deviation of eyes	Contralateral pontine lesion
Disconjugate deviation of eyes	Brainstem lesion
Lateral conjugate deviation of eyes with spontaneous movement	Contralateral irritative or epileptic focus
Spontaneous slow conjugate to and fro roving movements	Toxic or metabolic cause of coma
Normal purposeful eye movements	Locked-in syndrome, catatonia, pseudocoma

Table 9.3 Pupillary signs

Pinpoint Bilateral Unreactive	Opiate ingestion Metabolic disorders Pontine lesions
Small Bilateral Reactive	Metabolic disorders Medullary lesions
Midsize Bilateral Fixed	Midbrain lesion
Dilated Bilateral Fixed	Central brain stem herniation Anticholinergic drugs Sympathomimetic drugs
Dilated Unilateral Fixed	Uncal herniation IIIrd nerve palsy (Posterior communicating artery aneurysm)
Constricted Unilateral Reactive	Horner's syndrome

Fundal examination

Fundoscopy may be difficult to perform in the setting of an acutely unwell patient within the emergency department, however the presence of papilloedema and subhyaloid haemorrhages should be sought. Papilloedema is associated usually with non-acutely raised intracranial pressure but its absence does not imply a normal ICP. Subhyaloid haemorrhages are associated with acute rises in ICP, e.g. as occur in subarachnoid haemorrhage (SAH).

Ocular reflexes

The oculocephalic reflex (doll's head reflex) is assessed by turning the patient's head from side to side whilst observing the eye movements. For comatose patients with an intact brainstem, the eyes will appear to move in a direction opposite to that of the head movement (in fact the eyes remain staring at the ceiling whilst the head is turned). If, however, a comatose patient does not have an intact brainstem, the eyes stay in the mid-position on head turning, appearing to move with the head.

The oculovestibular reflex is tested by irrigating the ear canal with ice cold water producing nystagmus and vomiting in non-comatose patients, a tonic movement of the eyes towards the irrigated ear in comatose patients with an intact brainstem and no response in those with no brainstem reflexes. As it may elicit vomiting, it is rarely used for assessment other than in the diagnosis of brainstem death.

Both the oculocephalic and the oculovestibular reflexes involve movement of the neck and should therefore not be used in patients with suspected cervical injury.

Lateralizing signs

Differences between the two sides of the body in response to stimulation imply a unilateral focal brain lesion or diffuse supratentorial pathology with tentorial herniation and brainstem compression resulting in a IIIrd nerve palsy and an opposing hemiparesis.

Meningism

Neck stiffness, a positive Kernig's sign (extension of a flexed knee with the hip in flexion and the patient supine) or Brudzinski's sign (resistance to flexion of the thigh with the leg extended) imply a diffuse meningitic process due to either blood or inflammation. The value of these signs has been infrequently studied – Kernig's and Brudzinski's signs are thought to be of relatively low sensitivity but good specificity whereas neck stiffness is more sensitive but less specific (Thomas et al 2002). Illnesses such as pneumonia or upper respiratory tract infections may cause neck stiffness, which might also be confused with neck pain from diseases such as cervical spondylosis (Attia et al 1999, Oostenbrink et al 2001, Newman 2004). Care should obviously be taken with any history of neck trauma.

Diagnosis

It may be possible after an initial clinical assessment to make a presumptive diagnosis based on clinical findings. If this is not possible, a list of possible diagnoses may be shortened by considering the combination of signs found.

Altered consciousness level with focal brainstem or lateralizing cerebral signs:

- Cerebral infarction or haemorrhage
- Cerebral tumour/metastasis
- Cerebral infection/abscess
- Intracranial trauma
- Venous sinus thrombosis
- Epilepsy including a post-ictal state with a Todd's paresis.

Altered consciousness level without focal or lateralizing signs but with meningeal irritation:

- Subarachnoid haemorrhage (SAH)
- Meningitis
- Encephalitis.

Altered consciousness level without focal or lateralizing signs and without meningism:

- Drug intoxication
- Hypoxic-ischaemic conditions
- Metabolic and endocrine disturbances, e.g. particularly hypo- and hyperglycaemia as well as Addison's crisis, myxoedema coma, etc.
- Wernicke's encephalopathy
- Non-central nervous system (CNS) infections
- Epilepsy (post-ictal)
- Hypothermia/hyperthermia
- Hypertensive encephalopathy
- Carbon monoxide poisoning
- Psychiatric disturbance
- CO_2 retention
- Trauma.

Normal consciousness level with focal signs:

- Cerebrovascular disease
- Cerebral tumour or metastasis
- Trauma
- Cerebral abscess
- Migraine.

> **Tip**
> Keep an open mind, e.g. hypoglycaemia may present with focal neurological signs, and multifocal processes such as bilateral subdural haematomas may present with coma and no focal signs.

General examination

Examination of the rest of the body may give valuable information to aid in diagnosis.

General:

- The presence or absence of jaundice, cyanosis, anaemia
- Evidence of base of skull fracture (mastoid bruising, blood in external auditory meatus, periorbital bruising, cerebrospinal fluid (CSF) leak)
- Rash from meningococcal septicaemia
- Bruising or purpura indicating clotting disorder
- Needle marks suggesting drug abuse.

Respiratory:

- Odour of breath with alcohol, diabetic ketoacidosis, hepatic failure
- Respiratory pattern:
  - periodic Cheyne Stokes breathing due to ischaemic or metabolic hemispheric lesions (may also be caused by non-CNS problems such as heart failure)
  - Kussmaul breathing – deep sighing respiration due to acidosis
  - hyperventilation due to a hypothalamic/mid-brain lesion
  - slow and irregular apneustic breathing due to mid or lower pontine lesions
  - ataxic breathing due to medullary lesions.

Cardiovascular:

- Atrial fibrillation or carotid bruits as a source of emboli
- Cushing's reflex with high blood pressure and slow pulse.

CASE 9.3

A 23-year-old woman presented as an emergency. She was found collapsed on the street unconscious. On examination she was apyrexial with no neck stiffness. Her pupils were small, sluggishly reactive and equal. She did not open her eyes or make any noises in response to a painful stimulus and she had a bilateral decorticate posture. A diagnosis of a possible SAH was made and the decision to intubate her and perform a computed tomography (CT) scan was made.
   What essential piece of information is missing?

Answer
Her blood sugar level had not been measured.
It was immediately done and found to be 0.8 mmol/L. Within 2 min of being given 50 ml of 50% dextrose, she was fully conscious and orientated.

INITIAL MANAGEMENT

The assessment and management of the ABC take priority. Once dealt with, investigation and initial treatment of the patient may commence.

It is essential to perform a blood glucose measurement. Hypoglycaemia may mimic many presentations ranging from hemiparesis to coma with decorticate posture. Hyperglycaemia may cause coma (diabetic ketoacidosis or hyperosmolar non-ketotic coma), may also be an adverse prognostic marker of brain injury and should be corrected to maintain normoglycaemia.

Tip

Recent evidence from critical care patients suggests that the maintenance of normoglycaemia in any critically ill patient significantly improves outcome (Van de Berghe et al 2001).

If not already done so, temperature should be recorded, high-flow oxygen given and an intravenous line placed. Blood should be sent for tests as appropriate to the initial assessment.

Tip

If placing an IV line in a confused patient, always place two well-secured lines in case the patient pulls one out. This may also save someone being called to put one back in in the middle of the night and it could be you!

Consideration should be given to the use of naloxone if an opiate overdose is suspected, and this may help diagnostically, as well as the use of intravenous thiamine for those patients with a possible alcohol related presentation. The use of intravenous flumazenil is not usually recommended as this may precipitate fitting in someone with a benzodiazepine overdose (Seger 2004).

CASE 9.4

A 22-year-old known drug abuser, recently released from prison, is admitted as an emergency having sustained a respiratory arrest shortly after injecting himself with heroin. On arrival, he has an oropharyngeal tube in situ and is being ventilated by a paramedic using a bag and mask. He is GCS 3 (E = 1, V = 1, M = 1). You immediately administer IV naloxone after which he sits up, pulls his airway out and starts swearing profusely at you for waking him up. What is his GCS now?

Despite your attempts to reason with him, he immediately takes his own self-discharge. Shortly after, you receive a warning that a young male has been found collapsed near to the

Initial management

hospital and has sustained a respiratory arrest. What has happened?

Answer
After administration of IV naloxone, the patient's GCS is 15 (E = 4, V = 5, M = 6).

The half-life of parenteral naloxone is 1 h whereas the half-life of heroin is 2 h. To get around this problem, an intramuscular dose of naloxone or ideally an infusion may be given.

If an infective process is suspected or cannot be excluded, blind antibiotic therapy should be commenced after appropriate cultures. Risks of antibiotic administration are small and the consequences of not treating a CNS infection may be life threatening. Aciclovir to treat viral, usually herpes simplex encephalitis, should also be considered.

Finally, it may be difficult to exclude a traumatic process as the cause of a patient's presentation. Many neurological emergencies present in similar ways to a head-injured patient and may also cause the patient to collapse and injure their head. Think of any patient found unconscious in the house who may have fallen downstairs, or someone found unconscious in an alleyway who may have been assaulted with or without associated medical or drug-related problems in addition. Cervical spine immobilization and imaging should be considered in all patients with a depressed level of consciousness unless trauma can be excluded by the history.

Once the patient is stable and investigations are being arranged, a more detailed history should be obtained from both patient and witnesses/family if possible.

It would be usual for patients to undergo a range of blood tests as directed by their clinical state but this would likely include some or all of the following:

- Full blood count, clotting screen, glucose, urea and electrolytes
- Liver function tests, amylase, cardiac enzymes
- Arterial blood gases
- Venous blood cultures
- C-reactive protein and erythrocyte sedimentation rate (ESR)
- Urinalysis for Gram stain, microscopy and culture and sensitivity (C+S) for infection as well as for toxicology. Urine dipsticks are available which show recent (days to weeks) use of a range of illegal drugs but do not indicate whether the drug has been taken immediately before presentation
- Drug levels: in practice this is rarely of use. Occasionally a paracetamol or salicylate level may be indicated; similarly anti-epileptic drug levels may be useful for the management of patients with status epilepticus. A raised alcohol level is rarely clinically useful
- Electrocardiogram (ECG) and chest X-ray (CXR).

Although the approach described is sequential, in practice and particularly if a team approach is adopted, much of the initial assessment and management of the patient presenting with a neurological emergency takes place simultaneously.

NEUROLOGICAL INVESTIGATIONS

CT scanning (Fig. 9.1)

It is extremely likely that a CT scan will be performed early as part of the investigation of a patient with impaired consciousness as it enables rapid detection of intracranial blood, tumours and mass effect. They are less useful for the early detection of cerebrovascular accidents (CVAs) (as areas of infarction may not show up for several days) and inflammatory or infective processes such as anoxic brain injury or encephalitis. If cerebral venous thrombosis or an inflammatory process (such as meningitis or encephalitis) is suspected then a contrast-enhanced CT scan should be requested which will enhance areas of increased vascular perfusion. Modern CT scanners allow rapid scanning of the brain in minutes and should be accessible 24 h a day. If a patient undergoing a CT (or magnetic resonance imaging (MRI)) scan is thought to have impaired airway reflexes, anaesthetic consultation is required to consider securing the airway, thus preventing obstruction with hypoxia or vomiting with pulmonary aspiration whilst in the scanner. If trauma is suspected and the patient is unconscious, CT of the cervical spine should be considered at the same time as the head.

Magnetic resonance imaging (MRI)

MRI is able to detect inflammatory or infective conditions that may be undetected on CT scans as well as providing superior imaging of the

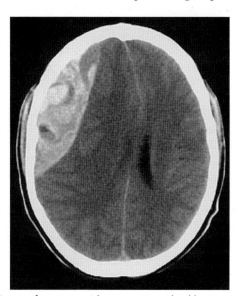

Figure 9.1 CT scan of a patient with massive extradural haematoma and mass effect requiring urgent neurosurgical decompression.

posterior fossa and brainstem. It is also useful for emergency imaging of the spinal cord. However MRI has limited availability and is very often impractical with a critically ill patient due to the prolonged time required for scanning: an MRI of the brain and spinal cord may take 45 min. It is difficult for many restless sick patients to lie still for this length of time. In addition access to the patient, e.g. to administer drugs, is very poor and the need for a metal-free environment limits monitoring to specific MRI compatible monitoring only and makes performing an MRI scan on ventilated patients or those on inotropes difficult. MRI in critically ill patients should therefore be undertaken only with early consultation with the MRI unit involving senior personnel with experience in this area.

Skull and spine X-rays (Fig. 9.2)

Since the publication of the NICE Head Injury Guidelines (NICE 2003), the use of skull X-rays has appropriately declined as they are of limited use. Spinal X-rays remain of use in traumatic conditions, although they are being superceded by rapid access to CT instead, and are of limited use in non-traumatic conditions, e.g. metastatic disease. They allow limited assessment of soft tissue abnormalities around the spine but cannot image the cord itself.

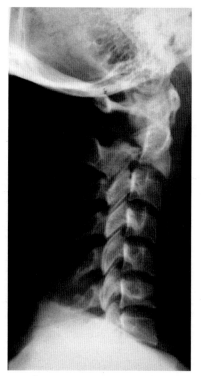

Figure 9.2 C-spine X-ray of an unconscious patient showing a typical Hangman's fracture of C2.

Lumbar puncture

Lumbar puncture (LP) to measure cerebrospinal fluid (CSF) pressure and to obtain a sample of CSF for analysis is a safe and straightforward technique. However, several safeguards apply and lessons may be learnt from anaesthesia to make this a safer and more comfortable procedure for the patient (see Ch. 13).

It is performed as an emergency for the investigation of possible meningitis and SAH. It may also be indicated on a semi-urgent basis for the evaluation and treatment of other disease processes such as Guillain-Barré syndrome, malignancy, demyelination and normal pressure hydrocephalus.

An absolute contraindication to performing an LP is skin sepsis at the site of the LP due to the risk of developing meningitis. A bleeding diathesis is a relative contraindication with a platelet count less than 80 or an INR > 1.5 as suggested cut off points.

An LP may precipitate brainstem herniation when performed in the presence of raised intracranial pressure. The exact incidence of this is unknown – it can be difficult to know whether brain herniation is directly due to the LP or progression of the disease (Archer 1993, Hasbun et al 2001). A CT scan is not infallible at predicting the presence or absence of raised ICP but should be performed pre-LP for the following reasons:

- Focal neurological findings (including altered level of consciousness, arm or leg drift, an inability to answer two consecutive questions correctly or follow two consecutive commands)
- Altered level of consciousness
- New onset seizures (within the last week)
- Papilloedema (this is unusual in acute bacterial meningitis despite raised ICP being common)
- Immunocompromise
- History of CNS disease.

CLINICAL QUESTION

List the structures that the LP needle sequentially passes through to reach, and the space it should penetrate to obtain, CSF. How far should your needle penetrate?

Answer
The needle should pass through skin, subcutaneous tissues, the supraspinous ligament, the ligamentum flavum, the epidural space, and the dura and the arachnoid mater, before encountering the subarachnoid space where CSF can be obtained.

The average distance from the skin to the epidural space is 4.5–5.5 cm and from the epidural space to the dura, it is approximately 7 mm (range 2 mm to 2.5 cm).

Table 9.4 CSF abnormalities according to type of infecting organism

CSF	Normal	Bacterial	Viral	Fungal	Tuberculous
Pressure cm/H$_2$O	5–20 clear, colourless	> 30	< 30	< 30	< 30
Protein g/L	0.15–0.45	> 1.0	< 1.0	Normal	Normal
Glucose mmol/L	2.5–3.5	Low	Normal	Low	Low
CSF:serum glucose ratio	0.6	< 0.4	Normal	< 0.4	< 0.4
WCC/mm^3	< 5 lymph. < 1 neutr. < 1eosin.	1000–10 000	< 1000	100–1000	100–5000
% PMN	0	> 90% neutrophils in 90% of cases	Potential neutrophilia in 1st 48 h then lymphocytes	Mainly lymphocytes	Mainly lymphocytes
Gram stain	Negative	Positive 80%	Negative (positive 1%)	Negative	Negative

The timing of an LP is important: for suspected meningitis, clinical need may dictate that antibiotics are given before an LP is performed. This will potentially alter the results of subsequent CSF analysis (Table 9.4) with CSF cultures becoming sterile in 2–6 h although biochemical and cellular parameters remain abnormal for up to 48 h. Detection of the infecting organism may still be made by Gram stain, use of polymerase chain reaction (PCR) techniques or isolation of the infecting organism from scrapings of any skin rashes.

For suspected SAH and where a CT scan has not been diagnostic, an LP should be delayed for at least 12 h to ensure the development and detection of xanthochromia within the CSF (Fig. 9.3). The sensitivity of an LP for the presence of xanthochromia post SAH is 96% if the LP is performed at least 12 h after the suspected SAH. Unlike CT scanning for suspected SAH, the sensitivity of a positive LP for xanthochromia remains high for a number of weeks, being 70% at 3 weeks and 40% at 4 weeks.

Complications of LP

Traumatic tap
The LP needle may cause bleeding that interferes with CSF analysis. There is no reliable method to determine whether the presence of red blood cells within the CSF is due to the disease process or to a traumatic tap. A traumatic tap is suggested by:

* the absence of xanthochromia
* presence of a blood clot

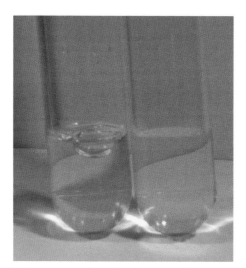

Figure 9.3 Xanthochromia – a yellow discolouration of the CSF due to the presence of bilirubin and oxyhaemoglobin.

- a decrease in the red blood cell count from the first to the last collection tubes either visually or by formal counting
- a WBC 'correction' factor may be applied. Some guidelines suggest that in traumatic taps you can allow 1 white blood cell for every 500 to 700 red blood cells and 0.01 g/L protein for every 1000 red cells. However, rules based on a 'predicted' white cell count in the CSF are not reliable. In order not to miss any patients with meningitis, guidelines relating to decisions about who not to treat for possible meningitis need to be conservative. The safest interpretation of a traumatic tap is to count the total number of white cells and disregard the red cell count. If there are more white cells than the normal range for age, then the safest option is to treat (adapted from Royal Children's Hospital Melbourne Clinical Practice Guidelines).

Infection
An LP should be performed under strict sterile conditions. Meningitis as a consequence of an LP can develop in a bacteraemic patient as well as by performing an LP at the site of skin infections. Other potential infective complications are epidural abscesses, osteomyelitis and a discitis.

Post-dural headache
This may occur in up to 50% of patients, developing in the hours or days following LP. The size of the needle used for performing an LP is the major risk factor, which may be corrected by the person performing the LP. A 22G needle is suggested as an adequate compromise between using too large a needle which increases the incidence of post-dural puncture headache and using too small a needle which will increase the failure rate of an LP and potentially alter manometric readings (American Academy of Neurology 2005). Anaesthetists often use a pencil point needle that does not cut the dura and is associated with a lower incidence of headache (Thomas et al 2000).

There is limited evidence that bed rest post LP reduces the incidence or severity of the headache – adequate hydration, caffeine and simple analgesics are reasonable treatments if headache develops.

Brainstem herniation

This is a rare but serious life-threatening condition that may occur up to an hour post LP, producing deteriorating consciousness level, with raised blood pressure and a bradycardia in its advanced stages. Its exact incidence as a complication of LP is unknown, but theoretically it occurs due to a sudden lowering of CSF pressure in the spinal canal in the presence of a raised ICP. CT is relatively insensitive for the detection of raised ICP, but the presence of hydrocephalus before LP would certainly be a contraindication. Treatment involves immediate sedation, intubation and ventilation, and manoeuvres on the critical care unit to protect the brain and lower ICP.

Other

These include failure to obtain CSF, the development of epidural haematomas, back pain and local nerve trauma. The development of progressively worsening low backache or signs of spinal cord compromise following LP is very rare but would necessitate immediate specialist opinion and radiological investigation.

Electroencephalogram (EEG)

EEG is one of the mainstay neurological investigations and is useful in the diagnosis and classification of epilepsy, exclusion of pseudoepilepsy and diagnosis of non-clinical status epilepticus. In addition, specific changes are seen with conditions such as herpes simplex, measles encephalitis and Creutzfeldt-Jakob disease. EEG is of limited prognostic value in coma, specific patterns being associated with a poor outcome, and may be useful taken in conjunction with a broader clinical picture in decision making. Continuous EEG monitoring is particularly useful in detecting intermittent non-clinical status epilepticus or status epilepticus in sedated or paralyzed critical care unit patients. Bispectral Index analysis is a cheaper and simpler form of EEG monitoring using a single forehead monitor strip which gives a statistically derived single number between 0 and 100, where 100 is an awake patient and 0 represents electrical silence. Developed predominantly for assessment of awareness during anaesthesia, it provides limited information in the critically ill about periods of cerebral ischaemia or fitting.

Electrophysiology studies

Electromyography

Electromyography (EMG) is the recording of muscular electrical activity by an electrode inserted into muscle with the muscle at rest and with minimal and maximal muscular contraction. Specific features looked for on EMG are spontaneous muscular activity, the response of the muscle to the insertion of the electrode, the muscle's individual motor unit action potentials and the speed with which additional motor units are recruited in response to an electrical signal. Muscle disease, denervation, or neuromuscular disease can all alter these components, giving rise to patterns that help in the diagnosis of the underlying pathology.

The usefulness of electromyography in the diagnosis of a patient with acute weakness can, however, be limited. This is due to the high degree of expertise necessary in the interpretation of EMG patterns, the limited availability of EMG in the acute situation, the time taken for EMG patterns to develop and the fact that primary muscular diseases often produce similar EMG patterns. However, EMG is most useful in distinguishing between muscular weakness and neurogenic weakness and some patterns may be diagnostic.

Nerve conduction studies

Nerve conduction studies (NCSs) involve the electrical stimulation of peripheral nerves and the recording of both nerve and muscular electrical responses that allow the calculation of latencies and nerve conduction times as well as identification of the site(s) of peripheral nerve damage.

Nerve conduction studies can distinguish between peripheral and central nerve damage, radiculopathies, entrapment neuropathies and peripheral neuropathies.

For peripheral neuropathies, NCSs may distinguish between generalized and focal neuropathies, sensory, motor or sensorimotor neuropathies and axonal or demyelinating neuropathies.

NCSs are abnormal earlier than with EMG studies, increasing their usefulness in the acute situation but again they may be of limited immediate availability.

EMGs and NCSs are often complementary and performed together. They should be viewed as an extension of a thorough history and examination and specific questions should be asked to maximize the usefulness of these studies, guide the operator and aid in their interpretation. It should also be asked, as with every diagnostic test, what additional information is to be gained from an EMG or NCS. For example, EMG studies will add little extra information for a patient with muscular weakness and raised inflammatory markers of muscle disease when a biopsy would be more useful. Similarly, for a patient with typical features of myasthenia and a positive test for acetylcholine receptor antibodies, NCS and EMG are unnecessary. However, they are of great use for the assessment and diagnosis of acute peripheral neuropathies and in the diagnosis of more unusual conditions such as botulism.

THE UNCONSCIOUS PATIENT – COMA

Background

Coma is defined as a GCS < 8. Normal consciousness is dependent upon bilaterally intact cerebral cortices, an intact reticular activating system (RAS)

Table 9.5 Causes of coma according to anatomical site

Bilateral cerebral hemisphere	Bilateral thalamus or hypothalamus	Brainstem
Metabolic	Haemorrhage	Supra- or infratentorial mass lesions
Hypoxia/ischaemia	Infarction	Haemorrhage
Drugs	Drugs	Ischaemia
Trauma	Metabolic	Drugs

located in the brainstem and an intact thalamus and hypothalamus through which the RAS connects to the cerebral cortices (Table 9.5 and Box 9.1). Unilateral cerebral cortical damage does not usually produce coma unless a mass effect leads to brain herniation and compression of the RAS. Similarly, lesions below the level of the pons do not usually result in coma.

Decorticate and decerebrate rigidity or flaccidity

Prognosis

Providing a prognosis for a patient in coma allows informed decisions to be made by family and carers. However, despite many studies on prognosis in coma, it remains extremely difficult to provide accurate prognostic information (Levy et al 1981). A small number of methodologically sound papers have determined that the overwhelming factors determining prognosis are the cause of coma, depth of coma and duration of coma as well as

---

Box 9.1   Clinico-anatomical correlation in coma (*adapted from Bateman 2001*)

Bilateral hemisphere damage/dysfunction

- Symmetrical signs (tone and flexor or extensor response to pain)
- May have fits or myoclonus
- Normal brainstem reflexes
- Normal oculocephalic response (OCR): normal caloric testing
- Normal pupils

Supratentorial mass lesion with secondary brainstem compression

- Ipsilateral third nerve palsy
- Contralateral hemiplegia

Brainstem lesion

- Early eye movement disorder: abnormal OCR or caloric testing
- Asymmetrical motor responses

Toxic/metabolic

- Normal pupils: single most important criterion (except opiate poisoning)
- Ocular motility: rove randomly in mild coma and come to rest in primary position with deepening coma
- Absent OCR and caloric testing

---

the presence or absence of brainstem reflexes such as the corneal reflex and pupillary reflexes (Bates 2001). Determining prognosis in the immediate post-resuscitation period is fraught with difficulty and should be discouraged especially when drugs given in the resuscitation period might interfere with clinical examination (CRSGBSIC 1988). Additional information may come from imaging studies and neurophysiological tests such as the EEG and, in the future, testing for proteins released by the damaged brain.

Despite this, it can be stated that:

- coma due to drug overdoses carries a very good prognosis
- coma due to vascular disease such as SAH or stroke carries a poor prognosis (only 7% make a moderate to good recovery), as does coma due to anoxia/hypoxia (11% making a good to moderate recovery) whereas coma due to metabolic disorders carries a relatively better prognosis (35% achieving a moderate to good recovery)
- the depth of coma as measured by the GCS correlates with outcome
- the longer the duration of coma, the worse the outcome with perhaps only 15% of patients with non-traumatic coma greater than 6 h making a good recovery
- the presence or absence of brainstem reflexes including the corneal and pupillary reflexes are useful in determining prognosis.

Brainstem death

Brainstem death usually results from either severe damage to the brain (usually trauma or SAH) with worsening ischaemia/infarction resulting in an inexorable rise in intracerebral pressure until the brainstem dies by being forced through the foramen magnum, during which process its blood supply is cut off. Less commonly, brainstem death may occur secondary to a direct insult, such as brainstem stroke. UK criteria for the diagnosis of brainstem death remain largely clinical, but the underlying pathology will usually be based on imaging. As this is a condition where consciousness and respiration are not possible because the brainstem has died, it equates to death. Indeed in the UK death is certified according to either brainstem or cardio-respiratory criteria. As such, if patients are apnoeic, they are by definition ventilated in the critical care unit and this is beyond the remit of this chapter. Further discussion of national criteria for the diagnosis of brain stem death and organ donation may be found at http://www.ics.ac.uk.

PROLONGED REDUCTION IN CONSCIOUSNESS LEVEL

Delirium

Background

Delirium is characterized by a variable combination of impaired consciousness and attention levels, psychomotor disturbance, (both hyper- and hypo-activity), alteration of sleep patterns and emotional disturbance.

Table 9.6   Risk factors and precipitating factors in delirium

Risk factors	Precipitating factors
Older age	Medications
Chronic cognitive impairment	Hypoxia
Chronic illness	Infections
Psychoactive drug use	Metabolic disturbance
Visual impairment	Neurological illness

It is frequently of acute onset with a fluctuating pattern occurring more commonly in the elderly. There are often a number of underlying risk factors (Table 9.6) such as chronic cognitive impairment and chronic illness that combine with an acute insult such as an alteration in medication (particularly drugs with anti-cholinergic activity), dehydration, malnutrition, alcohol withdrawal and metabolic disturbances.

It is important to recognize that delirium may be difficult to diagnose in its early stages, is associated with a significant mortality and may be the only feature of serious underlying disease such as myocardial infarction.

Management

Delirium should be recognized as early as possible, risk factors recognized and precipitating causes removed or treated. Patients with delirium should be nursed in as supportive an environment as is possible, e.g. well-lit, quiet rooms, whilst investigation and treatment are ongoing.

The patient with delirium may need sedation either to allow investigation or to relieve distressing symptoms and to prevent self-harm. Sedation should be avoided if possible but may be unavoidable despite expert nursing care. It is fraught with difficulty as all sedative drugs have the potential to worsen the condition of the patient, either by affecting the ABC or by having pharmacological side-effects that potentiate delirium. Drugs should be used in low doses and reviewed regularly.

First-line drugs for sedation are neuroleptics such as haloperidol orally, intramuscularly or intravenously.

Benzodiazepines such as lorazepam, or chlormethiazole may be useful alternatives particularly when delirium is thought to be due to alcohol withdrawal or the recent cessation of sedatives.

SUDDEN ONSET OF HEADACHE – SUBARACHNOID HAEMORRHAGE

Background

Headache is a distressing, potentially debilitating symptom that is commonly encountered in emergency medicine. The majority of patients will have a benign cause but a significant minority will have a potentially life-threatening secondary cause, in particular headache due to SAH. A careful history is extremely important in determining the cause of the headache, however, both minor and life-threatening diseases cause headaches that share certain characteristics. This overlap, combined with a low suspicion of significant illness in apparently well patients, contributes to patients with SAH being misdiagnosed.

CASE 9.5

A 47-year-old woman presented to A&E with a severe bilateral frontal headache that came on rapidly over a number of minutes. The headache had not settled with rest and paracetamol and she had not previously had headaches. Examination was normal. The diagnosis of a SAH was considered and a CT scan and LP were normal. She was reassured and discharged.

She returned 4 days later with a second severe, rapid onset headache similar to the previous headache. Again a CT scan was normal but an LP performed 14 h after admission showed marked xanthochromia. She was referred to the regional neurosurgical unit and underwent angiography which showed a small aneurysm that was successfully treated.

This case highlights some of the problems associated with the diagnosis of SAH. Traditional teaching to differentiate SAH from other more benign causes of headache has been that SAH presents with a 'thunderclap' headache. A recent more useful definition has expanded on this such that SAH should be considered for 'a sudden onset first or worst headache which is usually maximal within moments, but may sometimes develop over a few minutes and which lasts at least 1 h'. Problems also arose with this woman due to the negative initial CT and LP – you should be aware of the time-dependent nature of these investigations (Van Der Wee et al 1995). Beware also of the fact that a few laboratories still detect xanthochromia by eye rather than with the more sensitive spectrophotometer. Despite negative investigations, patients undergo angiography if there is a convincing enough history – this reinforces the importance of a thorough history in making the diagnosis of SAH.

Causes of headache

Primary

- Migraine
- Tension
- Cluster
- Thunderclap
- Benign exertional/sex headache
- Cough.

Secondary

- Vascular:
  - (ruptured) cerebral aneurysm/arteriovenous malformation
  - thrombo-embolic stroke/TIA

- – intracranial haemorrhage
- – cerebral venous thrombosis
- – carotid/vertebral arteries dissection
- – arteritis
- Traumatic
- CNS infection
- Hypertensive encephalopathy
- Other intracranial disease:
  - – tumour (primary or metastasis)
  - – intracranial hypertension
  - – hydrocephalus
  - – CSF hypertension (&BIH)
- Metabolic, e.g. hypoglycaemia, hypothyroidism, phaeochromocytoma
- Drug/toxin related, e.g. drug withdrawal, carbon monoxide
- Cervical spine disease
- Secondary to general medical conditions
- Ophthalmic, e.g. acute glaucoma
- ENT, e.g. sinusitis
- Dental, e.g. temporomandibular disease.

SAH is caused in the majority of cases by rupture of a cerebral aneurysm (Fig. 9.4). Additional causes include AV malformations, trauma, drug abuse, neoplasms and coagulopathies. Its incidence varies but is thought to cause approximately 15 deaths per 100 000 in the UK occurring most frequently between the ages of 40 to 60 years. Death rates from aneurysmal haemorrhage are of the order of 50% for the initial bleed, with the majority of deaths occurring in the first 24 h.

Aneurysmal haemorrhage accounts for up to 75% of SAH, depending on the case series and can itself be associated with a number of clinical

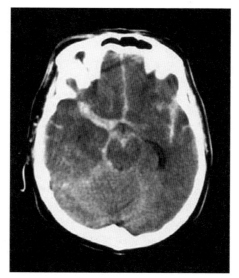

Figure 9.4 CT scan showing extensive SAH.

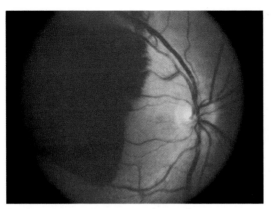

Figure 9.5 Subhyaloid haemorrhage in a patient with SAH.

conditions including polycystic kidney disease, aortic stenosis, infective endocarditis, aortic coarctation and Marfan's syndrome or Ehlers Danlos syndrome.

Clinical presentation

Headache occurs in almost all patients with SAH. This is classically of abrupt onset and severe in nature, commonly being described as 'the worst headache ever'. In severe SAH, there may be a brief period of unconsciousness followed either by a return to full consciousness or an altered level of consciousness. Pain often spreads to the cervical or occipital region as blood from the SAH tracks towards the spinal cord. Neck stiffness and even a positive Kernig's sign may be present. It is suggested that the severity and duration of headache and neck stiffness is dependent upon the severity of the bleed.

SAH may also cause photophobia, nausea and vomiting and focal neurological signs. Seizures occur in about 10% of patients. Ophthalmoscopy may reveal subhyaloid (Fig. 9.5), retinal and vitreous haemorrhages and can be useful in aiding in the diagnosis of SAH.

Additional systemic signs may include hypertension and hyperpyrexia.

Many patients (up to 50% in some series) retrospectively report a headache of brief duration, visual disturbance or dizziness in the days preceding SAH but it is unclear whether this represents a 'warning' bleed or 'recall bias' (Linn et al 2000).

Diagnosis

Investigation should be initially by CT scanning which makes the diagnosis in up to 85% of patients within the first two days following the haemorrhage. However, CT is a time-dependent process – 98% of CT scans are positive for SAH within 12 h, the sensitivity falling to 73% by the third day.

A negative CT scan does not exclude the diagnosis of SAH and patients should also undergo LP to look for xanthochromia which, whilst not specific for SAH, is a good indicator in the context of a patient presenting with

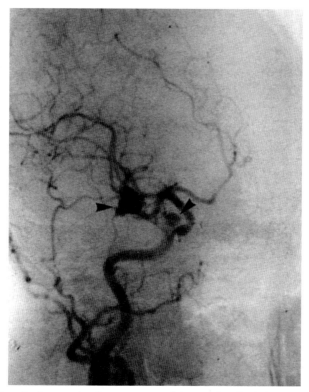

Figure 9.6 Angiogram showing aneurysms of the anterior circulation.

headache and collapse that SAH has occurred. The sensitivity of an LP for the presence of xanthochromia post SAH is 96% if the LP is performed at least 12 h after the suspected haemorrhage and remains high for weeks, being 70% at 3 weeks and 40% at 4 weeks.

A number of grading systems exist for the severity of a SAH, directing management and prognosis (Table 9.7).

Bizarre ECG abnormalities, echocardiographic changes and neurogenic pulmonary oedema are associated with SAH and thought to reflect catecholamine release (Fig. 9.7).

Repolarization, ischaemic-like ECG changes, and/or QT prolongation are found in approximately 75% of patients with SAH, irrespective of a history of heart disease.

Management

Once resuscitation has taken place, consultation with a neurosurgical team is mandatory so that the patient can be transferred for further investigation and treatment (Table 9.8, Fig. 9.6). Treatment before transfer should include: nimodipine, a calcium channel antagonist, either intravenously or nasogastrically to prevent vasospasm, and intravenous fluids to ensure hydration (patients with SAH develop a diuretic state). Deterioration may occur for a number of reasons:

Table 9.7   Grading systems for severity of SAH

	Hunt and Hess grading system for SAH	World Federation of Neurosurgeons grading system for SAH
Grade 0	Unruptured aneurysm without symptoms	
Grade 1	Asymptomatic or minimal headache and slight nuchal rigidity	GCS 15 Motor deficit absent
Grade 2	No acute meningeal or brain reaction but with fixed neurological deficit	GCS 14–13 Motor deficit absent
Grade 3	Drowsy, confused or mild focal deficit	GCS 14–13 Motor deficit present
Grade 4	Stupor, moderate to severe hemiparesis, possible early decerebrate rigidity and vegetative disturbances	GCS 12–7 Motor deficit present or absent
Grade 5	Deep coma, decerebrate rigidity, moribund appearance	GCS 6–3 Motor deficit present or absent

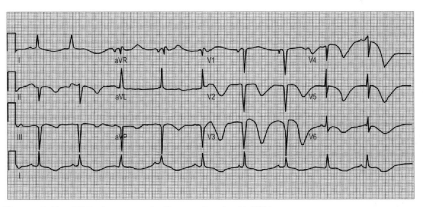

Figure 9.7   ECG changes typically associated with SAH.

Table 9.8   Suggested criteria for transfer of a patient with a SAH to a neurosurgical centre have been developed by the Society of British Neurosurgeons

Patient condition	CT findings	Action
Talking and obeying commands	CT scan positive for SAH or CT scan negative but LP positive	Transfer within 18 h (depending on bed availability)
No speech but localizing to pain	CT scan confirms SAH	Discuss with neurosurgery with view to transfer
Flexing, extending or no response to pain	CT scan confirms SAH	Defer transfer but discuss with neurosurgical unit

- Further SAH
- Vasospasm
- Cerebral oedema
- Hydrocephalus
- Brain herniation
- Seizures.

SUSPECTED CNS INFECTION

Infection of the CNS includes meningitis, encephalitis and focal infections/abscesses. It is not unusual for these to co-exist. These diseases frequently present in a non-specific manner to those who are least experienced in their management. Emphasis is placed upon early referral of patients with suspected meningitis to experienced clinicians.

Bacterial meningitis

Background

Despite advances in disease management, morbidity and mortality due to meningitis remains high (10–20%). Perhaps most importantly, this is due to patients being managed by relatively inexperienced clinicians, unfamiliar with the disease and its management. Emphasis is placed on early recognition of the disease, adherence to national guidelines, rapid referral to senior clinicians and involvement of critical care at an early stage.

The majority of cases of bacterial meningitis in adults are caused by *Neisseria meningitidis* or *Streptococcus pneumoniae*. In elderly people, there is an increased incidence of infection with *Listeria monocytogenes* as well as Gram-negative organisms such as *Escherichia coli*. There has been a reduction in the number of cases of *Haemophilus influenza* meningitis particularly in children as well as adults since the introduction of the haemophilus influenza type b vaccine.

Bacterial meningitis is often spontaneous in nature with no apparent predisposing factors. Predisposing factors to meningitis include sickle cell disease, diabetes mellitus, alcohol excess or immune suppression, either through congenital or acquired defects of the immune system, such as a neutropenia. It may be associated with sinusitis, mastoiditis, otitis media and may be associated with CSF leaks following trauma or neurosurgical procedures.

Diagnosis

Symptoms and signs are initially non-specific, including headache, malaise and fever. The triad of fever, neck stiffness and altered mental status appears in approximately 50% of patients, however, in a recent study, 95% of patients had two of the four symptoms of headache, fever, neck stiffness and altered mental status. Presentation may be atypical particularly in the very young, the very old and the immunocompromised.

Cranial nerve palsies may develop as the nerves emerge through the inflamed pustular meninges. Seizures occur in approximately 20% of cases. Focal signs, occurring in 15% of patients, suggest a vasculitis or the development of an intracranial abscess.

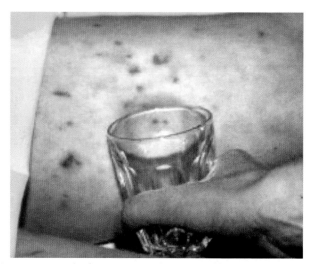

Figure 9.8   Purpuric rash of meningococcal sepsis not blanching to pressure.

Rashes are commonly found in patients with meningitis but may be extremely subtle, not present on initial presentation and be caused by a variety of infecting organisms. A petechial or purpuric rash is found most commonly with meningococcal meningitis (Fig. 9.8) occurring in about 50% of cases of, initially starting as a less obvious, less specific maculopapular rash.

The initial diagnosis of meningitis is made on clinical grounds – it can be further confirmed by LP and subsequent analysis of CSF and/or isolation of the causative organism either from CSF, blood or the rash. Raised intra-cranial pressure is commonly found with bacterial meningitis and LP is not without risk of cerebral herniation. However a CT scan before the LP does not reliably exclude raised intracranial pressure and certain clinical features may also be used to predict the presence of raised ICP. Some institutions limit CT scanning prior to LP to those patients with altered levels of con-sciousness, focal neurology, papilloedema, new onset seizures or those who are immunocompromised.

Bacterial meningitis is associated with typical CSF findings:

- Turbid fluid with neutrophilia and WCC > 1000 wbc/mL
- CSF glucose less than 40 mg/dL or less than 60% plasma glucose
- Elevated CSF protein.

Early bacterial meningitis, partially treated bacterial meningitis or certain causative organisms may limit the rise in the white cell count or produce a CSF lymphocytosis. Culture of CSF is positive in 75% of meningitis cases without prior antibiotic therapy but it may take up to 48 h before results are available. Gram staining of the CSF will show organisms in 60–90%. The yield will be approximately 20% lower if antibiotics are administered prior to LP. The specificity of a positive CSF Gram stain is 97%.

Rapid detection of bacterial antigen in CSF by latex agglutination is limited by a high false positive rate and has not been accepted as routine clinical practice. PCR techniques are increasingly available for rapid analysis of CSF and have been found to be both sensitive and specific in detecting common bacterial pathogens as well as enteroviruses but it is labour intensive, limited by its availability and has a high false positive rate. Gram staining of aspirates from skin rashes have a good yield for the diagnosis of meningococcal disease.

A number of complementary rapid diagnostic tests are available using either CSF or blood and include measurement of lactate levels, CRP and ESR and procalcitonin levels. These tests are inadequate when used in isolation but may provide useful information concerning prognosis and in distinguishing between viral and bacterial causes of meningitis.

Management

Antibiotics should be given immediately after an LP has been performed – if the LP will be delayed by more than 30 min, IV antibiotics should be given immediately. Current recommendations state that 2 g of IV cefotaxime or ceftriaxone should be used as a first-line agent with the addition of 2 g IV ampicillin for patients over 55 years of age.

Antibiotic therapy may be modified dependent upon clinical circumstance, local policy and sensitivities of isolated organisms if known. Discussion is encouraged with microbiologists or infectious disease specialists.

Dexamethasone at a dose of 0.15 mg/kg should be given before or with the first dose of antibiotics, particularly when the infecting organism is thought to be pneumococcus. Much of the morbidity associated with meningitis is thought to arise from bacterial lysis stimulating the inflammatory cascade.

If the patient fails to respond, additional diagnoses must be considered. There are a number of recognized complications of meningitis and a search for a continued source of infection and possible repeat CT scan and LP should be undertaken.

Complications of meningitis

Include:

- Cerebral abscess
- Subdural empyema
- Venous sinus thrombosis
- Hydrocephalus
- Hyponatraemia.

The mortality and morbidity from meningitis remains high – a number of prognostic scoring systems have been developed but none are in universal use. Prognosis has been found to be dependent upon a number of clinical and laboratory parameters and includes:

- level of consciousness at presentation as measured by the GCS
- time to administration of antibiotics
- age of the patient
- the infecting organism
- low CSF WCC, thrombocytopenia, raised ESR.

Tuberculous meningitis

There has been a resurgence of tuberculous disease in association with human immunodeficiency virus (HIV) infection, homelessness and immigration. Other risk factors include alcohol, drug abuse, immunocompromise and certain racial groups. It is typically of subacute onset, developing over a number of days to weeks rather than hours/days with malaise, low-grade fever and vague intermittent headaches. Tuberculous meningitis is especially likely to develop a vasculitis/endarteritis and present with focal neurological signs as well as cranial nerve palsies.

The CSF may show an initial neutrophilia but there is more usually a lymphocytosis within the CSF associated with a markedly raised CSF protein count and a moderately lowered CSF glucose.

Confirming the diagnosis of tuberculous meningitis is difficult; there is no rapid, sensitive test available. Whilst visualization of the tubercle on CSF microscopy or culture remains the gold standard, the mycobacterium is difficult to isolate from the CSF. Treatment may therefore have to be started on clinical suspicion alone.

Other diagnostic tests for the diagnosis of tuberculous meningitis suffer from being insensitive or non-specific. PCR techniques are increasingly available but may not be any more sensitive than CSF microscopy. A CXR looking for signs of tuberculosis may be of use; similarly a tuberculin skin test may occasionally be helpful.

Treatment will vary depending upon local policy and is made difficult by the emergence of multidrug-resistant tubercles. A multidrug regimen of isoniazid (with pyridoxine), rifampicin, pyrazinamide and one of either ethambutol or streptomycin is usually chosen with this being modified depending upon clinical response and drug sensitivities.

Fungal meningitis

This occurs in patients with impaired cellular immunity. Presentation is highly variable and may be overshadowed by the disease process that has led to impaired immunity.

Viral meningitis

Viral meningitis is a self-limiting illness occurring most typically in children and young adults. It is caused by enteroviruses such as Coxsackie as well as herpes simplex, varicella zoster and mumps. In its initial stages it may be confused with bacterial meningitis presenting with fever, malaise, headache, neck stiffness, photophobia and irritability. It is unusual for the disease to progress further than this and recovery takes place over a number of days. Its importance lies in its similarity with bacterial meningitis and occasionally SAH. CSF examination shows occasionally a CSF neutrophilia but more commonly a lymphocytosis as well as a slightly raised CSF protein and CSF glucose. It is frequently difficult to isolate a causative organism. PCR techniques are available and relatively sensitive and specific for the identification of enteroviruses. Other tests have been shown to be of limited use in distinguishing between bacterial and viral causes of meningitis. Treatment is symptomatic.

Encephalitis

Background

The vast majority of cases of encephalitis in the UK are due to viruses. However, depending on location, and in particular recent travel to certain locations, other infectious causes of encephalitis such as protozoa (malaria) and rickettsiae need to be considered. The epidemiology of encephalitis in the UK is also changing with the introduction of the measles, mumps and rubella (MMR) vaccine. Herpes simplex and other herpes viruses are now the leading cause of viral encephalitis in the UK with varicella zoster virus (VZV), Epstein-Barr virus, measles, mumps and enteroviruses accounting for the majority of other viruses causing encephalitis in immunocompetent individuals.

As with bacterial meningitis, the underlying pathophysiology explaining how viruses enter and attack the CNS are not known, nor why certain viruses such as herpes show a tendency to infect particular parts of the brain. Herpes infects preferentially the temporal lobe of the brain and this may be useful clinically.

Diagnosis

Patients often have a prodrome of a few days of non-specific symptoms such as lethargy and malaise as well as upper respiratory tract infection (URTI) type symptoms before developing headache, vomiting and possible meningism (due to frequent coexisting meningeal inflammation). Drowsiness develops with features of mental disturbance such as disorientation, abnormal behaviour and possible hallucinations. Coma will eventually supervene, seizures are common and focal neurological signs can develop.

Important clues to the diagnosis of encephalitis and the infecting virus may be found from the presence of gastrointestinal symptoms (enteroviruses), parotitis (mumps) and URTI symptoms (HSV-1). Rashes are also frequently found.

It is also important to ascertain the immune state of the patient as encephalitis is commoner in those with HIV, or those on immunosuppressant medication for organ transplantation.

Herpes simplex virus (HSV) preferentially infects the temporal lobe and features of this illness such as hallucinations, temporal lobe epilepsy and behavioural disturbance may point towards a herpes infection.

The gold standard for the diagnosis of viral encephalitis is increasingly recognized to be the detection of specific viral nucleic acid in CSF (or brain tissue) by PCR techniques. PCR is replacing the use of viral detection in cell cultures. PCR techniques are improving both in their sensitivities and specificities as well as the time taken to perform such techniques. The detection of viral nucleic acid is dependent upon the timing of the LP in relation to disease onset, for example, in HSV encephalitis, the sensitivity of PCR is 96% with a specificity of 99% if the CSF is studied between two and 10 days of disease onset.

LP itself will usually show a CSF lymphocytosis, red cells if there is a necrotising element to the encephalitis (particularly with herpes simplex infections), a normal CSF glucose, a moderately raised CSF protein and no organisms. A viral aetiology may also be strongly suggested by the measurement of antibodies in both CSF and serum (on acute and convalescing samples) and weakly suggested by the direct or indirect detection of virus from throat, stool or urine samples.

Diagnosis may occasionally be made by CT scanning although this is not a particularly sensitive or specific test in diagnosing viral encephalitis. It may, though, be useful when deciding to perform a LP and to exclude other diagnoses that may be confused with encephalitis.

Magnetic resonance imaging (MRI) is the most sensitive imaging test for viral encephalitis, however availability, duration of procedure and the need for a metal-free environment limits its use in the emergency situation.

An EEG will on occasion be useful as it may show cerebral involvement before its detection by neuroimaging techniques; specific features are present in HSV encephalitis and it can be of use in diagnosing other diseases confused with viral encephalitis.

Management

A high degree of suspicion is necessary and antiviral treatment with aciclovir may need to be given empirically before a diagnosis is reached. Aciclovir is of use particularly in the treatment of HSV encephalitis as well as VZV encephalitis. It is not active against cytomegalovirus (CMV); ganciclovir and foscarnet are recommended. Other newer antiviral drugs are under evaluation. Treatment is otherwise symptomatic and supportive. Mortality may be up to 30% with particular forms of encephalitis and there is also a significant morbidity with seizures, focal signs and alterations in mental function.

Intracranial abscess

Background

Intracranial abscesses may develop within the extradural and subdural spaces as well as within the brain parenchyma itself. This may be from local direct spread following an otitis media or sinusitis, distant spread from an endocarditis or direct innoculation following trauma or surgery. The underlying source of infection may not be identified.

Diagnosis

Presentation is often subacute and will depend upon the site of the abscess but often includes pyrexia, headache, vomiting, fever, alteration in mental state, focal neurological signs and seizures. An underlying cause may also be obvious clinically, such as signs of intravenous drug abuse. As with other CNS infections, symptoms and signs may be non-specific and be confused with other clinical conditions. Diagnosis is from CT scanning and neuro-surgical referral is mandatory.

Management

Antibiotics should be given after discussion with the neurosurgical team and transfer with symptomatic and supportive care made. Mortality is significant and may be up to 25%, as well as there being a significant long-term morbidity due to seizures.

SEIZURES – TONIC-CLONIC STATUS EPILEPTICUS

Background

Status epilepticus is defined as seizures lasting for more than 30 min, either in the form of one prolonged seizure, or multiple seizures without full recovery in between. There are a number of types of status epilepticus, tonic-clonic status being the commonest and easiest to recognize. Status epilepticus may also be classified by noting whether the seizures are partial or generalized.

The incidence of status epilepticus is approximately 20 per 100 000 and it most often occurs in patients without underlying epilepsy due to cerebral injury from infarction, infection, trauma, tumour or metabolic disturbance (including alcohol-related causes). The high mortality (up to 20%) reflects not only the systemic and local cerebral pathological changes that occur with status epilepticus but also the underlying disease process. When status occurs in known epileptics, it may be due to changes in drug levels, illness or progression of the underlying disease process.

The morbidity and mortality due to status epilepticus, separate from the underlying cause, is due to two distinct processes. Firstly, the massive physiological demands placed upon the body from prolonged seizure activity, and secondly, direct neuronal damage due to local seizure activity. The damage from both these processes increases as the duration of the seizures increases. This leads to the recognition that status epilepticus is a progressive condition with its management, response to treatment and outcome changing as time passes. Status epilepticus may therefore be classified into premonitory status, early status, established status and refractory status epilepticus.

Clinical presentation

Tonic-clonic seizures should be easily recognizable. Difficulty arises first in knowing how long seizures have been present for, and secondly, as seizures continue, muscular contractions become a less prominent part of the disease process. Additional clinical features such as excess salivation, sweating, impaired breathing and tachycardia should be noted and may support the diagnosis of ongoing seizure activity when muscular contractions become less prominent or when status occurs in the presence of coma.

It should not be forgotten that status occurs predominantly in those people without epilepsy and an underlying cause is sought. Features of alcohol abuse, infection, rashes or trauma may be present.

Management

Supportive therapy

Strict attention to the ABC is necessary. Seizures may prevent the jaw opening and the use of nasopharyngeal airways is important. Supplementary oxygen should be given and suction performed in response to excess salivation.

A blood glucose level should be taken and glucose given as necessary. If there is any suspicion of alcohol abuse, intravenous thiamine and vitamins should be given (pabrinex).

Both respiratory and cardiovascular support may be needed depending upon the stage and mode of presentation of a particular episode of status epilepticus.

Specific anti-epileptic therapy

There is only a small amount of evidence from high quality studies in adults to allow an evidence-based choice of the choice and timing of anti-epileptic medication for status epilepticus. Good quality trials exist showing that benzodiazepines in particular are effective for status epilepticus but the choice of subsequent medications, particularly for refractory status, is frequently guided by case series and expert consensus.

Benzodiazepines are the mainstay in treating patients in the early stages of status epilepticus. Benzodiazepines in common usage are diazepam (rectally or IV), lorazepam (increasingly the benzodiazepine of choice) and midazolam (buccal or IV). All benzodiazepines have the potential to cause respiratory depression and hypotension, particularly in older or sick patients.

If seizures are not terminated with benzodiazepines, phenytoin, which lacks the sedative effects of benzodiazepines, should be given. Phenytoin is associated with cardiac arrhythmias as well as phlebitis and hypotension. Fosphenytoin is a prodrug of phenytoin that can be given as a bolus and avoids the problems associated with phenytoin, but it is expensive. ECG monitoring is recommended during treatment with IV phenytoin.

Phenobarbital is often used as an alternative or in addition to phenytoin, especially when the patient may already be on phenytoin and drug levels are unknown. It may cause marked sedation and profound hypotension requiring treatment with vasopressors.

If tonic-clonic seizures are still continuing, the patient should be anaesthetized, ventilated and sedated with propofol or thiopental. Other anti-epileptic medication should be continued and expert advice sought.

Investigation should be performed to detect an underlying cause. An FBC, blood glucose, urea and electrolytes, calcium, magnesium and phosphate should all be taken. Anti-epileptic drug levels should be measured if possible. A CT scan should be performed to look for an underlying cause. Infection must not be forgotten, particularly meningitis, with antibiotics given and investigation performed as appropriate. If the patient is anaesthetized, an EEG, if available, should be performed to ensure seizure activity has been terminated by the anti-epileptic drugs given, and can also be of great help in investigating possible non-convulsive status epilepticus.

Non-convulsive status epilepticus (NCSE)

NCSE may be defined as ongoing seizure activity (as seen on an EEG) lacking in marked tonic-clonic activity associated with a variable and at

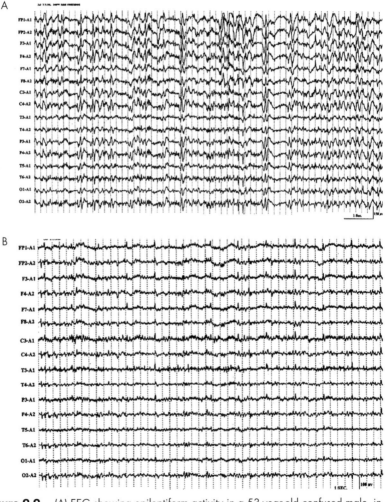

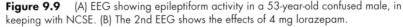

Figure 9.9 (A) EEG showing epileptiform activity in a 53-year-old confused male, in keeping with NCSE. (B) The 2nd EEG shows the effects of 4 mg lorazepam.

times fluctuating impairment of consciousness. Although less common than tonic-clonic status epilepticus, it may be more problematic due to the range of forms it may present with, the difficulty in its diagnosis, and the potential for direct neuronal damage from ongoing seizure activity.

NCSE should be considered in any patient with an unexplained altered level of consciousness – whilst it is impractical to order an EEG for every patient with an altered level of consciousness, certain features from the history (risk factors for epilepsy such as previous strokes, tumours, neurosurgery and meningitis) combined with features on examination (in particular nystagmus) have been suggested as pointers towards a diagnosis of NCSE (Fig. 9.9).

CASE 9.6

An unknown man, thought to be in his twenties, is found collapsed and fitting in the street. A paramedic ambulance is called – they administer 10 mg rectal diazepam with no effect. The patient is then brought to the emergency department, still fitting. In his wallet is a prescription for lamotrigine.

What are your priorities? Describe the initial management of this patient.

- ABC
- Glucose
- Treat seizures
- Establish a cause.

After 35 min in the emergency department and despite supportive therapy and two doses of lorazepam followed by a loading dose of intravenous phenytoin, the patient continues to fit. He is noted to be pyrexial and blood gas analysis shows a marked metabolic acidosis.

What are the possible causes of these abnormalities?

- Pyrexia due to fits, or underlying cause, e.g. infection or drugs
- Metabolic acidosis due to continued seizures or due to a possible underlying cause such as a drug overdose, e.g. salicylates.

What important investigations would you want to do and what additional drug therapy would you want to give?

- CT scan preceding an LP
- Antibiotics to cover possible infection, e.g. cefotaxime.

A decision is undertaken to intubate and ventilate this patient; this is undertaken successfully. He is transferred for a CT scan prior to the critical care unit.

CT shows hydrocephalus and a shunt in situ which had not been noted on general examination and he is transferred to the regional neurosurgical unit. LP is not undertaken due to the presence of hydrocephalus and flucloxacillin is given due to the possibility of a shunt-related infection.

He is therefore transferred to the critical care unit pending transfer where an EEG shows continuing seizure activity despite maintenance of anaesthesia/sedation with a propofol infusion.

What drugs are available to you to terminate this man's seizures?

The usual next step would be thiopental sodium to achieve burst suppression on EEG monitoring which would necessitate ventilation in ITU.

CASE 9.7

A 35-year-old alcoholic is brought to the emergency department in status epilepticus. His seizures settle after two doses of IV lorazepam and a phenytoin infusion. As his seizures settle, a blood gas is taken which shows a profound metabolic acidosis. Medical records show he has recently attended the emergency department after an assault six days previously. List the possible causes for this man's seizures.

Answer
- Alcohol withdrawal seizures
- Subdural haematoma
- Drug overdose, e.g. amitriptyline
- Methanol poisoning
- Meningitis
- Previous epilepsy unrelated to alcohol.

ACUTE NEUROLOGICAL DEFICIT ('STROKE' OR CEREBROVASCULAR DISEASE)

Background

Stroke is a syndrome defined by the acute onset of focal (or global) loss of cerebral function lasting more than 24 h (or less if death results), owing to a vascular cause. A transient ischemic attack (TIA) is defined as 'a brief episode of neurological dysfunction caused by focal brain or retinal ischemia, with clinical symptoms typically lasting less than 1 h, and without evidence of acute infarction'.

Stroke disease is a huge problem. It affects approximately 200 people per 100 000 population per annum in the UK. Its incidence increases markedly with increasing age and it occurs more commonly in men. It is associated with both a high mortality, with 20% of patients dying within 30 days of their first stroke, and a high morbidity with 30% of stroke patient survivors being disabled and dependent at 1 year.

Traditionally, stroke has been regarded as less of an emergency than other illnesses, such as myocardial infarction, owing perhaps to the lack of therapeutic options. With the advent of ready access to imaging and the emergence of effective new treatments, TIAs and stroke should be regarded as medical and neurological emergencies for which rapid assessment, diagnosis and treatment should occur.

The majority of strokes (70%) are due to thromboembolic disease of cerebral vessels, with the majority of thromboembolic strokes being due to atherothromboembolism from extracranial large vessels; 25% are due to intracranial small vessel disease, 20% to cardiac disease and 5% to other rarer causes.

Haemorrhagic stroke, accounting for 15% of strokes, is due to small vessel disease and underlying hypertension. Five percent of strokes are due to SAH.

Diagnosis

By its very definition, stroke may present with any neurological symptom or sign. In making a diagnosis of stroke, it is useful to establish that signs or symptoms are of sudden onset, focal in nature and maximal over minutes to hours, as well as attempting to establish the area of brain affected. A non-vascular cause is suggested if these conditions are not met, there are no vascular risk factors present and the patient is relatively young. Diagnosis may be difficult especially if presentation is atypical, e.g. stroke presenting with seizures, altered consciousness level or confusional state. There is no accurate clinical method of distinguishing between an ischaemic thrombo-embolic stroke, a haemorrhagic stroke or stroke due to other causes.

Stroke may lead to a range of systemic changes in both the short and long term that affect outcome:

- Hyperglycaemia – this may reflect the presence of underlying diabetes or reflect a stress response secondary to the stroke. Evidence suggests that a raised blood sugar is predictive of a poor outcome.
- Hyperpyrexia – this may be due to infection or be a consequence of the stroke where its presence is predictive of a poor outcome. It could also be a clue as to the cause of the stroke, e.g. infective endocarditis.
- Hypertension – this may be causal or result from the stroke.
- Loss of swallowing reflexes which leads to aspiration and possible poor hydration and nutrition.
- Increased risk of deep venous thrombosis and pulmonary embolus.

Management

The critical care team may be involved in the resuscitative phase; stroke patients may have a threatened airway due to a reduced consciousness level and/or loss of protective airway reflexes, breathing difficulties due to an aspiration pneumonia or circulatory difficulties due, for example, to a marked increase in blood pressure. In addition, input may be needed during CT scanning, and emerging therapies for stroke may necessitate management in a critical care area for cerebral oedema or the use of thrombolytic drugs.

Acute neurological deficit

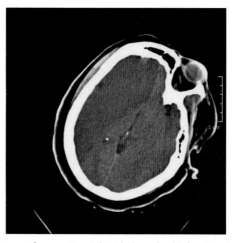

Figure 9.10 CT scan of a massive right-sided cerebral infarction due to carotid artery occlusion.

The treatment of stroke is rapidly changing and ideally a specialist multidisciplinary stroke team should manage patients. Admission to specialist stroke services has been proven to improve outcomes.

A CT scan should be performed ideally within 24 h to distinguish between occlusive (Fig. 9.10) and haemorrhagic strokes and to exclude conditions mimicking stroke. This scan should take place earlier if the patient has a severe headache, is on anticoagulants, has a bleeding tendency, an altered level of consciousness or other signs and symptoms suggestive of a non-vascular cause, e.g. neck stiffness, fever, papilloedema, fluctuating symptoms.

Patients with a TIA should ideally be seen and investigated in a specialist neurovascular clinic within seven days. If a patient has more than one TIA in a week, they should be admitted immediately to hospital for further care.

TIA and stroke patients (once a haemorrhagic event has been excluded) should be commenced on antiplatelet agents. Recent guidelines have stated that to prevent recurrent TIAs as well as strokes (and other occlusive vascular events), the combination of aspirin and modified release dipyrimadole should be prescribed. For those patients intolerant of aspirin, clopidogrel alone should be prescribed.

In addition to antiplatelet drugs, more simple measures for the treatment of acute stroke have been proven to be effective. Acute stroke units with ready access to services such as physiotherapy, speech therapy and occupational therapy are of proven benefit.

Abnormal blood sugars should be corrected, the patient adequately hydrated, paracetamol given for raised temperatures, thromboembolism prevented and the swallowing reflexes assessed. Longer-term risk factors such as hypertension should also be corrected.

A cause for the stroke must be looked for and an ECG, CXR, and blood tests including FBC, urea and electrolytes, a clotting screen, ESR and CRP are all routine. An ultrasound scan of the neck vessels may be necessary to assess a patient's suitability for a carotid endarterectomy as well as a transthoracic or transoesophageal echo to look for intracardiac thrombus or patent foramen ovale.

The use of thrombolysis is not yet part of UK routine practice and is limited to specialized stroke research centres. Studies so far have shown benefit for particular subtypes of stroke especially if given within 3 h of the onset of stroke. Further trials are ongoing to demonstrate the efficacy of stroke thrombolysis and its application to stroke management outwith specialist centres.

The use of heparin, either intravenous or subcutaneous low molecular weight heparin (LMWH), has not been shown to be of benefit if started early for the treatment of acute ischaemic stroke (they do, however, reduce the increased risk of deep vein thrombosis (DVT) or pulmonary embolism (PE) associated with stroke). Some physicians do prescribe heparin for specific indications including basilar artery thrombosis, where stroke is due to intracardiac thrombus or if there is an evolving CT proven ischaemic stroke thought to be due to ongoing thromboembolism. The evidence for such an approach is lacking.

Surgery may be an option for selected patients with haemorrhagic stroke, however, the neurosurgical management of patients with intracerebral haemorrhage varies widely with there being no good evidence for improved outcomes after surgery.

The treatment of raised blood pressure in the acute phase of stroke is a difficult area. Blood pressure is raised following a stroke and there is no good evidence to guide treatment. Concern is due to the potential loss of cerebral autoregulation of blood flow following a stroke and perfusion of the ischaemic brain being directly dependent on an adequate systemic blood pressure – if this is lowered, the ischaemic brain is inadequately perfused and the infarct size is increased. Treatment of raised blood pressure should therefore only be undertaken when it is likely to be harmful, e.g. hypertensive encephalopathy.

ACUTE RESPIRATORY FAILURE DUE TO NEUROMUSCULAR DISEASE

Neuromuscular diseases occasionally present with acute respiratory failure either de novo or through deterioration of pre-existing neuromuscular disease. All neuromuscular diseases have the potential to cause acute respiratory failure hence their relevance to critical care. Respiratory failure develops either through respiratory muscle weakness or paralysis resulting in hypoventilation or through the failure of protective airway reflexes leading to airway obstruction and/or pulmonary aspiration or super-added infection (Table 9.9).

The incidence of acute respiratory failure varies according to the disease process, e.g. approximately 15–20% of patients presenting acutely with Guillain-Barré require ventilation.

The decision to initiate mechanical ventilation will depend upon an accurate clinical assessment, in particular to the underlying diagnosis if

Table 9.9 Causes of neuromuscular weakness potentially leading to acute respiratory failure

Central	Spinal cord	Peripheral neuropathies	Disorders of neuromuscular transmission	Disorders of muscle
Drugs, e.g. opiates	Cord compression	Guillain-Barré syndrome	Myasthenia gravis	Hypokalaemia
Central transtentorial herniation	Motor neuron disease	Critical illness polyneuropathy	Botulism	Polymyositis
Metabolic disorders	Tumours	Poisons, e.g. organophosphates	Hypermagnesaemia	Rhabdomyolysis
Vascular (infarction, haemorrhage)	Poliomyelitis Transverse myelitis	and heavy metals Diptheria	Envenomations Drugs, e.g. anticholinesterase	Hypo-phosphataemia Acid maltase deficiency
Tumours		Chronic idiopathic	overdose	
Motor neuron disease		demyelinating polyneuropathy	Eaton-Lambert Syndrome	
Infection		(CIDP)		
Extrinsic compression		Lymphoma Drugs, e.g. vincristine Metabolic		

known, the speed of progression of muscular weakness and the wishes of the patient, particularly for those with pre-existing, long-standing, neuromuscular disease.

The patient with muscle weakness and imminent respiratory failure will appear exhausted and is likely to be unable to talk other than in short sentences with a rapid shallow respiratory pattern using the accessory muscles of respiration. Whilst clinical assessment is important, it must be recognized that it may be misleading and falsely reassuring. Although the respiratory rate will probably be raised, patients may present in acute respiratory failure with a normal or slow respiratory rate. Oxygen saturations and carbon dioxide levels may also be misleading, as they are poor late indicators of acute respiratory failure and the need for critical care intervention.

For these reasons, the forced vital capacity used in conjunction with the patient's clinical state is perhaps the best method to decide upon the need for mechanical ventilation. If the FVC falls below 15 mL/kg, ventilation should be initiated. Therefore, frequent regular monitoring of the FVC is critically important for any patient with muscle weakness presenting as an emergency. Measurement of the FEV1 may not be possible in the acute situation; it would therefore seem reasonable to use the PEFR as a proxy for the FEV1, although no data based on the PEFR is available as to when ventilation should be initiated.

If there is any doubt as to the presence or absence of acute respiratory failure or the ability of the patient to protect the airway, the patient should be transferred to and monitored in a critical care area.

Guillain-Barré syndrome is an acute peripheral neuropathy, the most common subtype being an inflammatory demyelinating polyradiculoneuropathy. It presents with progressive weakness over a number of days to weeks. Diagnosis can be made by examination of the CSF which shows a typically elevated CSF protein content, and through neurophysiological studies. Specific treatment, aside from acute respiratory failure, is by intravenous immunoglobulin therapy or plasma exchange. Prophylaxis of thromboembolism, pain management and urinary catheterization are important. Despite advances in therapy, 5–10% of patients die, with deaths due to respiratory failure, cardiovascular failure and thromboembolism. Up to 20% of patients are disabled.

Myasthenia gravis is an autoimmune disorder characterized by antibodies that act against the acetylcholine receptor of the neuromuscular junction. It presents with (fluctuating) fatiguable muscular weakness. Diagnosis is made by detecting the presence of antibodies against the acetylcholine receptor, neurophysiological studies and, less commonly, the use of edrophonium (Tensilon test). Treatment includes pyridostigmine, steroids, steroid-sparing agents and thymectomy in select cases. Acute respiratory failure may develop with a myasthenic crisis precipitated by infection or surgery as well as through cholinergic drug excess.

Critical care polyneuropathy is a polyneuropathy of uncertain aetiology and variable recovery, occurring in patients who have been critically ill. Many drugs and factors have been implicated as possible causes, but sepsis and the use of inotropes is almost universal. Although presenting as a tetraparesis following recovery on the critical care unit, recovery can be complete.

SPINAL CORD DISEASE

Background

The spinal cord may be injured by a number of traumatic and non-traumatic processes that may present acutely or subacutely. All of these processes may lead to acute respiratory failure if the level of spinal cord damage involves the nerves that supply the respiratory muscles.

In addition, spinal cord damage at any level may result in a need for critical intervention for control of the ABC, transport and specific therapies.

It is important to realize that failure of prevention of secondary injury of the spinal cord, similar to secondary injury of the brain, may result from poor management of the ABC. It can easily be imagined that failure to perform simple manoeuvres such as provision of oxygen and maintenance of the airway may be sufficient to cause secondary injury of the spinal cord, resulting in a dependent existence for a patient who might otherwise have become relatively independent.

The symptoms and signs of a patient with a spinal cord injury will vary depending on the underlying cause and level at which the cord is injured but will involve a particular combination of:

- back pain
- motor deficit
- sensory deficit
- abnormal reflexes
- urinary dysfunction.

Whilst a number of classic syndromes or patterns of spinal cord injury are recognized, patients almost never present with precise combinations of motor and sensory symptoms. Both the history and in particular the neurological examination may be baffling and inconsistent. Spinal cord disease is therefore frequently overlooked or misdiagnosed, with patients potentially being labelled as 'hysterical', or inappropriately observed, delaying referral for definitive diagnosis and management. All complaints possibly related to the spinal cord should therefore be treated seriously with appropriate emergent investigation.

Management

Initial investigation will be with plain films of the spine that are of particular use in patients with trauma or suspected malignancy or infection. CT scanning delineates bony pathology and soft tissue abnormalities as well as narrowing of the spinal canal. Imaging of the spinal cord requires MRI.

Additional non-radiological investigations of potential use are full blood count, ESR/CRP and blood cultures as well as more specialized blood tests for particular diseases such as systemic lupus erythematosus (SLE) and X-rays, e.g. to detect a primary malignancy.

Management of the spinal cord injury itself should include maintenance of the ABC, stabilization of the spine as necessary and the provision of analgesia, as well as prevention of thromboembolism, temperature control, hydration, pressure area care and urinary catheterization. Further treatment will depend upon the underlying pathology.

Neoplasms

These are predominantly found in the thoracic spine (70%), are frequently non-contiguous and are more likely to be metastatic in origin. Although frequently presenting as an emergency, a detailed history can often reveal a process that has been developing over a number of weeks, with pain as a central early component and bladder involvement as a late component. Decompression or radiotherapy as well as steroids may be of use.

Trauma

The clinical context suggests this diagnosis. 15% of patients have an injury at more than one level of the spine. Spinal shock is due to transection of the cord resulting in a flaccid paralysis with absent reflexes below the level of the injury of varying duration. Similar to brain injuries, it is important to maintain the ABC to prevent secondary injury of the cord. Spinal cord injury itself may cause hypotension through loss of sympathetic innervation of the blood vessels and heart, resulting in a shocked patient with warm peripheries, a slow pulse and little response to intravenous fluids (i.e. neurogenic shock). Invasive monitoring and the use of vasopressors (e.g. ephedrine) may be required. The use of intravenous steroids for the treatment of traumatic spinal cord injury continues to be debated.

Degenerative disease

Disc herniation leading to a central cord syndrome is an emergency that again is frequently overlooked. Red flags for this condition are severe low back pain with unilateral or bilateral sciatica, bladder or bowel dysfunction, anaesthesia or paraesthesia in the perineal or buttock region, lower limb weakness, sexual dysfunction and gait disturbance. Treatment is surgical decompression.

Multiple sclerosis

This is a chronic demyelinating disease affecting the brain and spinal cord, particularly in the cervical region. Therapy includes steroids, other immunosuppressive therapy and plasmapheresis.

Transverse myelitis

This is an inflammatory condition affecting the whole cross-section of the spinal cord at a particular level of the cord, interfering with all neurological function distal to the level affected. It is commonly associated with diseases such as systemic lupus erythematosus, sarcoidosis, acquired immune deficiency syndrome (AIDS) and multiple sclerosis.

Infection

This may be of the structures surrounding the cord such as osteomyelitis of the vertebral bodies, pedicles or laminae, or a discitis, as well as infections within the spinal canal such as an epidural abscess. Severe pain localized to the level of infection is a characteristic of this condition and may be elicited by tapping over the spine. Antibiotics and possible surgical management will be needed.

Vascular injury

- Spinal cord infarction resulting from hypoperfusion of the cord, thrombosis or embolism. There is sudden progressive development of neurological deficits, in particular weakness with associated loss of touch and temperature sensations and loss of bladder and bowel control. Therapy is supportive.
- Haemorrhage into the epidural, subdural and subarachnoid spaces or into the cord parenchyma characterized by sudden onset of severe back

pain with progressive development of neurological deficits. Treatment may require neurosurgical intervention.

REFERENCES AND FURTHER READING

AHA/ASA (American Heart Association and American Stroke Association) 2005 Scientific statement guidelines for the early management of patients with ischaemic stroke. Stroke 36:916

Albers G W, Caplan L R, Easton J D et al 2002 Transient ischemic attack – proposal for a new definition. New England Journal of Medicine 347:1713–1716

Alldredge B K, Gelb A M, Isaacs S M et al 2001 A comparison of lorazepam, diazepam, and placebo for the treatment of out-of-hospital status epilepticus. New England Journal of Medicine 345(9):631–637

Appleton R, Martland T, Phillips B 2003 Drug management for acute tonic clonic convulsions including convulsive status epilepticus in children. Cochrane Review in the Cochrane Library, Issue 3

Archer B D 1993 Computed tomography before lumbar puncture in acute meningitis: a review of the risks and benefits. Canadian Medical Association Journal 148:961–965

Armon C, Evans R W 2005 Addendum to assessment: Prevention of post-lumbar puncture headaches. Report of the Therapeutics and Technology Assessment Subcommittee of the American Academy of Neurology. Neurology 65:510–512

Attia J, Hatala R, Cook D J et al 1999 The rational clinical examination: does this patient have acute meningitis? Journal of the American Medical Association 282(2):175–181

Bamford J, Sandercock P, Dennis M et al 1991 Classification and natural history of clinically identifiable subtypes of cerebral infarction. Lancet 337:1521–1526

Bateman D 2001 Neurological assessment of coma. Journal of Neurology, Neurosurgery and Psychiatry 71(suppl l):i13–i17

Bates D 2001 The prognosis of medical coma. Journal of Neurology, Neurosurgery and Psychiatry 71:20–23

Begg N, Cartwright K A V, Cohen J et al 1999 Consensus statement on diagnosis, investigation, treatment and prevention of acute bacterial meningitis in immunocompetent adults. Journal of Infection 39:1–15

British Geriatric Society. Clinical guidelines for the diagnosis and management of delirium. Online. Available: http://www.bgs.org.uk

Broderick J P, Adams H P Jr, Barsan W et al 1999 Guidelines for the management of spontaneous intracerebral hemorrhage: a statement for healthcare professionals from a special writing group of the Stroke Council, American Heart Association. Stroke 30:905–915

Calssen J, Hirsch L J, Emerson R G et al 2002 Treatment of refractory status epilepticus with pentobarbital, propofol or midazolam: a systematic review. Epilepsia 43:146–153

CRSGBSIC (Cerebral Resuscitation Study Group of the Belgian Society for Intensive Care) 1988 Predictive value of the Glasgow Coma Score for awakening after out-of-hospital cardiac arrest. Lancet 1:137–140

Davenport R 2002 Acute headache in the emergency department. Journal of Neurology, Neurosurgery and Psychiatry 72:33–37

Edlow J A, Caplan L R 2000 Avoiding pitfalls in the diagnosis of sub-arachnoid haemorrhage. New England Journal of Medicine 342:29–36

Gabbe B J, Cameron P A, Finch C F 2003 The status of the Glasgow Coma Scale. Emergency Medicine 15(4):353–360

Gentleman D, Jennett B 1981 Hazards of inter-hospital transfer of comatose head-injured patients. Lancet 2(8251):853–854

Goldstein L B, Simel D L 2005 Is this patient having a stroke? Journal of the American Medical Association 293:2391–2402

Hasbun R, Abrahams J, Jekel J et al 2001 Computed tomography of the head before lumbar puncture in adults with suspected meningitis. New England Journal of Medicine 345:1727–1733

Heyderman R S, Lamber H P, O'Sullivan I et al 2003 Early management of suspected bacterial meningitis and meningococcal septicaemia in adults. Journal of Infection 46:75–77

Hill M D, Buchan A M for The Canadian Alteplase for Stroke Effectiveness Study (CASES) Investigators 2005 Thrombolysis for acute ischemic stroke: results of the Canadian Alteplase for Stroke Effectiveness Study. Canadian Medical Association Journal 172:1307–1312

Hogan Q H 1998 Epidural anatomy: new observations. Canadian Journal of Anaesthesia 45:R40–48

Holtkamp M, Masuhr F, Harms L et al 2003 The management of convulsive and complex partial status epilepticus in three European countries: a survey among epileptologists and critical care neurologists. Journal of Neurology, Neurosurgery and Psychiatry 74:1095–1099

Jorgensen E O, Malcohw-Moller A 1981 Natural history of global and critical brain ischaemia. Resuscitation 9:133–191

Leppik I E, Derivan A T, Homan R W et al 1995 The intensive care treatment of convulsive status epilepticus in the UK. Results of a national survey and recommendations. Anaesthesia 50:130–135

Levy D E, Bates D, Carona J J et al 1981 Prognosis in non-traumatic coma. Annals of Internal Medicine 94:293–301

Liebenberg W A, Worth R, Firth G B et al 2005 Aneurysmal SAH: guidance in making the correct diagnosis. Postgraduate Medical Journal 81:470–473

Linn F H H, Rinkel G J E, Algra A et al 2000 The notion of 'warning leaks' in sub-arachnoid haemorrhage: are such patients in fact admitted with a rebleed? Journal of Neurology, Neurosurgery and Psychiatry 68:332–336

Maurice-Williams R S, Richardson P L 1988 Spinal cord compression: delay in the diagnosis and referral of a common neurosurgical emergency. British Journal of Neurosurgery 2:55–60

Mendelow A D, Gregson B A, Fernandes H M et al; STITCH Investigators 2005 Early surgery versus initial conservative management in patients with spontaneous intracerebral haematomas in the International Surgical Trial in Intracerebral Haemorrhage (STITCH) a randomised trial. Lancet 365:387–397

Mills K R 2005 The basics of electromyography. Journal of Neurology, Neurosurgery and Psychiatry 76:32–35

National Institute for Health and Clinical Excellence 2003 Guidelines. Triage, assessment, investigation and early management of head injury in infants, children and adults. National Institute for Health and Clinical Excellence. Online. Available: http://www.nice.org.uk

National Institute for Health and Clinical Excellence 2005 Guidelines. Clopidogrel and dipyrimadole for the prevention of atherosclerotic events. National Institute for Health and Clinical Excellence. Online. Available: http://www.nice.org.uk

Neil-Dwyer G, Lang D 1997 'Brain attack' – aneurysmal subarachnoid haemorrhage: death due to delayed diagnosis. Journal of the Royal College of Physicians London 31:49–52

Newman DH 2004 Clinical assessment of meningitis in adults. Annals of Emergency Medicine 44:71–73

Ninis N, Phillips C, Bailey L et al 2005 The role of healthcare delivery in the outcome of meningococcal disease in children: case-control study of fatal and non-fatal cases. BMJ 330:1475–1478

Oostenbrink R, Moons K G, Theunissen C C et al 2001 Signs of meningeal irritation in the emergency department: how often bacterial meningitis? Pediatric Emergency Care 17(3):161–164

Richards P J 2005 Cervical spine clearance: a review. Injury 36(2):248–269

Rinkel G J E, Feigin V L, Algra A et al 2005 Calcium antagonists in aneurysmal subarachnoid haemorrhage. Stroke 36:1816–1817

Rinkel G J E, Feigin V L, Algra A et al 2005 Hypervolaemia in aneurysmal subarachnoid haemorrhage. Stroke 36:1104–1105

Rothwell P, Giles M, Flossman E et al 2005 A simple score to identify individuals at high early risk of stroke after transient ischaemic attack. Lancet 366(9479):29–36

Sandercock P, Counsell C, Stobbs S L 2005 Low-molecular weight heparins or heparinoids versus standard unfractionated heparin for acute ischaemic stroke. The Cochrane Database of Systematic Reviews, Issue 3

Seger D L 2004 Flumazenil – treatment or toxin. Journal of Toxicology. Clinical Toxicology 42(2):209–216

Shaner D M, McCurdy S A, Herring M O et al 1988 Treatment of status epilepticus: a prospective comparison of diazepam and phenytoin versus phenobarbital and optional phenytoin. Neurology 38(2):202–207

Steinera I, Budkab H, Chaudhuric A et al 2005 Viral encephalitis: a review of diagnostic methods and guidelines for management. European Journal of Neurology 12:1–13

Stroke Unit Trialists' Collaboration 2000 Organised inpatient (stroke unit) care for stroke. The Cochrane Library, Issue 1

Teasdale G, Jennett W B 1974 Assessment of coma and impaired consciousness: a practical scale. Lancet ii:81–84

The Intercollegiate Stroke Working Party 2004 National clinical guidelines for stroke, 2nd edn. Royal College of Physicians, London

Thomas K E, Hasbun R, Jekel J et al 2002 The diagnostic accuracy of Kernig's sign, Brudzinski's sign and nuchal rigidity in adults with suspected meningitis. Clinical Infectious Diseases 35:46–52

Thomas S R, Jamieson D R S, Muir K W 2000 Randomised controlled trial of atraumatic versus standard needles for diagnostic lumbar puncture. BMJ 321:986–990

Treiman D M, Meyers P D, Walton N Y et al 1998 A comparison of four treatments for generalized convulsive status epilepticus. Veterans Affairs Status Epilepticus Cooperative Study Group. New England Journal of Medicine 339(12):792–798

Tunkel A R, Hartman B J, Kaplan S K et al 2004 Practice guidelines for the management of bacterial meningitis. Clinical Infectious Diseases 39:1267–1284

Van de Beek D, de Gans J, Spanjaard L et al 2004 Clinical features and prognostic factors in adults with bacterial meningitis. New England Journal of Medicine 351:1849–1859

Van de Berghe G, Wouters P, Weekers F et al 2001 Intensive insulin therapy in the critically ill patient. New England Journal of Medicine 345(19):1359–1367

Van der Wee N, Rinkel G J, Hasan D et al 1995 Detection of sub-arachnoid haemorrhage on early CT: is lumbar puncture still needed after a negative scan? Journal of Neurology, Neurosurgery and Psychiatry 58:357–359

Van Gijn 1999 Pitfalls in the diagnosis of sudden headache. Proceedings of the Royal College of Physicians Edinburgh 29:21–31

Vilches A, Narro M, Singh I 2005 Delirium in the elderly. British Journal of Hospital Medicine 66(8):474–476

Walker M C, Smith S J, Shorvon S D 1983 Double-blind study of lorazepam and diazepam in status epilepticus. Journal of the American Medical Association 249(11):1452–1454

Wardlaw J M, Sandercock P A G, Berge E 2003 Thrombolytic therapy with recombinant tissue plasminogen activator for acute ischaemic stroke. Stroke 34:1437–1432

Weir C J, Murray G D, Adams F G et al 1994 Poor accuracy of scoring systems for differential diagnosis of intracranial haemorrhage and infarction. Lancet 344:999–1002

Whitehead M A, McManus J, McAlpine C et al 2005 Early recurrence of cerebrovascular events after TIA. Stroke 36(1):1

Widjaja E, Salam S N, Griffiths P D et al 2005 Is the rapid assessment stroke clinic rapid enough in assessing transient ischaemic attack and minor stroke? Journal of Neurology, Neurosurgery and Psychiatry 76:145–146

Gastrointestinal emergencies

10

C.E. Johns

OBJECTIVES

After reading this chapter you should be able to:

- *Recognize the varied presentation of patients with gastrointestinal pathology*
- *Optimize initial treatment and resuscitation*
- *Understand the advantages of different imaging modalities*
- *Understand appropriate and timely surgical referral*
- *Understand the use of non-surgical interventions*

INTRODUCTION

The presentation of gastrointestinal pathology is often obvious, e.g. in a patient with witnessed haematemesis, but the signs and symptoms can be more subtle. Elderly patients are often particularly difficult to diagnose as they present more frequently with very non-specific complaints such as confusion or decreased mobility. Comorbidities such as cognitive impairment, diabetes or psychiatric illness can add to the difficulties of reaching a diagnosis. Prior treatment with steroids and antibiotics in hospital and in the community may also mask signs and symptoms.

Physicians are often also involved in the care of postoperative surgical patients when complications such as renal or respiratory failure prompt a referral, and treatment may include surgical intervention, e.g. sepsis caused by anastomotic leak.

Appropriate and timely treatment of patients with gastrointestinal pathology has a significant effect on prognosis. Urgent surgery or endoscopic therapy may be necessary. Radiological procedures are invaluable. This chapter will discuss the medical management of intra-abdominal sepsis, intestinal obstruction, perforation and ischaemia. Relevant aspects of liver failure, acute inflammatory bowel disease and gastrointestinal haemorrhage are also covered.

INTRA-ABDOMINAL SEPSIS AND PERFORATION

Intra-abdominal sepsis develops following obstruction, inflammation or perforation of the gastrointestinal tract. Abcesses can form as a result of local inflammation or perforation. Generalized peritonitis leads to abscess formation, usually in the subphrenic space, paracolic gutters and pelvis because of the effects of gravity and intra-abdominal pressure.

Biliary sepsis

Gallstone obstruction of the cystic duct causes acute cholecystitis which classically presents with right upper quadrant or epigastric pain, vomiting and fever. Common bile duct obstruction causes jaundice. Cholangitis occurs if the bile ducts become infected and the patient develops high fevers and rigors. Ultrasound is frequently sufficient to demonstrate gallstones and/or common bile duct dilatation. Magnetic resonance (MR) will give more detailed imaging of the bile ducts and can detect stones not seen at ultrasound. Broad-spectrum antibiotics are given, usually ciprofloxacin with or without metronidazole and the biliary obstruction relieved at endoscopic retrograde cholangiopancreatography (ERCP). Biliary sepsis can be associated with a degree of pancreatitis that may be exacerbated following ERCP and should be looked for. Percutaneous or surgical drainage should be considered if ERCP is unsuccessful. Biliary sepsis following gallstone impaction can occur with poorly localized pain or no pain. If a patient presents with sepsis without an obvious source or pyrexia of unknown origin, an abdominal ultrasound is frequently useful to detect biliary dilatation and gallstones.

Intra-abdominal abscess

Intra-abdominal abcesses may present with little abdominal pain, general malaise and anorexia. Patients will usually have a fever and often rigors. There may be nausea, vomiting and constipation or diarrhoea, and pain can be severe. Subphrenic abscesses are associated with dyspnoea, cough and chest or shoulder tip pain. Systemic sepsis leads to multiple organ failure. Renal or respiratory impairment may be the most obvious features of the patient's presentation. Paralytic ileus can develop. If there are features of systemic sepsis and other causes are excluded there must be a strong index of suspicion to reach the diagnosis of intra-abdominal abscess. When the diagnosis is suspected, abdominal imaging, usually computed tomography (CT), should be performed early so surgical or radiological drainage can be planned. Radiological drains are minimally invasive but have the disadvantage of a narrower lumen than those placed surgically. Broad-spectrum antibiotics should be prescribed. The abscess fluid should be cultured so that antibiotic therapy can be refined. Adequate fluid resuscitation is vital and if organ failure is developing the patient is best managed in a critical care environment. Early fluid resuscitation, antibiotic therapy, surgical or radiological drainage and nutritional support, preferably via the enteral route will improve outcome.

Intra-abdominal perforation

Perforation of an intra-abdominal viscus usually causes severe abdominal pain, although this can be poorly localized. The elderly, diabetics and those who have received prior treatment with steroids may present with little or no pain. Leakage of bowel fluids into the peritoneum causes peritonitis and abscess formation can occur. Patients become shocked with hypotension and tachycardia. Young patients can maintain their systolic blood pressure despite significant fluid loss and the presence of a postural drop in blood pressure is an important sign of fluid loss. Patients treated with beta-blockers may not develop a tachycardia despite hypotension. Fluid resuscitation will be inadequate if factors that mask the degree of shock are overlooked. The signs of peritonitis are a rigid abdomen and absent bowel sounds. Plain X-rays are frequently sufficient to detect an intestinal perforation. An abdominal X-ray may show Wriggler's sign (Fig. 10.1) and an erect chest X-ray (CXR) may show air under the diaphragm (Fig. 10.2). Wriggler's sign describes the presence of air outside the bowel lumen. This means that both sides of the bowel wall can be seen; normally only the inner wall is visible on X-ray.

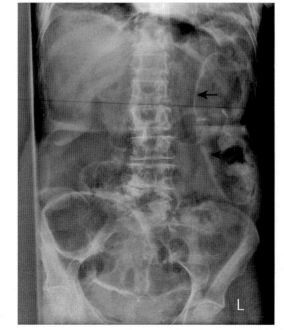

Figure 10.1   Wriggler's sign (arrowed) gas visible on both sides of the bowel wall. (Courtesy of Dr Anand Reddy).

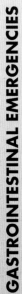

A

B

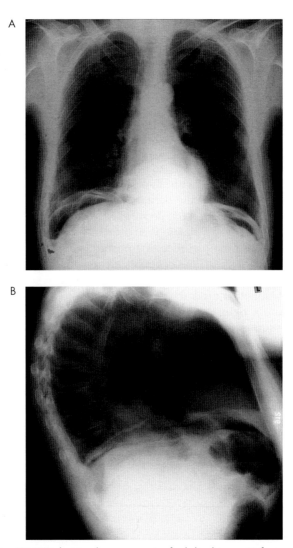

Figure 10.2 (A) CXR showing large amounts of subdiaphragmatic free gas indicating a perforated viscus. This patient had a perforated gastric ulcer in combination with a hiatus hernia as may be seen on the lateral CXR (B).

There are many causes of perforation. Peptic ulceration can lead to duodenal or, less commonly, gastric perforation. The gallbladder may perforate following empyema. Bowel perforation can be due to obstruction, diverticulitis, or appendicitis. Iatrogenic perforation can be caused be endoscopic procedures, particularly colonoscopy and ERCP. Placement of suprapubic catheters or ascitic drains can cause bowel trauma. Breakdown of a surgical anastomosis will present as a bowel perforation. It is vital to suspect an iatrogenic perforation if abdominal pain, hypotension or tachycardia occur after an invasive procedure. Chest and abdominal X-rays should be obtained.

If abscess formation is suspected in addition to perforation this may be seen on ultrasound, or CT scanning. The latter is more sensitive especially in cases of left-sided subphrenic abscess when the spleen, gas-filled stomach and splenic flexure make ultrasound more difficult. The retroperitoneal space is best imaged by CT scanning. Gas can sometimes be seen on abdominal X-ray outside the bowel lumen in retroperitoneal abcesses and the psoas muscle outline can be lost.

INTESTINAL OBSTRUCTION

Intestinal obstruction classically presents with abdominal pain, distension, vomiting and a lack of flatus per rectum. The vomiting may be bilious or faeculant depending on the level of the obstruction. However, high small bowel obstruction can present with vomiting alone. Partial obstruction may present with diarrhoea and vomiting which could be misinterpreted as gastroenteritis. Examination of the patient will sometimes reveal the cause of obstruction, e.g. a strangulated hernia, or give clues, e.g. scars suggesting that post-surgical adhesions could be the cause of the obstruction.

Plain supine abdominal X-ray will usually determine whether obstruction is present. In small bowel obstruction gas is present in the small bowel, which may be dilated. The small bowel usually lies centrally and has valvulae conniventes that completely encircle the bowel lumen. No gas is seen in the more peripheral large bowel. In large bowel obstruction no air is present in the rectum and the gas-filled bowel proximal to the blockage may be dilated. The large bowel haustra do not completely cross its lumen.

Causes of intestinal obstruction

Mechanical obstruction is normally associated with abdominal pain and active bowel sounds. Sigmoid volvulus and faeces cause large bowel obstruction. A preceding history of weight loss or rectal bleeding may raise the possibility of an obstructing colonic tumour. Small bowel obstruction is caused by hernia, Crohn's inflammatory mass, adhesions, and less frequently by tumour, foreign body ingestion, gallstone ileus or intussusception.

Functional obstruction is caused by ileus or pseudo-obstruction. In ileus the bowel is paralyzed with no pain and bowel sounds are absent. Causes include electrolyte disturbances including low potassium, magnesium and phosphate, surgery and intra-abdominal sepsis. Pseudo-obstruction resembles mechanical obstruction, but no cause is found. It is associated with anticholinergic drug use and recumbence.

Treatment of intestinal obstruction

Initial treatment of bowel obstruction is fluid resuscitation and electrolyte replacement. A nasogastric tube should be passed to avoid aspiration. Urgent surgery is required if the small bowel is obstructed by a strangulated hernia, to avoid gangrene. Large bowel obstruction with bowel dilatation of more than 8 cm also requires urgent surgical intervention to avoid caecal perforation which carries a high mortality. In less urgent cases of large bowel obstruction a water-soluble contrast enema is useful to distinguish mechanical and pseudo-obstruction. Pseudo-obstruction is managed conservatively and decompression with a colonoscope is useful. Volvulus usually has a classical X-ray appearance and responds to decompression with a flatus tube.

INTESTINAL ISCHAEMIA

Bowel ischaemia occurs when the superior or inferior mesenteric artery is blocked by thrombosis or emboli. Hypoperfusion, for example, due to hypotension or low output cardiac failure, also leads to ischaemia. Bowel infarction and gangrene then follow. Venous thrombosis can occur but is less common. The superior mesenteric artery and small bowel are more commonly affected by ischaemia.

Acute intestinal ischaemia

Acute intestinal ischaemia carries a mortality rate of 80%. It usually presents in older patients with sudden severe generalized abdominal pain. Bloody diarrhoea occurs if the inferior mesenteric artery is blocked. Patients often have diffuse abdominal tenderness which is followed by abdominal distension, absent bowel sounds and shock. Early in the presentation the patient is classically much more unwell than the physical signs suggest. There may be clues to the cause of this, such as atrial fibrillation. Investigations reveal a metabolic acidosis, elevated white cell count and the bowel may be dilated on abdominal X-ray. There is often mild pyrexia, tachycardia and a raised white cell count. Serum amylase may be mildly raised.

Chronic intestinal ischaemia

Chronic ischaemia usually affects the 'watershed' area at the splenic flexure and causes recurrent ischaemic colitis. Patients suffer from lower left-sided abdominal pain, particularly after eating, bloody diarrhoea and weight loss. Submucosal colonic oedema can be seen as 'thumbprinting' on barium enema and abdominal X-ray.

Treatment of intestinal ischaemia

The treatment of acute ischaemia requires fluid resuscitation, oxygen, and broad-spectrum antibiotics. The possibility of resecting the infarcted portion of bowel should be discussed when the diagnosis is suspected. Perioperative mortality is high as patients are extremely ill by the time they present and usually have comorbid disease, especially cardiovascular disease. If extensive bowel infarction has occurred, resection may be inappropriate as the condition is frequently fatal despite surgical intervention.

Ischaemic colitis usually responds to supportive therapy with fluids and antibiotics, although strictures can develop. Mesenteric 'angina' may respond to vascular surgical repair.

KEY POINT
- Symptoms of intra-abdominal pathology are often non-specific, especially in the elderly, diabetics and those who have received steroids, analgesia or antibiotics.

GASTROINTESTINAL HAEMORRHAGE

Upper gastrointestinal haemorrhage is a common cause for hospital admission. The mortality in patients admitted with acute upper gastrointestinal haemorrhage has been reported as 11%. Mortality is three-fold higher when gastrointestinal bleeding occurs in patients already in hospital with other diagnoses. Peptic ulceration is the commonest cause for upper gastrointestinal haemorrhage but other causes include gastric erosions, oesophagitis, varices, Mallory Weiss tear or malignancy.

Initial treatment of acute upper gastrointestinal bleeding is resuscitation. Adequate intravenous access must be obtained with two large bore (at least 16G) cannulae and fluid losses replaced. Saline or colloid may be used until cross-matched blood is available, unless the patient has liver failure, in which case saline should be avoided. Rarely the blood loss is severe enough to warrant the use of O negative blood. In less severe cases type-specific blood should be transfused if the haemoglobin is less than 10g/dL. Pulse, blood pressure and urine output must be monitored to ensure resuscitation is sufficient and to detect rebleeding early. The patient's haemoglobin must also be monitored closely so further blood loss is detected. Comorbidities such as heart failure or airways disease must be treated. Coagulopathies caused by comorbid disease or the use of anticoagulants must be reversed with vitamin K and/or fresh frozen plasma. Non-steroidal anti-inflammatory drugs must be stopped. It is important to identify patients with liver disease as they may be bleeding from oesophageal or gastric varices (see below).

Non-variceal upper gastrointestinal haemorrhage

Patients should be discussed with an endoscopist at an early stage so that endoscopic therapy can be performed. Haemostasis can be achieved at endoscopy with the injection of adrenaline (epinephrine), and application of heater probe or endoscopic clips. Endoscopy is safest when performed after adequate resuscitation, although when bleeding is severe this may not be possible. If the patient has severe blood loss, anaesthetic input is important and intubation should be considered pre-endoscopy to prevent pulmonary aspiration. Once the source of haemorrhage is known, appropriate medical therapy can be given. Intravenous proton pump inhibitor therapy reduces the risk of further bleeding from a peptic ulcer. More than 90% of duodenal ulcers are associated with *Helicobacter pylori* infection and eradication

Table 10.1 Rockall score

Score	0	1	2	3
Age	< 60	60–79	> 80	
Shock	None, systolic BP > 100, pulse < 100	Tachycardia pulse > 100, systolic BP > 100	Hypotension systolic BP < 100, pulse > 100	
Comorbidity	None		CCF, IHD, other major comorbidity	Renal failure, liver failure, disseminated malignancy
Endoscopic diagnosis	Mallory Weiss tear, no lesion	All other diagnoses	Upper gastrointestinal tract malignancy	
Stigmata of recent haemorrhage	None or dark spot		Blood in upper gastrointestinal tract, adherent clot visible of spurting vessel	

CCF – congestive cardiac failure, IHD – ischaemic heart disease

significantly reduces the risk of rebleeding. Proton pump inhibitors can be commenced prior to endoscopy but do not negate the need for a diagnostic and therapeutic endoscopic procedure.

The prognosis from acute upper gastrointestinal bleeding depends on the patient's age, comorbidities, degree of haemodynamic compromise and the cause of bleeding found at endoscopy. Rockall et al defined a scoring system that identifies those patients at high risk of dying from their gastrointestinal bleed (Table 10.1).

Patients with a Rockall score over 8 have a high risk of death, while those with a score of less than 3 have an extremely good prognosis. A modified Rockall score, without endoscopic findings, has been used to identify those who warrant urgent endoscopy but has not yet been validated.

An episode of rebleeding from a source other than varices requires repeat endoscopy. At this stage, further management should be discussed with the on-call surgical team. The patient's age, comorbid diseases and endoscopic findings will influence the decision to proceed to surgery or to continue with medical therapy. Anaesthetic review is necessary prior to surgery and is helpful at an earlier stage if haemodynamic compromise or poor oxygenation persist despite treatment.

Variceal haemorrhage

The blood loss in variceal haemorrhage is usually large and the overall mortality approaches 50%. The highest mortality is seen in patients with more advanced liver disease. Adequate fluid resuscitation and early endoscopy are necessary. Blood should be transfused with the aim of keeping the patient's haemoglobin above 9 mg/dL. Coagulopathy is corrected with intravenous vitamin K and fresh frozen plasma. Patients should be managed in a unit familiar with variceal haemorrhage.

Intubation prior to endoscopy is important if the patient has severe uncontrolled bleeding, severe encephalopathy, aspiration pneumonia or oxygen saturations below 90% despite oxygen therapy.

Oesophageal varices can be treated endoscopically by variceal banding. If this is not possible. injection sclerotherapy can be used. If adequate haemostasis cannot be achieved bleeding can be temporarily controlled with balloon tamponade. A Sengstaken tube should be passed via the mouth and into the stomach. The gastric balloon should be inflated and the tube put on traction. The oesophageal balloon should be inflated if the gastric balloon fails to control bleeding. Both balloons will cause pressure necrosis after 48 h and should be deflated to allow a further attempt at endoscopic therapy after 12 to 24 h. In uncontrolled variceal bleeding a transvenous interventional portosystemic shunt (TIPSS) can be performed and rapidly controls bleeding because of the reduction in portal pressure. Gastrooesophageal varices should be treated in the same manner as oesophageal varices. Haemorrhage from isolated gastric varices is more difficult to control endoscopically and rebleeding after injection sclerotherapy occurs in 50–90% of patients. Band ligation is not recommended. A Linton tube with a single large gastric balloon is more effective than a Sengstaken tube although these can be used. TIPSS or shunt surgery is frequently required for long-term control of haemorrhage from gastric varices.

How to insert a Sengstaken-Blakemore tube

Uncontrolled variceal bleeding can be stopped by inserting a Sengstaken-Blakemore tube. If the patient's consciousness level is impaired such that they cannot protect their airway, the airway should be secured with a cuffed endotracheal tube first. A known oesophageal stricture or recent oesophageal surgery increases the risk of oesophageal damage, but if bleeding is uncontrolled there may be no option but to insert the tube.

- The tube should be kept in the fridge; this makes it stiffer and easier to pass.
- Check the balloons are patent and identify the aspiration and inflation ports.
- Check you have:
  – 4 tube clamps (without serrated edges)
  – suction
  – a padded gag
  – 2 60 mL bladder syringes
  – 2 or 3 assistants.
- If a Sengstaken tube is placed after an endoscopy the patient will still be sedated which makes the procedure easier.

- Lubricate the Sengstaken tube and pass it via the mouth. The patient will usually vomit; have suction ready.
- Insert the tube to at least 60 cm and check it has not coiled in the mouth.
- Suction on the gastric aspiration port should produce blood if the tube is in the stomach.
- Inflate the gastric balloon with up to 300 mL of air or water. Clamp the inflation port.
- Stop and deflate the tube if inflation is difficult or if the patient develops pain.
- Pull the tube back until the resistance of the gastrooesophageal junction is felt.
- Or if you prefer, inflate to 100 mL and pull the tube back until the resistance is felt and then inflate further to reduce the risk of accidental inflation in the oesophagus.
- The position should be checked on CXR (Fig. 10.3). Traction should be provided by attaching a bag of fluid to the end of the tube (e.g. 500 mL).
- If it is necessary to inflate the oesophageal balloon (i.e. if haemorrhage continues) do so with air or water to a pressure of 40 mmHg and check the pressure hourly. Use a 3-way tap and a standard sphygmomanometer to do this. Some authorities recommend deflating the oesophageal balloon every 8 h for 30 min.
- Attach low pressure suction to the oesophageal aspiration port to prevent blocking.
- Document in the patient's notes the position of the tube and the volume and pressure in the balloons.
- The Sengstaken tube should not be inflated for more than 24 h and ideally less than 12 h. Definitive treatment (endoscopy or TIPPS) should be arranged prior to deflation of the tube.

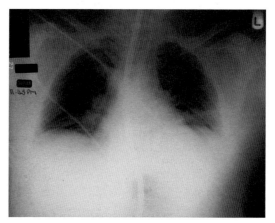

Figure 10.3 CXR with a Sengstaken-Blakemore tube in situ. Note the gastric balloon inflated in the stomach below the diaphragm.

Once endoscopic therapy has been performed the risk of rebleeding is reduced by medical therapy. Intravenous glypressin is given at a dose of 2 mg 6 hourly with high dose intravenous proton pump inhibitors, e.g. pantoprazole 40 mg 12 hourly and intravenous antibiotics. The reduction in bacterial infections with prophylactic antibiotics has been shown to improve short-term survival. The choice of antibiotic therapy will depend on local guidelines but cefuroxime or ciprofloxacin are frequently used. Repeat endoscopy should be performed after successful treatment of variceal haemorrhage so that varices can be obliterated by banding. Beta-blockers, usually propranolol at a dose of 40 or 80 mg twice daily, are used for primary and secondary prophylaxis of variceal bleeding. If band ligation and beta-blocker therapy cannot be used, isosorbide mononitrate 20 mg twice daily is used. Selective gut decontamination may also be considered.

Lower gastrointestinal haemorrhage

Lower gastrointestinal haemorrhage is frequently less severe than upper gastrointestinal haemorrhage and can settle spontaneously. Usually red blood is passed per rectum, but caecal bleeding can present as melaena and massive upper gastrointestinal bleeding can present as fresh red rectal bleeding.

The initial management is fluid resuscitation, blood transfusion and treatment of comorbidities including coagulopathy. If bleeding is uncontrolled the patient is best managed in a critical care unit but this is more commonly required in acute upper gastrointestinal bleeding. Haemostasis can be achieved endoscopically or angiographically and surgical intervention is rarely required.

Diverticular disease is the commonest cause of lower gastrointestinal haemorrhage. Other causes are colonic neoplasia and polyps, ischaemia, inflammatory or radiation-induced colitis, Meckel's diverticulum, aorto-enteric fistula and arteriovenous malformations. Bleeding can occur after colonoscopy particularly if polypectomy has been performed. Arteriovenous malformations include angiodysplasia and congenital malformations, e.g. in hereditary haemorrhagic telangiectasia (HHT), or Peutz-Jegher's syndrome. Portal colopathy and varices can occur in patients with portal hypertension.

Haemorrhoids cause rectal bleeding but this is rarely severe and obvious on examination. Surgical treatment, usually banding, is required.

Investigation and treatment of lower gastrointestinal haemorrhage

Colonoscopy is the investigation of choice if the patient can be stabilized. Bowel preparation is necessary but will increase the volume of fluid replacement required by the patient. Colonoscopy will be able to detect bleeding from diverticulae, colonic tumours, polyps and angiodysplasia. Endoscopic thermal treatment and adrenaline (epinephrine) injection can be performed. Bleeding is localized to the right colon in 60% of cases so colonoscopy is superior to sigmoidoscopy.

Gastrointestinal haemorrhage

Mesenteric angiography is the best investigation in an unstable patient and does not require bowel preparation. Digital subtraction angiography is used with glucagon to decrease peristalsis during episodes of bleeding and can detect bleeding that occurs at 0.5 mL/min or faster. The superior mesenteric artery is examined first as the right colon is more frequently the source of bleeding. The inferior mesenteric artery is then examined. If these examinations are negative the coeliac axis is catheterized to look for vascular anomalies such as a coeliac origin or the middle colic artery. This will also examine the arterial supply of the upper gastrointestinal tract. Embolization of the feeder artery can be performed using microcoils with or without polyvinyl alcohol or gelfoam. Superselective embolization is necessary as the colon and small bowel does not have an extensive collateral blood supply. Early use of non-selective embolization is associated with mesenteric ischaemia and bowel infarction.

Labelled red cell scans performed with radiolabelled technetium (^{99m}Tc) can accurately localize the site of active lower gastrointestinal bleeding. They have a sensitivity of 90% when more than 500 mL of blood is lost over 24 h. Atypical activity or a 'blush' is seen at the site of bleeding. An early blush suggests more rapid blood loss than a late blush and localization will guide angiographic therapy or, rarely, surgical resection.

Colonoscopy, angiography and ^{99m}Tc scintography scanning are useful in excluding the lower gastrointestinal tract as the source of bleeding and upper gastrointestinal endoscopy is frequently useful if lower gastro-intestinal investigations are negative. In stable patients, small bowel wireless capsule endoscopy will detect bleeding not found by upper and lower gastrointestinal investigation with a sensitivity of 50 to 70%. Meckel's diverticulae contain ectopic gastric mucosa which can bleed. They are detected using technetium-99m-pertechnetate scintiscanning which is taken up and excreted by gastric mucoid cells. Meckel's scintiscanning has a sensitivity of 80%. If the cause of gastrointestinal haemorrhage is difficult to detect, combined laparoscopic and endoscopic procedures may be required and blind right hemicolectomy is occa-sionally performed if blood loss is life-threatening with no identifiable source.

FULMINANT LIVER FAILURE

Acute liver failure is defined as rapidly developing synthetic liver failure. Coagulopathy occurs and, in later stages, hepatic encephalopathy. Patients can decompensate very quickly with multiorgan failure and specialist hepatology advice and critical care review is extremely important. Acute liver failure has been subdivided on the time interval from onset of jaundice to the development of encephalopathy. In hyperacute liver failure, encephalo-pathy develops within a week of jaundice. The interval in acute liver failure is 8 to 28 days and in subacute liver failure, 4 to 12 weeks. The incidence of cerebral oedema is higher in hyperacute liver failure but the prognosis is better than in subacute liver failure.

Causes of acute liver failure

The commonest cause for hyperacute liver failure in the UK is paracetamol overdose. Jaundice and encephalopathy usually occur at least 48 h after the ingestion of tablets. Hepatitis B and A are the commonest viral infections causing acute liver failure. Hepatitis D is only pathogenic as a co-infection with hepatitis B and increases the risk of fulminant liver failure. Cytomegalovirus, Epstein-Barr virus, herpes simplex virus and hepatitis viruses E, and less commonly C, have also been demonstrated to lead to acute liver failure. Idiosyncratic drug reactions can result in liver damage. Chlorinated hydrocarbons found in industrial cleaning agents are hepatotoxic as are toxins present in *amanita* or *galerina* mushrooms. In a significant proportion of patients, no causal agent will be found.

Chronic liver diseases present as subacute liver failure rather than liver failure, with a short interval between jaundice and encephalopathy. Causes include autoimmune liver disease hepatitis, Wilson's disease, alcoholic liver disease and non-alcoholic fatty liver disease, or steatohepatitis. Ischaemic damage caused by hypotension or low cardiac output and venous occlusion can also lead to liver injury.

Treatment of acute liver failure

Supportive medical therapy involves fluid management, monitoring and treatment of hypoglycaemia and electrolyte disturbance. Severe metabolic acidosis should be corrected with continuous veno-venous haemofiltration (CVVH) if necessary. Intravenous dextrose is used as fluid replacement and saline should not be given. An aggressive search for infection must be performed and should include blood cultures, mid-stream urine, CXR, and ascitic tap if ascites is present. Broad-spectrum antibiotics should be given if there is evidence of infection. Antifungal therapy should also be considered.

It is important to prevent gastrointestinal bleeding as this represents a protein load to the gut. Proton pump inhibitors should be used and coagulopathy can be corrected with vitamin K (10 mg intravenously for 3 days), platelets and fresh frozen plasma if there is active bleeding. Coagulopathy will also need to be corrected prior to invasive procedures, e.g. central line insertion. Potentially hepatotoxic drugs must be withdrawn. B vitamins should be replaced with intravenous pabrinex in those who drink alcohol to excess.

Complications of liver failure

Hepatic encephalopathy carries a very poor prognosis. Preventative treatment with lactulose, enemas and gut decontamination should be commenced, with the aim of ensuring that the patient passes 2–3 soft stools per day. If the patient cannot take lactulose orally it should be given via a nasogastric tube. Patients with grade 2 encephalopathy should be observed in a critical care unit. If grade 3 or 4 encephalopathy is present lactulose and gut decontamination will not improve consciousness level. The patient

KEY POINTS

Grades of encephalopathy

1 Mild confusion, sleep disturbance, personality change
2 Drowsiness, disorientation, short attention span
3 Sleepy but arousable, gross disorientation
4a Coma, arousable by pain
4b Unresponsive

should be intubated and intracerebral pressure monitoring considered. Sepsis, dehydration, electrolyte disturbance, gastrointestinal haemorrhage and uraemia can all precipitate encephalopathy and should be treated. Sedative drugs must be withdrawn.

Cerebral oedema is seen most frequently in hyperacute liver failure. Hyperventilation, muscular rigidity, systemic hypertension and abnormal papillary reflexes develop. If untreated, worsening cerebral oedema will cause decerebrate posturing. Hypoxia, hypoglycaemia, and hypercapnia must be corrected to treat cerebral oedema. The patient should be nursed with the head of the bed raised at 10% and with minimal tactile and auditory stimulation. Mannitol should be given intravenously in a bolus dose of 0.5 mg/kg until cerebral perfusion pressure improves. If repeated doses are required it is necessary to monitor plasma osmolality to prevent a significant hyperosmolar state developing. If renal failure is present, haemofiltration is required in addition to mannitol therapy for this to be effective. Hyperventilation can be helpful in advanced coma. Cerebral oedema is the commonest cause of death in fulminant liver failure.

Renal failure is frequently seen in association with acute liver failure. Patients require fluid replacement if hypovolaemic, and central venous pressure monitoring is extremely useful to guide this as patients may be intravascularly depleted but may be fluid overloaded with significant peripheral oedema. Once the patient's circulation is well filled, intravenous glypressin (0.5–2 mg every 6 hours) and albumin infusions have been shown to improve prognosis. If ascites is present, paracentesis of 2–4 L will improve renal perfusion. Haemofiltration can be used prior to transplantation. Respiratory failure may be due to infection, aspiration pneumonia, pulmonary haemorrhage or acute respiratory distress syndrome (ARDS) and will require ventilation in addition to antibiotic therapy.

Specific medical therapy for the underlying cause of liver failure

N-acetyl cysteine is the antidote for paracetamol poisoning and is given at a dose of 150 mg/kg in 200 mL 5% dextrose over 15 min followed by 50 mg/kg in 500 mL over 4 h and then 100mg/kg in 1 L over 16 h. If the patient has a hypersensitivity reaction to N-acetyl cysteine, oral methionine is the alternative which is given at a dose of 2.5 g every 4 h to reach a total dose of 10 g. Both antidotes are effective if given within 12 h of paracetamol ingestion and N-acetyl cysteine can be effective up to 24 h after overdose. *The hepato-protective effects of N-acetyl cysteine have also led to it being administered in other causes of hepatic failure and this option should be discussed with a hepatologist.*

The criteria for transfer to a specialist liver unit following paracetamol overdose are:

- prothrombin time (PT) > 50 s
- encephalopathy
- pH < 7.3
- creatinine > 200 μmol/L
- oliguria
- systolic hypotension < 100 mmHg
- lactate > 3.5
- acidosis unresponsive to fluid resuscitation.

Autoimmune hepatitis usually presents as chronic liver disease but can cause fulminant liver failure. It is associated with a raised IgG and positive antinuclear antibody and is diagnosed by liver biopsy. The treatment is high-dose steroids. Herpes simplex virus and cytomegalovirus can cause liver failure in immunocompromised patients and are treated with intravenous aciclovir and ganciclovir respectively. If liver function does not improve with supportive therapy, patients should be considered for transplantation (see below).

Patients should be managed in a critical care unit if there is concern over the safety of their airway or grade 2 or 3 encephalopathy is present. Hypoxia with a PaO_2 of less than 9 kPa on air, hypercapnia with a $PaCO_2$ of more than 6.5 kPa, or acidosis with a pH of less than 7.25 or a lactate greater than 3.5 also require critical care unit management. Renal replacement therapy, if appropriate, should be performed in the critical care unit. Transplantation should be discussed if the patient has features associated with a poor prognosis and no contraindications to the procedure. In paracetamol overdose the indicators of a poor outcome are a pH less than 7.3 or a PT greater than 100 s and a creatinine greater than 300 μmol/L and grade 3 coma. When liver failure is due to causes other than paracetamol overdose the poor prognostic features are:

- prothrombin time > 100 s

  or three of the following:

- bilirubin greater than 300 μmol/L
- age less than 10 years or greater than 40 years
- prothrombin time > 50 s
- > 7days between the onset of jaundice and encephalopathy
- non-A, non-B hepatitis or idiosyncratic drug reaction as the cause of liver failure.

Contraindications to liver transplantation are ongoing drug or alcohol abuse, cerebral damage, septic shock, multiorgan failure, inability to oxygenate due to ARDS or underlying cardiopulmonary disease, widespread mesenteric vein thrombosis or a major comorbidity. Usually a period of abstinence from alcohol of six months is required although this may be shorter if the patient is clearly deteriorating. Irreversible cerebral damage may result if cerebral perfusion pressure is less than 40 mmHg for more than 2 h or there is sustained intracranial pressure more than 50 mmHg. Patients whose liver function shows an improvement are no longer eligible for transplantation.

ACUTE INFLAMMATORY BOWEL DISEASE

Inflammatory bowel disease (IBD) presents acutely when patients suffer a flare-up of their disease. This can occur in well-diagnosed ulcerative colitis or Crohn's disease or in previously undiagnosed patients. The real emergency is to avoid bowel perforation or deterioration of the patient's condition to such a degree that surgical resection of inflamed bowel becomes more dangerous because the patient is extremely ill and malnourished. There should be early liaison with a colorectal surgeon to plan surgery; it is often useful to agree a date by which treatment is deemed to have failed. This also allows the patient time to adapt to a decision of surgery, especially if a stoma is necessary.

Severe inflammatory bowel disease presents with diarrhoea, nausea, vomiting, abdominal pain and rectal bleeding. The Truelove-Witts criteria that identify severe IBD are:

- fever > 37.5°C
- passage of more than 6 loose stools per day
- macroscopic blood in stool
- pulse > 90 bpm
- ESR > 30
- Hb < 9 g/dL.

Infectious causes of diarrhoea must be excluded, including a stool sample for *Clostridium difficile* toxin in patients who have received previous antibiotic therapy. Sigmoidoscopy should be performed to assess the severity of colitis present. If severe inflammation is seen there is a high risk of perforation and sigmoidoscopy should not proceed further. In toxin-negative *Clostridium difficile* infection, a pseudomembrane is seen at sigmoidoscopy. Colonic biopsies may help distinguish ulcerative colitis from Crohn's disease. There may also be macroscopic features that favour a diagnosis of Crohn's disease such as deep apthous ulcers or the presence of perianal disease. It is extremely important to perform an abdominal X-ray to detect bowel distension and impending perforation which requires urgent surgical intervention. Treatment with steroids and immunosuppression will mask the symptoms and signs of bowel perforation.

Treatment of acute IBD

Fluid resuscitation must be commenced and electrolyte disturbance corrected. Blood transfusion is required if anaemia is present. As acute colitis is a prothrombotic state, prophylactic subcutaneous heparin is frequently given unless there are contraindications. Antidiarrhoea agents are avoided. Once infection has been excluded, high-dose intravenous steroids are given (e.g. 100 mg, 6–8 hourly). If patients fail to improve, intravenous ciclosporin can be effective in ulcerative colitis and anti-TNF drugs such as infliximab in Crohn's disease. Prolonged medical therapy which causes a significant delay to surgery can be detrimental. Patients frequently become malnourished during a severe flare-up of inflammatory bowel disease and nutritional support is important.

CASE 10.1

A 78-year-old woman presents with vague abdominal discomfort and vomiting. She has a pulse of 110 bpm, blood pressure of 94/60 mmHg and a respiratory rate of 28. What does her abdominal X-ray and subsequent CT show (Figs 10.4 and 10.5)? The cause of this condition was discovered on examination. What was it? What is the initial treatment that she requires?

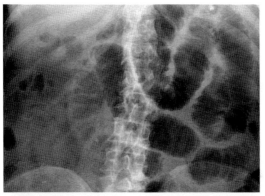

Figure 10.4   Abdominal X-ray.

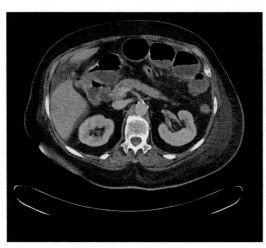

Figure 10.5   Abdominal CT scan.

Answer

The abdominal X-ray shows small bowel obstruction. Dilated small bowel is present in the centre of the X-ray with valvulae conniventes that encircle the lumen. The CT shows fluid-filled dilated loops of small bowel. The cause was a femoral hernia. She is significantly shocked and requires resuscitation with crystalloid or colloid, oxygen therapy and correction of any electrolyte disturbance (most commonly low potassium) prior to surgery. Cardiovascular fluid filling according to CVP in a critical area before theatre (preoptimization) may improve outcome.

CASE 10.2

A 73-year-old man presents with haematemesis and melaena. He has had a previous myocardial infarct and takes aspirin but is otherwise well. On admission he has a pulse of 120 bpm, and a systolic blood pressure of 110 bpm with a postural drop of 20 mmHg.

What should be his initial management? His endoscopic findings are shown in Figure 10.6. What is his Rockall score and how does this influence further management?

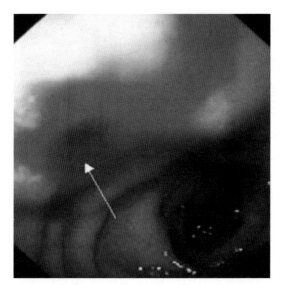

Figure 10.6   Endoscopic view (with acknowledgement to University of Hong Kong).

Answer

Initial management is fluid replacement. Despite a systolic blood pressure of 110 this patient has significant fluid loss demonstrated by his tachycardia and postural drop. He requires crystalloid and/or colloid via two large cannulae. Blood should be cross-matched urgently and given quickly. Once he is haemodynamically stable, an urgent endoscopy should be performed. Critical care input would be required if there was difficulty in improving his pulse and blood pressure, airway compromise or continued uncontrolled bleeding. His aspirin must be stopped. The endoscopic image shows a bleeding duodenal ulcer. This makes his Rockall score 7 and puts him at high risk of a further bleed. Intravenous proton pump inhibitor therapy should be commenced and empirical *Helicobacter pylori* eradication. If further bleeding occurs a second endoscopy could be performed by an experienced endoscopist but the threshold for proceeding to surgery is low.

CASE 10.3

A 63-year-old man presented with severe right upper quadrant pain, nausea and a temperature of 38.2°C. On examination he was tender in the right upper quadrant, had a pulse of 112 bpm, and blood pressure of 108/64 mmHg. An ultrasound was performed and subsequently a CT (Fig. 10.7). What does this show? What is the appropriate management? An endoscopic procedure was unsuccessful. In Figure 10.8, what procedure has been performed?

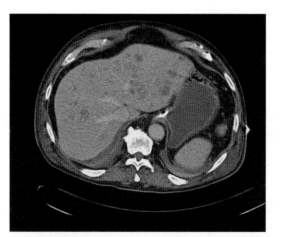

Figure 10.7 Abdominal CT scan.

Answer
The CT demonstrates ascending cholangitis due to gallstones and probable multiple small abscesses in the liver. He requires aggressive fluid resuscitation and antibiotic therapy with ciprofloxacin and metronidazole. A drainage procedure to relieve the common bile duct obstruction is needed. An ERCP could be performed or, as in this case, a stent placed at a percutaneous transhepatic cholangiogram (PTC). Figure 10.8 is a still from a PTC showing a dilated biliary duct with a guidewire being passed into the duodenum prior to stenting.

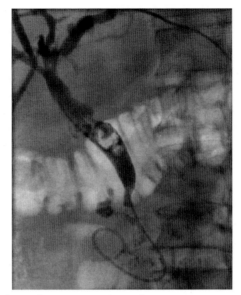

Figure 10.8   What endoscopic procedure is this?

FURTHER READING

British Society of Gastroenterology Endoscopy Committee 2002 Guidelines for the management of non-variceal upper gastrointestinal haemorrhage (correspondence K R Palmer). Gut 51 (suppl IV): iv1–iv6

Carter M J, Lobo A J, Travis S P L (on behalf of the IBD section of the British Society of Gastroenterology) 2004 Guidelines for the management of inflammatory bowel disease. Gut 53 (suppl V):v1–v16

Jalan R, Hayes P C (on behalf of the British Society of Gastroenterology) 2000 Guidelines for the management of variceal upper haemorrhage in cirrhotic patients. Gut 46 (suppl III): iii1–iii15

O'Grady J G, Williams R, Calne R 1986 Transplantation in fulminant hepatic failure. Lancet 22:2(8517):1227

Metabolic emergencies

Jonathan Louden

11

OBJECTIVES

After reading this chapter you should be able to:

● *Assess the patient with acute renal failure (ARF)*

● *Anticipate and manage associated risk factors of ARF*

● *Understand the important strategies to reverse ARF and prevent acute tubular necrosis*

● *Assess and manage hyponatraemia and hypernatraemia*

● *Manage the important endocrine disturbances that result in cardiovascular instability, shock or neurological disturbance (diabetic ketoacidosis, non-ketotic hyperglycaemia, hypoadrenal crisis, severe hypothyroidism and thyrotoxic crisis)*

ACUTE RENAL FAILURE

Definition

Acute renal failure (ARF) describes the rapid deterioration in solute excretion by the kidneys, over a period of days or weeks – there is no universal definition. In ARF, urine output usually decreases markedly, but

KEY POINTS
- ARF is common in hospitalized, critically ill patients and may be associated with iatrogenic factors.
- ARF is potentially reversible in the early stages. The patient should be assessed to identify causative factors.
- Patients with ARF often require intensive care due to multi-organ failure, sepsis, or multisystem disease.
- ARF has a high mortality rate, partly as a result of other critical illness, although isolated ARF usually recovers fully.

may be maintained in many cases. The term *oliguric renal failure* is used if urine output falls below approximately 400 mL/24 h.

Pre-renal failure is by far the most common form of ARF, particularly as a complication of hospitalized, critically ill patients (Table 11.1). Numerous surveys at large tertiary centres show that ARF is most commonly associated with intravascular volume depletion, recent surgery, sepsis and nephrotoxins. Nephrotoxins include nephrotoxic drugs (aminoglycoside antibiotics, the renin angiotensin system (RAS) blocking agents – angiotensin coverting enzyme (ACE) inhibitors and angiotensin receptor antagonists, non-steroidal anti-inflammatory drugs (NSAIDs)), exposure to radio-contrast agents (especially in the presence of volume depletion) and haem protein toxicity (myoglobin or haemoglobin). Pre-existing renal impairment increases the risk of a complicated course in ARF.

Table 11.1 Common causes of ARF

Pre-renal failure (often due to a combination of these factors)	Impaired perfusion from hypotension or shock, frequently due to sepsis Depletion of circulating blood volume Nephrotoxic drugs Renal arterial occlusion (thrombosis)
Intrinsic renal failure	Glomerulonephritis – including vasculitis (e.g. Wegener's granulomatosis; see Fig. 11.1), antiGBM antibody disease (Goodpasture's disease), systemic lupus erythematosus Acute tubular necrosis – ischaemic insult resulting in established tubular injury Toxic – myoglobin in rhabdomyolysis, light chains in myeloma Drug-induced injury, e.g. gentamicin Interstitial nephritis – allergic, drug induced – NSAIDs, penicillins
Obstructive renal failure (post-renal failure)	Bladder outflow obstruction – prostatic hyperplasia or carcinoma Ureteric – TCC, prostatic carcinoma or gynaecological malignancies, retroperitoneal fibrosis, intra-abdominal lymphadenopathy, other intra-abdominal malignancies

Assessment of the patient

Frequently you will not know that the patient has renal failure when conducting the initial assessment. Patients are often referred non-specifically unwell or with features of the underlying cause of ARF, which is often only recognized with biochemistry. Vigilance for evidence of renal failure including hyperkalaemia should be exercised in all acutely ill patients, particularly those who are already hospitalized. Most cases of ARF arise in hospital and are, at least in part, iatrogenic.

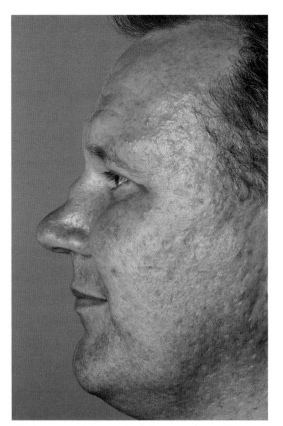

Figure 11.1   This patient presented with malaise and dipstick haematuria. He was found to be in ARF and gave a history of sinusitis and epistaxis. These are characteristic features of Wegener's granulomatosis, a systemic vasculitis characterized by granulomatous inflammation in a variety of organs and a positive C-ANCA. Destructive nasal inflammation resulted in collapse of the nasal septum which is a classical but unusual clinical sign.

Priorities in assessment of the patient with ARF (after airway, breathing and circulation (ABC))

- In all acutely ill patients, look for *clues to the presence of ARF* (see Box 11.1).
- The most important need is to *identify the patient at risk* (see Box 11.2).
- Establish whether the patient is being nursed in the correct area – is a high dependency area needed?
- Are there any *features of hyperkalaemia?* Obtain an ECG immediately, even if you have to do this yourself; you can continue assessment and take a history as you do this.
- Take a blood gas sample – *is the patient acidotic?*
- Is the patient *haemodynamically* stable? Is fluid resuscitation or inotropic support needed? Are there signs of *shock?* (see Table 11.2).
- Are there any signs of *volume overload* or *pulmonary oedema?*

Box 11.1   Clues that ARF might be present

- *Features of hyperkalaemia on ECG:* tall and tented T waves, small P waves, prolonged PR interval, prolonged QT interval, broad QRS complexes, ventricular arrhythmias, bradycardia (and ultimately a sinusoidal wave or asystole or ventricular fibrillation)
- *Kussmaul's respiration* – a deep sighing form of respiration indicating metabolic acidosis
- *Hypotension* – this often results in ARF, whatever the cause of the hypotension. Review the TPR or EWS charts
- *Sepsis*
- *Oliguria*
- Confusion or inability to give a coherent and detailed history
- A *multisystem* presentation
- *Blood or protein on dipstick urinalysis* – urine should be dipped for all acutely ill patients and this should be repeated when the diagnosis remains unclear. Blood or protein might indicate the presence of intrinsic renal failure

---

Box 11.2   Immediately life-threatening complications of ARF

- Hyperkalaemia with resulting cardiac arrest (see Box 11.3)
- Pulmonary oedema with resulting respiratory failure (see Box 11.4)
- Severe acidosis which can result in circulatory collapse and death
- Sepsis or shock: both commonly cause ARF and can lead to circulatory collapse and death
- Severe illness due to the multisystem diseases which can cause ARF (e.g. systemic vasculitis, systemic lupus erythematosis and haemolytic uraemic syndrome)

Essential points in the history

- Take a careful and comprehensive drug history including any drugs taken recently which might have been discontinued.
- Search for any indication of sepsis or multisystem disease.
- Are there any symptoms to suggest obstruction, particularly prostatic disease or gynaecological malignancy?
- Is there a history of cardiac or vascular disease (clues to the possibility of athero-occlusive renal arterial disease or leaking aortic aneurysm)?
- If the patient is confused, seek additional information from companions or relatives, even if you have to make a telephone call to do so.

Essential points on examination

- Check the blood pressure yourself on both arms.
- Assess the patient's fluid status – paying particular attention to the vascular compartment. Does the patient need fluid resuscitation? (see Table 11.2).
- Is there evidence of cardiac or vascular disease?
- Is there evidence of obstruction of the urinary tract – palpable bladder, tender loins, abdominal or pelvic mass; conduct a digital rectal and a bimanual vaginal examination.

Tip

If the patient is not breathless *tip the bed head down (as you would when inserting a central venous pressure (CVP) line)*. If you need to do this in order to make the external or internal jugular veins fill, the patient's intravascular compartment is very likely to be under-filled indicating the need for fluid resuscitation.

Table 11.2 Assessment of fluid status

Skin	The skin and mucous membranes are poor indicators of fluid status. Reduced skin turgor is a relatively late sign and can be misleading from middle age onwards
Blood pressure	Careful measurement and intensive monitoring of BP is vital in ARF. However, BP also can be misleading
	A postural fall in BP is usually an indication of volume depletion but the patient is often too sick to undergo measurement of BP while standing. (A postural fall in BP can also occur in autonomic neuropathy and with sympatholytic drugs)
	In chronically hypertensive patients, the BP might appear to be satisfactory (e.g. 120/70) but if the patient's usual BP is higher (e.g. 170/90), such a relative fall in BP might be sufficient to decrease renal perfusion. (This is because the autoregulation curve for renal blood flow moves to the right in chronic hypertension)
Jugular venous pressure	The bulk of the circulating volume is contained within the venous compartment. Assessment of the JVP plays a pivotal role in determination of the cause of ARF, in selection of the correct approach to fluid management and in monitoring progress
	The internal jugular vein is typically assessed with the patient at 45 degrees. Jugular venous pressure reflects central venous pressure leading to a normal range of approximately 1–8 cm water above the sternocleidomastoid or a value of 1–6 mmHg measured with CVP monitoring
	If the JVP cannot be seen easily, consider whether it is very high:
	Sit the patient upright
	The JVP might now be visible near the ear lobe. The internal and external jugular veins should be distended in such cases
	If this does not answer the question, the JVP might be low (see Tip box on p. 241)

Table 11.2 Assessment of fluid status – *continued*

Listen to the chest *Record respiratory rate*	Are there signs of pulmonary oedema or consolidation?
	CXR appearance can help to confirm the clinical impression, but the appearance of alveolar oedema can be caused by ARDS and by pulmonary haemorrhage (systemic vasculitis and Goodpasture's syndrome)
	Elevation of respiratory rate might indicate metabolic acidosis or impending respiratory failure. If the patient is acidotic, contact the renal unit. Dialysis might be needed. If respiratory failure is developing, contact the critical care team
Consider use of central venous pressure monitoring	This is both to assess fluid status and guide therapy, but remember that central venous catheterization is not wise until adequate peripheral fluid resuscitation has taken place in volume deplete patients. Insertion of a central venous catheter can consume considerable time, diverting efforts from appropriate fluid resuscitation and can result in dangerous complications if attempted in severe volume depletion

Initial investigations and treatment

Look for evidence of hyperkalaemia

Perform an ECG (if necessary, do this yourself while taking the history).

If hyperkalaemic, initiate treatment (Box 11.3). This can be done while you take the history and perform an examination.

Is the patient acidotic?

Take an arterial blood sample for gas analysis. Most analyzers provide an estimate of potassium also (this might be inaccurate if the machine has not been calibrated recently).

If severely acidotic, discuss management with renal and critical care teams.

Correct hypoxaemia

Look for signs of pulmonary oedema and arrange a chest X-ray (CXR). Treatment of pulmonary oedema is described in Box 11.4.

Provide fluid resuscitation if indicated

Patients with ARF are often fluid depleted (causing pre-renal failure) but patients with obstruction of the urinary tract (post-renal failure) become overloaded with fluid. Cardiac failure and hepatic failure result in a decrease

Box 11.3 Management of hyperkalaemia

- *The priority is to protect the patient from fatal arrhythmia*
  Give calcium gluconate 10%, 10 mL or calcium chloride 10%, 10 mL IV as a slow push
  If hyperkalaemic ECG features are present this should result in an improvement in the ECG monitor trace with a reduction in the QRS complex width. If there is no improvement, this can be repeated up to three times (i.e. 40 mL in total)
- After this, you can lower the potassium concentration, temporarily, by infusing 50% glucose. A small dose of insulin is usually added:
  Give 50 mL of 50% glucose and add 10 IU short acting insulin (usually Actrapid) unless the blood sugar is low. This must be infused IV slowly – usually over 20–30 min and if given peripherally, flush the cannula to minimize thrombophlebitis
  Check the blood sugar at approximately 10-min intervals until 20 min after the infusion is complete
  Remember that this will have only a transient effect on serum potassium by transferring potassium into cells
- Ion exchange resins can remove potassium from the body but they work slowly and are best administered by retention enema
  Give 30 g calcium resonium rectally
- Bicarbonate may also help reduce serum potassium and will work in the presence or absence of acidosis
  Give sodium bicarbonate 8.4% 50 mL if pH < 7.0 or the patient is in cardiac arrest

These measures can allow time for more definitive treatment to be organized. Many patients will require urgent dialysis, but, if fluid resuscitation is needed and a good urine output can be established, the need for dialysis might be avoided.
It is always prudent to discuss cases with the local renal unit at an early stage.

Box 11.4 Management of pulmonary oedema

- Administer enough oxygen to achieve normal oxygen saturation; if in doubt give 100% oxygen and consider facial CPAP
- Stop IV fluid
- Monitor the ECG rhythm
- Patients with ARF may not respond to small doses of diuretic and might not respond at all. Give furosemide 250 mg IV over 60 min if smaller doses have no effect
- If BP permits (if BP > 100 mmHg systolic) IV nitrate can be used. This will reduce preload by venodilation. A sublingual or buccal dose can help while the infusion is being prepared. Monitor BP per 5 min and start at a slow infusion rate
- Haemodialysis at the renal unit or haemofiltration on ICU might be the only way to control the pulmonary oedema. Discuss with the renal unit and the critical care team at an early stage
- Diamorphine may help to offload the left ventricle but should only be administered in a low dose and with extreme care, monitoring closely for respiratory depression
- Always maintain vigilance for the early signs of pulmonary oedema, especially when giving fluids (rising respiratory rate, tachycardia, falling oxygen saturations)

in cardiac output. This produces an apparent decrease in 'effective arterial blood volume'. These three situations require very different actions. For this reason, careful assessment of fluid status is very important in ARF (see Box 11.5). Careful attention should be paid to assessing the intravascular compartment.

Hypotension in the face of normovolaemia or fluid overload

Contact the critical care team and the renal unit. The patient requires more intensive monitoring (CVP +/- PA catheter), probably needs vasopressors or inotropes and might require dialysis or haemofiltration soon.

Exclude obstructon of the urinary tract (post-renal failure) by means of urgent ultrasound imaging

Identify indications for referral to critical care or dialysis
(See Table 11.3).

Box 11.5   Fluid resuscitation when the patient's intravascular compartment is under-filled

- Give 250 mL of IV colloid. This can be given as a rapid infusion or via a pump over a few minutes
- Following this, recheck the BP and heart rate; look for the JVP – has it become visible or risen? Can you now see the external jugular veins? Is the urine output increasing?
- This manoeuvre should then be repeated until these parameters respond
- A fall in oxygen saturation, rise in respiratory rate or the development of new crackles or wheezes suggest pulmonary oedema. At this point stop the infusion, order a chest X-ray and re-evaluate the patient frequently (every few minutes)
- Change to crystalloid if you have already had to give 1 L of colloid. There is no evidence that colloid offers any mortality benefit over crystalloid in fluid resuscitation of critically ill patients with ARF (Roberts et al 2005)
- Remember that you must re-evaluate the patient frequently. You cannot set a prescription covering several hours for a patient requiring fluid resuscitation. It is unlikely to be correct and might be unsafe

---

Table 11.3   Indications for referral to the critical care team and the local renal unit

Contact the critical care team if there is:	Severe or persistent hypotension
	Severe or resistant acidosis
	A respiratory rate of > 40/min or < 8/min
	Deterioration in consciousness level or GCS
Contact the renal unit as urgent dialysis might be needed if there is:	Severe hyperkalaemia (particularly if oliguria persists)
	Persisting oliguria or anuria
	Severe acidosis
	Evidence of an intrinsic renal disease (on history or urinalysis)
	Worsening ARF despite adequate filling of the vascular compartment

Additional investigations (Table 11.4)

Many texts describe investigations to help distinguish between reversible pre-renal failure and established acute tubular necrosis (ATN). These tests can mislead if a diuretic has been administered. Attention to reversible factors (as detailed above) is more important in the hope that ATN can be avoided.

The fractional excretion of sodium (FE Na) is the percentage of the filtered sodium load that is excreted in the urine:

$$\text{FE Na (\%)} = \frac{\text{urine [sodium]} \times \text{plasma [creatinine]}}{\text{plasma [sodium]} \times \text{urine [creatinine]}} \times 100$$

Investigations for glomerulonephritis and multiple myeloma
Serum should be sent for anti-neutrophil cytoplasmic antibody (ANCA), anti-GBM antibodies, anti-nuclear antibodies and complement components C3 and C4 in order to look for evidence of glomerulonephritis.

If the cause of ARF is not clear after a thorough clinical assessment, plasma and urine should be sent for electrophoresis to look for evidence of *multiple myeloma*.

Rhabdomyolysis
Consider rhabdomyolysis which usually causes muscular pain and tenderness. This can be related to drug therapy, strenuous exercise, prolonged immobility or unconsciousness, illicit drug use and (rarely) metabolic myopathy. Measure serum *creatine kinase* if there is any suspicion or if the cause of ARF is not immediately obvious.

Renal biopsy
If ARF progresses despite adequate intravascular volume and exclusion of obstruction, specialist investigations such as renal biopsy might be needed urgently (Figs 11.2 and 11.3). This is an indication for urgent referral to the renal unit.

Consider whether imaging of renal arterial supply is needed
Atherosclerotic renal arterial disease can cause bilateral renal artery occlusion which usually causes the patient to present with sudden onset of anuria, pulmonary oedema and severe renal failure.

Table 11.4 Additional investigations

	Pre-renal failure	Established ATN
Urine sodium (mmol/L)	< 10	> 20
Urine osmolality (mosmol/L)	> 400	< 300
Fractional sodium excretion (%)	< 1	> 2

Acute renal failure

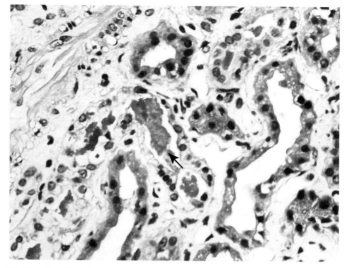

Figure 11.2   Red blood cells on urine microscopy strongly suggest an underlying glomerulonephritis. Red cell casts are said to be pathognomonic of glomerulonephritis (but are also seen, rarely, in ATN). Red cell casts are formed in the renal tubules as seen in this renal biopsy.

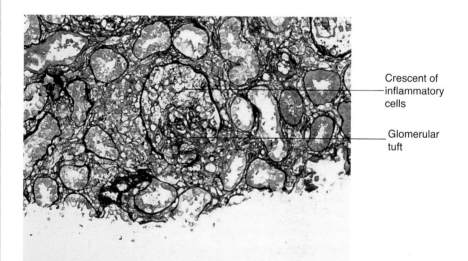

Crescent of inflammatory cells

Glomerular tuft

Figure 11.3   This methenamine-silver stained renal biopsy shows compression of the glomerular capillary tuft by a cellular 'crescent' of inflammatory cells. This is the classic appearance of the extracapillary glomerulonephritis seen in systemic vasculitis.

KEY POINT

- Even a modest fall in blood pressure can result in ARF in some patients due to a fall in renal perfusion.

Prevention of acute renal failure

Most cases of ARF develop in hospitalized patients and are associated with *haemodynamic compromise* due to intravascular volume depletion, sepsis or a low effective arterial blood volume (as in cardiac failure or liver failure). Attention to correcting volume deficit, control of sepsis and maintenance of blood pressure (using vasopressors if necessary) are essential.

Such relative hypotension carries a risk of ARF in those with chronic hypertension and in arteriopathic patients with stenosed renal arteries, particularly bilaterally.

Avoidance of *nephrotoxic drugs* and appropriate modification of drug doses is equally important. Nephrotoxic agents have been implicated in up to 25% of cases of hospital-acquired ARF (Hatala et al 1996). Important nephrotoxins are shown in Box 11.6.

Single daily dosing of aminoglycoside appears to reduce nephrotoxicity as compared with multiple daily dosing (Hatala et al 1996). Careful monitoring of blood levels is essential and consideration should be given to the use of alternative antimicrobial agents as a single dose of aminoglycoside can result in severe renal failure. It is wise to seek expert microbiological and nephrological advice if considering use of an aminoglycoside in a patient with renal impairment.

Maintenance of adequate hydration helps to protect against radiocontrast nephrotoxicity.

Box 11.6 Common nephrotoxic drugs

Antimicrobials

- Aminoglycosides (e.g. gentamicin/tobramicin/amikacin)
- Tetracyclines (not doxycycline)
- Pentamidine

Haemodynamic agents

- Non-steroidal anti-inflammatory agents:
  Decreased synthesis of vasodilatory prostaglandins causes relative vasoconstriction of afferent arterioles; this causes GFR to fall in the presence of systemic hypotension or volume depletion (Fig. 11.4)
- Renin-angiotensin system blockade:
  – ACE inhibitors
  – Angiotensin receptor antagonists
  Blockade of angiotensin II-mediated vasoconstriction of efferent arteriole; efferent arteriolar constriction is important to maintain GFR in systemic hypotension or volume depletion

---

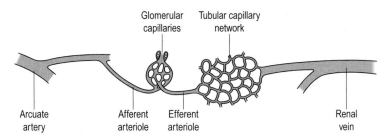

Figure 11.4 This diagram shows the glomerular blood supply. Angiotensin II vasoconstricts the efferent arteriole. It is not involved in day-to-day tonal regulation of GFR but is important in maintenance of glomerular filtration when afferent arteriolar pressure is compromised. Blockade of the action of angiotensin II by ACE-inhibition or by a receptor antagonist can cause GFR to fall during volume depletion or hypotension. (Adapted from Lemley K V, Bayliss C 1997.)

NSAIDs cause relative vasoconstriction of the afferent arteriole by inhibiting synthesis of vasodilatory prostaglandins (Fig. 11.4) and can compromise glomerular filtration, especially in combination with volume depletion, aggressive diuresis, ACE-inhibition or angiotensin receptor blockade.

Radiocontrast nephropathy

Adequate hydration must be maintained prior to radiocontrast exposure. When attention is paid to this, the incidence of radiocontrast nephropathy is very low.

Renal dose dopamine

Dopamine has been used in an attempt to prevent progression of pre-renal failure to established ATN. In healthy animals, low dose (3–5 µmol/kg/min) dopamine infusion has been shown to increase renal blood flow ('renal-dose dopamine') due to arterial and afferent arteriolar vasodilatation. Efferent arterioles respond similarly so there is no effect on glomerular filtration rate (GFR). Higher doses decrease renal blood flow.

Much of our understanding of the actions of dopamine comes from studies in healthy volunteers and we cannot presume that its effects are the same in the presence of ARF. Dopamine clearance is usually decreased in ARF. This has called many to question the safety of dopamine infusion even at low dose.

Potential harmful effects of dopamine at higher plasma concentrations:

- Increased left ventricular afterload
- Tachyarrhythmia
- Intrapulmonary shunting of blood
- Unpredictable effects on splanchnic circulation
- Depression of respiratory drive
- Complications of administration (a central venous catheter is required as extravasation causes tissue necrosis).

Increased left ventricular afterload and tachyarrhythmia increase cardiac work, carrying the risk of ischaemia.

Evidence base for dopamine administration in ARF

Dopamine use has been commonplace in the management of ARF and many older texts advise on dosage regimens. The efficacy and safety of dopamine in management of ARF and in prophylaxis of ARF for those undergoing high-risk intervention have been the subject of scrutiny in recent years.

Improvement in urine output with low-dose dopamine has been reported in several small uncontrolled series but dopamine appears to have no significant effect on renal function in those with severe ARF. No effect has been demonstrated in terms of patient survival or avoidance of the need for long-term dialysis.

Given the potential risks of dopamine administration, many reviews have advocated caution (Burton & Tomson 1999). Consequently, renal physicians in the UK generally advise against the use of dopamine in ARF. There is no evidence to support the use of dopamine prophylactically.

Furosemide

Furosemide is used widely in oliguric ARF. There are several potential benefits:

- Decreased oxygen requirement in tubular epithelium (due to inhibition of active sodium and chloride reabsorption in the thick ascending limb of the loop of Henle)
- Increased renal blood flow (due to increased PgE_2 synthesis)
- Increased urine flow which can limit tubular toxicity (e.g. from myoglobin in rhabdomyolysis)
- Similarly, by improving urine flow, furosemide can relieve tubular obstruction by casts.

Evidence base and recommendations for use of furosemide

There are numerous reports that furosemide converts an oliguric to a non-oliguric state. However, there is no convincing evidence of reduction in requirement for dialysis or in mortality (Gambaro et al 2002).

Most renal physicians would use furosemide only when there is evidence of pulmonary oedema in a volume-replete patient but it is important to recognize that many such patients will need urgent dialysis and attempts to achieve a diuresis should not delay nephrology referral.

Some authorities believe that furosemide sometimes has a place in promoting diuresis in patients subject to tubular toxicity (myoglobinuria, haemoglobinuria, light chain toxicity in myeloma) but there is no general agreement.

Mannitol

Mannitol has been used in the treatment of ARF and in attempts to prevent ARF in high-risk populations undergoing surgery. There are several potentially beneficial effects including volume expansion, establishment of an osmotic diuresis, flushing out of intratubular casts, relief of cell swelling which causes vascular congestion and a free-radical scavenging action. However, it is also potentially harmful due to excessive volume expansion, and there are no controlled trials showing convincing benefit in treatment or prevention of ARF.

Nutrition and metabolic managment

Patients with ARF are at particularly high risk of becoming malnourished. The pathogenesis involves several factors which are prevalent in renal failure, including a catabolic state, metabolic acidosis, altered metabolism of amino acids and insulin-resistance.

There is no evidence that intensive nutritional support improves prognosis but it makes sense to attempt to correct negative nitrogen and caloric balance, which is strongly associated with mortality. Early introduction of supplemental nutrition, preferably by the enteral route, is generally considered important from an early stage in ARF. Nutritional management in critically ill patients has already been discussed in Chapter 5.

Insulin resistance and hyperglycaemia

Hyperglycaemia with features of insulin resistance is common in the critically ill and is associated with increased mortality in non-diabetic patients. Intensive insulin therapy to maintain tight control of blood glucose has been shown to reduce morbidity and mortality among critically ill patients in a surgical intensive care unit (Van den Berghe et al 2001). In an observational study of 618 adult critical care unit patients with ARF in the USA, insulin resistance was significantly associated with in-hospital mortality (Basi et al 2005).

Prognosis in ARF

Mortality rates in patients with ARF who require dialysis are approximately 50% (with variation according to differences in definition and severity). Bhandari & Turney studied the outcome of 1095 patients with severe ARF admitted to a single centre in the UK during a 10-year period. Overall survival was 59.5% and 16.2% remained dialysis dependent (Bhandari & Turney 1996). In another study, development of contrast-associated ARF in hospitalized patients increased mortality five-fold (Levy et al 1996).

Some studies suggest that there has been little change in mortality of ARF during the last few decades. This is presumed to be the result of increased comorbidity of critically ill patients associated with increased willingness on the part of physicians to treat sicker patients. There is, however, some evidence suggesting improvement in outcome during the last two decades (Nolan & Adamson 1998).

However, survivors of ARF cannot always be expected to recover independent renal function. The rates of end-stage renal failure in survivors of ARF appear to be increasing (Bhandari & Turney 1996).

HYPONATRAEMIA

Introduction and definition

Hyponatraemia is one of the most common electrolyte disorders and is often induced by intravenous fluid therapy or medication. It exists when serum sodium concentration falls below 135 mmol/L. Concern tends to arise when serum sodium reaches 125 mmol/L or lower. However, the severity of the clinical consequences of hyponatraemia is related more to the rate of fall of serum sodium rather than the precise level.

Important facts

- Acute hyponatraemia can cause seizures and coma due to cerebral oedema, while over-enthusiastic correction in the wrong circumstances can result in permanent neurological disability or death due to osmotic demyelination (central pontine myelinolysis).
- Hyponatraemic patients might present in shock (due to volume depletion, sepsis, cardiac failure or hypoadrenalism).
- The syndrome of inappropriate secretion of anti-diuretic hormone (SIADH) is well recognized but it must be remembered that this condition is not the most common cause of hyponatraemia. SIADH must be confirmed and other more common causes excluded.

Consequently, hyponatraemia demands great care in its assessment and treatment.

Causes of hyponatraemia

Assessment of the hyponatraemic patient and selection of the correct therapy can be challenging. It is helpful to examine the possible causes and the mechanisms by which they produce hyponatraemia. Causes can be classified according to whether there is volume depletion or alternatively according to whether antidiuretic hormone (ADH) is elevated but this classification is of limited clinical utility.

Conditions in which ADH is elevated

Many of the conditions causing hyponatraemia are associated with elevation of antidiuretic hormone (ADH). This impairs ability to excrete a water load and in these conditions hyponatraemia is due to water excess.

Hyponatraemic states with hypovolaemia

In these conditions, ADH secretion is stimulated appropriately (via the baroreceptors in the great arteries) due to depletion of water with or without salt loss also. (Sodium loss can be classified as renal or non-renal.)

Renal sodium loss

- Hypoadrenalism (Addison's disease)
- Salt-losing nephropathies
- Diuretic therapy (commonest).

Non-renal salt and water loss

- Gastrointestinal
- Third space (pancreatitis)
- Haemorrhage.

Hyponatraemic states with decreased effective arterial blood volume

- Cardiac failure
- Hepatic cirrhosis
- Nephrotic syndrome.

In these conditions also, baroreceptor-mediated stimulation of ADH secretion attempts to correct a perceived volume deficit caused by decreased cardiac output in cardiac failure and by vasodilation in hepatic failure. (The ADH secretion could be considered inappropriate, but these conditions should not be confused with those causing the syndrome of inappropriate ADH secretion (SIADH)):

Hyponatraemic states with normovolaemia

This group generally comprises SIADH and drugs causing either ADH release or increased sensitivity to ADH.

Causes of SIADH
These can be classified as malignant neoplasms, pulmonary diseases and central nervous system (CNS) disorders:

- Malignant neoplasms:
  - small cell lung cancer
  - pancreatic carcinoma
  - prostatic carcinoma
  - lymphomas
  - leukaemias
- Pulmonary diseases:
  - bacterial pneumonia
  - tuberculosis

- abscess
- vasculitis
- CNS disorders:
  - trauma and surgery
  - infection
  - subarachnoid haemorrhage
  - cerebral vasculitis.

Drugs causing hyponatraemia

Thiazide diuretics (e.g. bendrofluazide) cause renal salt wasting; additionally, volume depletion owing to either thiazide or loop diuretics results in ADH release which may worsen hyponatraemia.

Some other drugs also increase ADH release or potentiate its action in the kidney:

- Chlorpropamide
- Amitriptyline and selective serotonin reuptake inhibitors
- Carbamazepine
- Haloperidol, thioridazine
- Opiates
- Oxytocin
- Cisplatin, cyclophosphamide, vinblastine, vincristine.

Psychogenic polydipsia (compulsive water drinking)

Such patients can dilute their serum sufficiently to lower osmolality below the normal range but they produce an appropriately dilute urine (unlike SIADH).

Hyponatraemic states with elevated osmolality

Hyperglycaemia (as in diabetic ketoacidosis) causes dilutional hyponatraemia due to the movement of water out of cells down an osmotic gradient.

Assessment and management of hyponatraemia

Priorities

Ensure that you have excluded artefactual hyponatraemia

- Check lipid profile and ask the laboratory whether the serum appeared lipaemic.
- Is it possible the blood sample was taken proximal to an IV infusion?
- Is blood glucose elevated?

Identify the patient at risk

Rapidly falling serum sodium: In cases where serum sodium is falling rapidly, neurological symptoms including seizures and coma can occur due to

KEY POINT
- Over-enthusiastic correction of serum sodium in a patient who has adapted to hyponatraemia can cause osmotic demyelination which is frequently fatal. One rule of thumb is to try and correct the hyponatraemia at the same rate as it developed, as long as no life-threatening complications exist.

cerebral oedema. Monitor GCS closely. *Neurological deterioration is an indication to transfer the patient into a high dependency or intensive care bed immediately. In these circumstances, appropriate therapy to correct hyponatraemia will require expert assistance.*

Rate of correction of serum sodium: Consider carefully the rate of correction needed. Try to identify the cause of hyponatraemia. Correction of an underlying fluid deficit or elimination of an offending drug will often rectify serum sodium. In the absence of symptoms of hyponatraemia, serum sodium should not be allowed to rise by more than 10 mmol/L/day.

Try to assess fluid status accurately

Ultimately, this assessment is important because hyponatraemia can occur in the presence of salt and water deficit (volume depletion), water excess (SIADH) or salt *and* water excess (e.g. cardiac failure) with very different treatment pathways. However, clinical examination and laboratory parameters are poor at predicting whether a patient is normovolaemic or volume depleted in hyponatraemia (Spital 1988).

Consider adrenal insufficiency

The features suggesting adrenal insufficiency are reviewed below. Pay close attention to blood pressure. Is there a postural fall? Remember that a normal serum potassium does not exclude hypoadrenalism (Hoorn et al 2005). Like SIADH, it is therefore essentially a diagnosis of exclusion. If in doubt, seek confirmation by a short synacthen test. Dexamethasone can be administered immediately if the patient is haemodynamically compromised as it does not interfere with the assay for cortisol.

Look for evidence of SIADH

Ensure that you have sent serum and (unless the patient has received a diuretic) urine for osmolality. Excretion of inappropriately concentrated urine in the presence of a low serum osmolality suggests SIADH which results in water retention in excess of salt.

SIADH requires restriction of water intake. This treatment can cause cardiovascular collapse if used mistakenly in adrenal insufficiency. Remember that fluid restriction for SIADH should be used only if adrenal insufficiency has been excluded.

Drug-induced hyponatraemia

Find out which drugs are being prescribed and which have been prescribed recently. As in acute renal failure you might need to enquire of the patient's

KEY POINTS

- It is essential to make a distinction between acute and chronic hyponatraemia and to consider the rate of correction of serum sodium needed.
- Rapid fall in serum sodium can cause cerebral oedema. *Clinical features of neurological deterioration should prompt urgent transfer to a high dependency or intensive care bed. Seek expert senior assistance to guide correction of serum sodium.*
- Adaptation to hyponatraemia occurs rapidly by accumulation of osmolytes within brain cells; rapid correction then carries a risk of osmotic demyelination with permanent neurological damage or death.
- *In the absence of symptoms of hyponatraemia, serum sodium should not be allowed to rise by more than 10 mmol/L/day.*
- During infusion of hypertonic saline, there is an abrupt increase in plasma osmolality, which falls subsequently when excess sodium is excreted. This fluctuation in osmolality increases the risk of neurological deterioration.
- Any active intervention undertaken to correct hyponatraemia must be considered carefully and should be directed by a senior physician.
- **Monitor the rate of correction of serum sodium.**
- **Monitor GCS and clinical condition during treatment.**
- **Consider adrenal crisis if the patient becomes hypotensive.**

family or contact the general practitioner's surgery directly. Drugs such as bendrofluazide may take months to cause hyponatraemia.

Clinical algorithms and calculations

Numerous clinical algorithms exist to assist in assessment and management of hyponatraemia. There are also several approaches which can be employed to estimate the sodium deficit, to guide choice of fluid and to calculate the appropriate rate of fluid administration and the effect on serum sodium. *These must be used with caution, monitoring serum sodium, clinical well-being and GCS frequently during treatment.*

HYPERNATRAEMIA

Definition

Hypernatraemia describes a serum sodium concentration above 145 mmol/L but symptoms are unusual unless serum sodium exceeds 155 mmom/L. High serum sodium and osmolality causes water to move out of cells. This results in shrinkage of brain cells, potentially resulting in permanent neurological damage. Like hyponatraemia, the clinical features are determined by the rate at which hypernatraemia develops.

Causes of hypernatraemia

Thirst should protect against the development of hypernatraemia. Therefore this disorder occurs when there is a significant fluid deficit together with either of the following:

...gical disease affecting the thirst mechanism ... to fluid consumption (e.g. in the very elderly or in the critically ill ... d replacement is inadequate).

...ical features

...in hyponatraemia, chronic hypernatraemia is accompanied by few symptoms, due to adaptation of brain cells (see below). If serum sodium continues to rise, initial lethargy and irritability can progress to agitation, seizures and coma.

Adaptation of brain cells

Brain cells adapt rapidly to hypernatraemia, initially by uptake of electrolytes and, within days, by accumulation of osmolytes (mirroring the adaptation to hyponatraemia). Consequently, correction of hypernatraemia must be undertaken slowly. Brain cells are unable to lose osmolytes rapidly. Rapid correction of serum sodium causes water movement into brain cells and cerebral oedema, leading to seizures and coma. The maximum advisable rate of correction of hypernatraemia is 12 mmol/L per day.

DIABETIC KETOACIDOSIS AND NON-KETOTIC HYPERGLYCAEMIA

Introduction

Severe hyperglycaemic decompensation of diabetes mellitus occurs in two forms: diabetic ketoacidosis (DKA) and hyperosmolar non-ketotic form (HONK) – a form of non-ketotic hyperglycaemia (NKH). These conditions are both characterized by severe volume depletion and a risk of potentially fatal neurological complications.

Definitions

DKA is characterized by:

- hyperglycaemia
- ketonaemia
- acidosis
- dehydration which is usually of a severe degree (except in patients with end-stage renal failure).

DKA is a common complication of diabetes and is frequently the presenting feature in type 1 diabetes mellitus. It occurs in type 2 diabetes also.

HONK/NKH is characterized by a lesser rise in glucose than DKA but generally a much greater degree of fluid depletion and a high risk of thrombosis.

Causes of DKA

Insulin deficiency

- Newly diagnosed diabetes
- Non-adherence to insulin therapy.

Increased insulin requirement

Increased insulin requirement is due to increased secretion of counter-regulatory hormones. Causes are:

- infection
- myocardial infarction
- CVA, etc.

Assessment of the patient and diagnosis

Diagnosis is usually made soon after presentation with findings of:

- hyperglycaemia
- acidosis with a raised anion gap (> 16 mmol/L)
- ketonaemia/ketonuria.

Remember to ensure that admitting staff check blood glucose in all patients with an acute illness; DKA occurs in type 2 diabetes as well as type 1 and can be the first presentation of the condition.

Plasma glucose is not always markedly elevated in DKA, particularly in malnourished patients and in chronic liver disease.

Essential points in assessment of the hyperglycaemic patient

- Take a blood gas sample – you need to know the *acid base status if the patient is severely hyperglycaemic.*
- Always remember to look for the underlying precipitant of DKA or NKH. This might be clinically silent and often requires urgent attention in its own right.
- Search for evidence of sepsis. Culture urine and blood.
- Perform an ECG – look for evidence of myocardial infarction, even in young adults as diabetic people are at increased risk of cardiovascular disease.
- Initial hyperkalaemic ECG changes require urgent attention (calcium gluconate infusion and urgent insulin administration if this has not yet happened).
- If vomiting, insert a nasogastric tube due to the risk of aspiration.

Diabetic ketoacidosis and non-ketonic hyperglycaemia

- Make a careful initial assessment of consciousness level and neurological state. Monitor closely for deterioration in consciousness level which might indicate development of cerebral oedema (see complications).
- Establish whether the patient is being nursed in the correct area – is a high-dependency area needed?

Important risks for the patient with DKA

- Severe dehydration resulting in circulatory collapse, oliguria and shock.
- The precipitating illness must not be ignored (commonly sepsis or myocardial infarction).
- Cardiac arrest due to presenting hyperkalaemia or secondary to hypokalaemia during insulin therapy (initial hyperkalaemia is due to insulin deficiency, however insulin treatment causes plasma potassium to fall, usually revealing a state of severe potassium depletion due to chronic urinary loss during the hyperkalaemic stage – see potassium replacement in DKA).
- Cerebral oedema causing raised intracerebral pressure which rarely may progress to brain stem coning and death.

Treatment of DKA

Fluid replacement

The mean volume deficit in DKA is in the range of 3–7 L.

In NKH, patients tend to have a much larger deficit of up to 10 L but such large volume losses must be replaced over several hours, while monitoring for early signs of cerebral oedema.

This deficit is mainly a result of osmotic diuresis driven by hyperglycaemia. For this reason, patients with end-stage renal disease tend to have a much smaller volume deficit as the GFR is insufficient to sustain such a diuresis. Care must be taken to avoid over-aggressive fluid replacement in such patients.

The osmotic diuresis is also responsible for large urinary losses of sodium and potassium.

Dangers associated with incorrect fluid replacement prescription in DKA

- Fluid overload/pulmonary oedema – this is mainly a risk in end-stage renal disease (ESRD).
- Cerebral oedema – this is probably caused by rapid lowering of plasma osmolality.
- Hypokalaemia – this can arise despite initial hyperkalaemia, if potassium supplementation is inadequate during insulin therapy.

Which fluid?

Normal (0.9%) saline should be used rather than half normal (0.45%) saline despite hyperosmolality. This is because normal saline is hypo-osmolar in relation to the patient's plasma.

Serum osmolality usually falls at an acceptable rate because rehydration brings about an increase in GFR with ensuing clearance of urea.

Colloid should be used to deal with a hypotensive crisis but crystalloid with potassium supplementation as appropriate (see below) is the mainstay of fluid therapy.

Rate of fluid replacement

The initial rate must be determined by clinical judgement (see fluid resuscitation in ARF for general principles). A general guide is provided below.

General guidance on fluid replacement in DKA

- If there is shock/severe hypotension (systolic BP < 90 mmHg)/oliguria – colloid might be needed. A rapid initial rate (up to 1000 mL/h or greater) might be required during the first hour but *fluid administration must be guided by clinical response.*
- Use *haemodynamic response* to guide treatment. Use 0.9% saline initially (unless severe hypotension indicates the need for colloid). Typically, a rate of approximately 1000 mL/h is needed for the first hour then 500 mL/h for the following 2 h. Subsequent rate should be guided by clinical examination.
- *Add potassium* to fluid, guided by *regular monitoring of serum potassium*, except in severe renal failure or ESRD.
- Observe closely for features of cerebral oedema. *Confusion or deterioration in consciousness level indicate urgent transfer to a critical care or intensive care bed and adjustment of the rate of insulin and fluid administration under the guidance of a senior physician.*
- Consider use of central venous pressure monitoring after initial fluid resuscitation.

Potassium replacement

Potassium replacement is needed almost invariably in DKA, despite initial hyperkalaemia. The only common exception is in ESRD patients and some patients with a severe degree of chronic renal failure.

Initial hyperkalaemia is due to insulin deficiency and consequent movement of potassium out of cells but potassium is mainly an intracellular ion and there is a large whole-body deficit due to high urinary potassium loss. Serum potassium falls rapidly when insulin therapy is commenced due to re-entry into cells.

Start intravenous potassium supplementation at the initiation of insulin therapy if serum potassium is not > 5 mmol/L and urine output is good (Lebovitz 1997).

Diabetic ketoacidosis and non-ketonic hyperglycaemia

> **KEY POINT**
> * Frequent monitoring of serum potassium is essential in the treatment of DKA. Check at least every 2 h in the early phase of treatment to avoid dangerous hypokalaemia. Serum magnesium may also fluctuate and may contribute to arrhythmias, and should be corrected.

Potassium replacement should be given on a sliding scale according to frequent measurement of serum concentration (at least 2 hourly):

If serum potassium is < 3 mmol/L, give 40 mmol/h
If K^+ is 3–4 mmol/L, give 30 mmol/h
If K^+ is 4–5 mmol/L, give 20 mmol/h
If K^+ is > 5 mmol/L, stop potassium supplementation.

High rates of potassium supplementation will only be possible with central venous access due to risks of peripheral thrombophlebitis with concentrated potassium infusions.

Insulin therapy

* Administer soluble human insulin by infusion with an initial loading dose of 6 units.
* Set up an intravenous insulin infusion, 6 units/h initially.
* Aim to lower blood glucose by 5 mmol/L/h.
* Measure blood glucose hourly and adjust the insulin infusion rate accordingly.

Switch the intravenous fluid to 5% dextrose with potassium supplementation as appropriate when blood glucose falls below 14 mmol/L and recommence standard insulin treatment or change to glucose and insulin infusions. Resolution of ketoacidosis may be implied by normalization of the anion gap (Lebovitz 1997).

Complications of DKA

It is important to be aware of the risks associated with DKA and its treatment. Vigilance must be exercised throughout treatment.

Cerebral oedema

Headache or a deteriorating consciousness level should raise suspicion of cerebral oedema. This potentially devastating complication is more common in children and adolescents and can occur despite careful management.

Ultimately, intracranial pressure may rise (hypertension and bradycardia) and in these patients there is a high rate of death or permanent injury. Likely causative factors include:

* endothelial dysfunction with consequent breakdown of the blood–brain barrier

- fluid shift into brain cells due to hyponatraemia or rapid lowering of serum osmolality
- ischaemic cerebral injury in shocked patients.

Risk factors have been defined in children and adolescents, which largely indicate greater severity of disease or delay in presentation (Dunger et al 2004):

- Younger age
- New presentation of diabetes
- Persistence of hyponatraemia
- Higher initial blood urea
- Administration of sodium bicarbonate.

The rate of fluid and insulin administration and rate of correction of hypoglycaemia have not been shown to be risk factors.

> **Tip**
> Vigilance for early features and attention to careful fluid management is paramount. If suspicion of cerebral oedema arises, decrease rate of fluid and insulin administration and organize assessment by the critical care team as intubation might be needed.

Pulmonary aspiration

Vomiting is an indication for nasogastric tube insertion and aspiration. Some authorities insist on nasogastric tube insertion as a matter of routine as gastroparesis is common and pulmonary aspiration a risk.

Hypokalaemia

Life-threatening arrhythmias can be precipitated by hypokalaemia if intravenous potassium supplementation is insufficient. Frequent monitoring to ensure adequacy of supplementation is essential.

Hypomagnesaemia

Hypomagnesaemia is common and may also contribute to arrhythmias. 20 mmol of magnesium is commonly required in the first 24 h.

Hypoglycaemia

This was a devastating complication in the past when large subcutaneous doses of insulin were used. It is rarely encountered with modern infusion pumps, regular monitoring of blood glucose and close observation of patients during the initial hours of therapy.

Complications of the precipitating event

The precipitating illness and its complications must not be ignored. Underlying sepsis is frequently the cause of DKA and the infective focus might not be obvious. In adults, myocardial infarction should be excluded (remember that diabetic people are at much greater risk of cardiovascular disease and this might be clinically silent).

NKH in contrast to DKA

In NKH, volume depletion and hyperosmolality are usually severe. Consequently there are some differences in the approach, which are covered by numerous texts:

- 0.45% saline should be used if serum sodium is above 145 mmol/L.
- There is a very high risk of thrombosis; heparinization is required if there is no obvious contraindication.
- Insulin sensitivity is greater than in DKA.
- Serum potassium is more erratic and demands frequent monitoring as in DKA.

ADRENAL INSUFFICIENCY AND HYPOADRENAL CRISIS

Introduction

Adrenal insufficiency usually arises insidiously, subsequently presenting with shock as *adrenal crisis* at times of stress due to intercurrent illness. It is mineralocorticoid deficiency that tends to provoke hypotension and shock, as opposed to glucocorticoid deficiency.

Clues to the presence of adrenal insufficiency

- Hyperpigmentation (due to long-term hypersecretion of ACTH)
- History of pre-existing anorexia, fatigue, weight loss or vomiting (try to question the patient's family or companions)
- Hypotension and hypovolaemia
- Hyponatraemia (+/− hyperkalaemia)
- Features of an acute precipitating illness (frequently infection).

Normal serum potassium does not exclude the diagnosis (Hoorn et al 2005).

Diagnosis and treatment

Adrenal crisis is a potentially fatal condition. Treatment is urgent and should be commenced before definitive laboratory confirmation.

- Replace volume deficit by 0.9% saline – this effectively corrects the effects of mineralocorticoid deficiency.
  (Hyponatraemia can cause adrenal crisis to be mistaken for SIADH; incorrect therapy by water restriction as opposed to volume replacement may lead to fatal circulatory collapse.)
- Administer *dexamethasone* while a short synacthen test is performed. (Dexamethasone does not interfere with laboratory assay for cortisol).
- Search for the underlying precipitant. This is frequently infective and must not be neglected.
- Acute bilateral adrenal haemorrhage can cause adrenal crisis to develop in patients without pre-existing adrenal dysfunction.

  Risk factors for bilateral adrenal haemorrhage:

  – meningococcal septicaemia (Waterhouse-Friederichsen syndrome)
  – coagulation disorders and therapeutic anticoagulation
  – recent surgery.

  Long-term glucocorticoid and mineralocorticoid replacement can be commenced subsequently, on receipt of confirmatory laboratory results.

HYPOTHYROIDISM AND MYXOEDEMA COMA

Introduction

Severe hypothyroidism can present with hypothermia, severe hypotension and deteriorating mental status or coma. Fortunately this presentation is now rarely encountered.

Clinical features

- Mental obtundation
- Hypothermia
- Bradycardia
- Severe hypotension
- Typical hypothyroid facies.

Priorities

- Check blood glucose – hypoglycaemia may result from hypothyroidism or co-existing adrenal insufficiency.

- Look for a precipitating illness – infection, myocardial infarction.
- Summon expert help – the assistance of the critical care team and endocrinological advice will usually be needed.

Diagnosis and treatment

Treatment is urgent and cannot await laboratory results for thyroid function. Hence, diagnosis is effectively based on clinical features. *Administration of thyroid hormones, which will usually require intravenous T3, is potentially dangerous and should always be directed by a senior physician.* The patient usually requires admission directly to the intensive care unit.

THYROTOXIC CRISIS (THYROID STORM)

Definition

These terms describe extreme hyperthyroidism. Diagnostic criteria based on a scoring system for individual symptoms have been suggested (Burch & Wartofsky 1993). It is an uncommon condition which occurs in patients with Graves' disease or multinodular goitre and is usually precipitated by infection, surgery, trauma or pregnancy. With adequate preconditioning of the thyroid, it is unusual for this condition to be precipitated by thyroid surgery.

Clinical features and diagnosis

Symptoms and signs are those of extreme thyroid overactivity. Pyrexia and profuse sweating are almost invariable. Cardiovascular features include tachycardia sometimes in excess of 140/min and high output cardiac failure. Restlessness progresses to agitation and ultimately to delirium, stupor and coma. Nausea, vomiting and abdominal pain are also common.

Diagnosis is dependent on clinical suspicion when compatible clinical features develop in a patient who has a goitre or ophthalmic signs of Graves' disease or who is known to have pre-existing hyperthyroidism. If control is not established the condition is fatal, so treatment must not be delayed while waiting for laboratory results.

Treatment of thyrotoxic crisis

Initially, many patients are in need of fluid resuscitation but subsequently there is a risk of pulmonary oedema as cardiac failure develops. Attention

> **Tip**
> Supportive therapy is vital; patients suspected of having thyrotoxic crisis should be referred to the critical care unit as mortality is high. Treatment should always be guided by a senior physician.

must be paid to the precipitating illness in addition to establishing control of hyperthyroidism.

There are several elements to controlling thyroid overactivity. The principal elements of the drug therapy of thyrotoxic crisis are outlined below.

Thionamides

These drugs inhibit de novo synthesis of thyroid hormone.

Propylthiouracil is short acting but also inhibits peripheral conversion of T4 to T3.

Methimazole is an alternative with a longer duration, but does not inhibit peripheral conversion of T4 to T3.

Iodine-containing solutions

These inhibit release of T4 and T3 from the thyroid gland but can provide a substrate for synthesis of new hormone so thiomamide must be given at least 1 hour before iodine.

Glucocorticoids

Many physicians use glucocorticoids in thyrotoxic crisis because they act synergistically with propylthiouracil to inhibit peripheral conversion of T4 to T3. There is some evidence that glucocorticoids improve outcome.

Dexamethasone 2 mg orally at 6 hourly intervals or hydrocortisone 100 mg intravenously at 8-h intervals can act synergistically with propylthiouracil to inhibit peripheral conversion of T4 to T3.

Beta-blockade

Beta-blockade has an important role in many thyrotoxic patients. Control of severe tachycardia can optimize cardiac output and reduce myocardial oxygen consumption. Caution is required, however, as rarely, high-output cardiac failure may be worsened when treated with beta-blockade, and cardiac output monitoring as well as invasive cardiac pressure monitoring may be required during treatment of a thyrotoxic crisis.

Some protocols use propranolol intravenously whilst concurrently loading orally.

A short-acting agent such as esmolol may also be used intravenously.

High pyrexia can be treated pharmacologically by acetaminophen. However, salicylates must be avoided as they increase circulating free T4 and T3 due to competition for binding sites on carrier proteins.

CASE 11.1

A 56-year-old man is admitted directly to the coronary care unit with the ECG shown below (Fig 11.5). He lives alone and had been found by relatives lying unconscious on the floor of his home. Clinical examination shows him to be severely dehydrated, confused and he is anuric.
  Serum creatinine is 1500 μmol/L.

1. Which laboratory investigations should be undertaken most urgently?
2. What is the most likely cause of the ECG abnormality and what immediate treatment is required?
3. Which condition is most likely to be responsible for the renal failure?

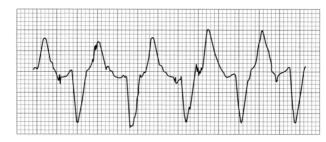

Figure 11.5   ECG.

Answers

1. Check the serum potassium urgently. (Most blood gas analyzers will give an estimate of serum potassium on a heparinized sample but this might be inaccurate if the analyzer has not been calibrated regularly.) Also check serum creatine kinase and serum calcium (rhabdomyolysis can cause severe hypocalcaemia).
2. Broad complex tachycardia should be regarded as ventricular tachycardia but in this case the underlying cause is almost certainly hyperkalaemia. The serum creatinine concentration of 1500 μmol/L indicates ARF or CRF. Immediate cardioprotection with 10 mL of 10% calcium gluconate is indicated whilst more definite treatment is prepared. His rhythm strip following this is shown in Figure 11.6.
3. The history suggests that he might have been unconscious on the floor for many hours resulting in rhabdomyolysis. Following fluid resuscitation he produced urine, deep red in colour (Fig. 11.7) from the presence of myoglobin.

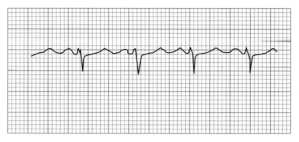

Figure 11.6 ECG following calcium gluconate.

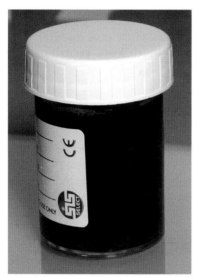

Figure 11.7 Deep red urine indicative of myoglobinuria.

Rhabdomyolysis results in a toxic form of intrinsic acute renal failure with severe hyperkalaemia due to lysis of myocytes. Fluid resuscitation is needed urgently. Establishment of a good urine output reduces the toxicity of myoglobin during its transit through the renal tubules. Tubular toxicity is exacerbated by acidosis but the role of bicarbonate in therapy is not clear. Sodium bicarbonate is potentially harmful in hypocalcaemia as a rise in pH can lower serum ionized calcium concentration and intravenous bicarbonate should be used with caution. There are several good reviews of this subject (Holt & Moore 2001).

CASE 11.2

A 65-year-old man is referred to the acute medical intake with a three-day history of left-sided chest pain which is pleuritic in nature. He underwent coronary artery bypass grafting three weeks earlier. He knows that he has been receiving anti-hypertensive medication but has not brought his medication with him.

Examination reveals crackles at the left lung base and his BP is 122/68. CXR shows left basal consolidation and a small effusion. Serum creatinine is 217 μmol/L.

He is admitted to the ward. It is Friday afternoon.

48 h later he is described by the nursing staff as clammy. His BP is 100/60. JVP is not elevated. Serum creatinine is now 675 μmol/L and serum potassium is 7.2 μmol/L. The medication card indicates that he received a single dose of an NSAID 2 days before for pleuritic chest pain. It is also noted that an ACE-inhibitor was added to his chart on the evening of his admission to hospital.

1. Summarize the immediate management.
2. List all the factors which have contributed to the development of ARF.

Answers

1. He requires urgent management of hyperkalaemia. You should organize an ECG immediately and, if there are hyperkalaemic features, administer calcium gluconate intravenously (10 mL of calcium gluconate 10% by slow intravenous injection over 5 min). Assess fluid status. He might have cardiac failure but it is more likely that he is volume deplete (as he has been admitted with a post-operative pneumonia). A CVP line is likely to be needed if fluid challenge is to be initiated. If he is over-loaded he requires urgent dialysis. You should contact the renal unit anyway to alert them to the case.
2. This case is a classic example of hospital-acquired ARF. The patient has four of the most important and common risk factors (Nolan & Adamson 1998):

- Recent surgery
- Infection/sepsis
- Volume depletion
- Nephrotoxic drug therapy.

This patient was volume deplete and demonstrated relative hypotension, having been chronically hypertensive. There was no response to fluid therapy initially and he required urgent dialysis for hyperkalaemia. Following this, renal function improved, which is usually the case in ARF.

His medications, which included an ACE-inhibitor had been brought in by his wife and written up by the house officer on call.

Intensive monitoring of biochemistry and haemodynamic parameters is essential in such patients. The risk factors for ARF should be identified and highlighted at admission. Nephrotoxic and antihypertensive therapy should be modified accordingly.

Institution of dietary potassium restriction can help avoid development of life-threatening hyperkalaemia when serum potassium starts to rise. (Dietary potassium should not be restricted if serum potassium is normal or low.)

A 20-year-old woman is referred to the acute medical intake by her general practitioner due to malaise, cough and shortage of breath on exertion. She gives a history of haemoptysis and polyarticular arthralgia during the preceding two months.

A CXR is performed (Fig 11.8). Dipstick urinalysis shows blood ++++ and protein +++. The serum creatinine is 550 μmol/L.

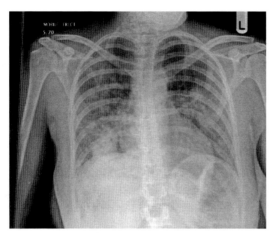

Figure 11.8   Chest X-ray.

1. What type of renal failure is she likely to be suffering from? Suggest a possible diagnosis.

2. Why is she in danger of respiratory failure and how should she be monitored on the ward?

Answers

1. This patient is very likely to have an intrinsic renal disease on the basis of both the history, which suggests a multisystem inflammatory condition, and the urinalysis which is compatible with an active glomerulonephritis. Her CXR and history suggest pulmonary haemorrhage. She probably has a systemic vasculitis such as Wegener's granulomatosis or microscopic polyangiitis.

2. She gives a history of haemoptysis and shortage of breath on exertion. Her CXR shows an alveolar pattern of shadowing and the haemoglobin is falling. This indicates pulmonary haemorrhage which can result in respiratory failure and is sometimes fatal. Monitor respiratory rate and oxygen saturation closely with vigilance for the onset of respiratory failure.

Pulmonary haemorrhage in the context of a vasculitis is a clear indication for immunosuppression and plasma exchange. Such patients must be referred to the local renal unit urgently and might require critical or intensive care.

Respiratory rate and oxygen saturation must be monitored closely with a daily CXR. Pulmonary haemorrhage can precipitate respiratory failure requiring ventilation. C-ANCA was positive in this case, with a high titre, indicating a diagnosis of Wegener's granulomatosis. She received plasma exchange and immunosuppression by corticosteroid and cyclophosphamide. Renal function recovered.

CASE 11.4

A 58-year-old man is referred to the medical unit with a 5-day history of vomiting, dizziness and headache. Ten days earlier, he had attended the accident and emergency department complaining of severe frontal headache of sudden onset but had been discharged home following CT scan of the head which showed no abnormality.

There is a family history of subarachnoid haemorrhage. He is taking no medication.

Clinical examination reveals no neurological deficit and no meningism. He is apyrexial but mildly confused. BP is 138/78 and heart rate 60 bpm. Investigations show a serum sodium of 106 mmol/L, potassium of 5.4 mmol/L and blood glucose of 4.7 mmol/L. Repeat CT scan shows no abnormality.

1. Suggest three possible causes for hyponatraemia in this case.
2. Which investigations should now be undertaken to identify the cause of the low serum sodium?

Answers

1. If artefactual hyponatraemia is excluded, the likely cause is either SIADH associated with subarachnoid haemorrhage, cerebral salt wasting, or pituitary apoplexy.

Subarachnoid haemorrhage has not been excluded with a normal CT scan; both SIADH and cerebral salt wasting (CSW) are associated with a variety of intracranial disorders including subarachnoid haemorrhage, infection, tumours, head injury and following neurosurgery. CSW is believed to be caused by the presence of salt-losing factors which might include atrial natriuretic peptide and ouabain-like factors secreted by the hypothalamus. Laboratory investigations compatible with these diagnoses are outlined below.

Pituitary apoplexy results from infarction in a pituitary tumour, causing headache with or without a visual field defect. This condition is important because loss of pituitary function is sudden and profound, sometimes resulting in hypoadrenal crisis and cardiovascular collapse.

Secondary (pituitary) and tertiary (hypothalamic) adrenal insufficiency do not usually cause hypoadrenal crisis as mineralocorticoid production is unaffected but glucocorticoids have a role in maintaining sympathetic tone and sudden loss can cause hypotension. Pituitary apoplexy should always be considered in a patient with headache and hyponatraemia.

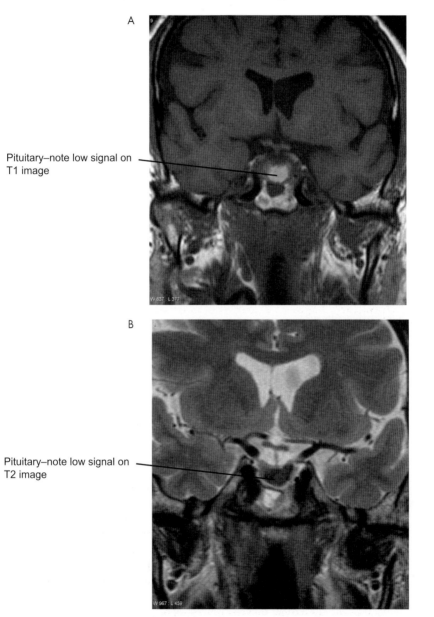

A

Pituitary–note low signal on T1 image

B

Pituitary–note low signal on T2 image

Figure 11.9   Coronal T1 and T2 weighted images demonstrate hyperintensity on T1 and hypointensity on T2, indicating subacute haemorrhage with the formation of intracellular deoxyhaemoglobin. This is indicative of pituitary haemorrhage and pituitary apoplexy. (A) High signal on T1 weighted image. (B) Low signal on T2 weighted image. (Courtesy of Dr N. Bradey.)

2. Lumbar puncture should be performed and a sample analyzed by photospectrometry for xanthochromia helps to exclude a diagnosis of SAH. If doubt remains due to ongoing symptoms or a convincing history, a neurosurgical opinion should be sought as cerebral angiography might be indicated.

Serum and urine osmolality and urine sodium concentration should be measured to look for evidence of SIADH or CSW. Both conditions are associated with a urine to plasma osmolality ratio of > 1 due to an inappropriately high urine osmolality. Urine sodium is usually > 20 mmol/L. Differentiation between SIADH and CSW can be very difficult (Albanese et al 2001).

A complete anterior pituitary profile should be ordered to look for evidence of pituitary apoplexy. Magnetic resonance imaging (MRI) is required in order to image the pituitary satisfactorily.

In this case, hypopituitarism was demonstrated and MRI scan (Fig. 11.9A,B) revealed features of pituitary apoplexy. He received glucocorticoid replacement and intravenous rehydration using 0.9% saline. Thyroid hormone replacement should be commenced only following glucocorticoid replacement.

REFERENCES AND FURTHER READING

Acute dialysis quality initiative (4th consensus conference). Online. Available: http://www.adqi.net

Albanese A, Hindmarsh P, Stanhope R 2001 Management of hyponatraemia in patients with acute cerebral insults. Archives of Diseases of Childhood 85:246–251

Basi S, Pupin L B, Simmons E M et al 2005 Insulin resistance in critically ill patients with acute renal failure. American Journal of Physiology. Renal Physiology 289:F259–F264

Bell J I, Hockaday T D R 1996 Diabetes mellitus. In: Weatherall D J, Ledingham J G G, Warrell D A (eds) Oxford textbook of medicine, 3rd edn. Oxford Medical Press, Oxford, p 1498–1503

Bhandari S, Turney J H 1996 Survivors of acute renal failure who do not recover renal function. QJM 89(6):415–421

Burch H B, Wartofsky L 1993 Life threatening thyrotoxicosis. Thyroid storm. Endocrinology and Metabolism Clinics of North America 22:263

Burton C J, Tomson C R V 1999 Can the use of low-dose dopamine for treatment of acute renal failure be justified? Postgraduate Medical Journal 75:269–274

Dunger D B, Sperling M A, Acerini C L et al 2004 ESPE/LWPES consensus statement on diabetic ketoacidosis in children and adolescents. Archives of Diseases of Childhood 89:188–194

Dunger D B, Sperling M A, Acerini CL et al 2004 European Society for Pediatric Endocrinology/Lawson Wilkins Pediatric Endocrine Society consensus statement on diabetic ketoacidosis in children and adolescents. Pediatrics 113:e133–140

Firth J D 1998 The clinical approach to the patient with acute renal failure. In: Davison A M, Cameron S, Grunfeld J P et al (eds) Oxford textbook of clinical nephrology, 2nd edn. Oxford University Press, Oxford, p 1557–1582

Gambaro G, Bertaglia G, Puma G et al 2002 Diuretics and dopamine for the prevention and treatment of acute renal failure: a critical reappraisal. Journal of Nephrology 15:213–219

Hatala R, Dinh T, Cook D J 1996 Once-daily aminoglycoside dosing in immuno-competent adults: a meta-analysis. Annals of Internal Medicine 124: 717–725

Holt S G, Moore K P 2001 Pathogenesis and treatment of renal dysfunction in rhabdomyolysis. Intensive Care Medicine 27:803–811

Hoorn E J, Halperin M L, Zietse R 2005 Diagnostic approach to a patient with hyponatraemia:traditional versus physiology-based options. QJM 98(7):529–540

Larsen P R, Davies T F, Hay I D 1998 The thyroid gland. In: Wilson J D, Foster D W, Kroenberg H M et al (eds) Williams textbook of endocrinology, 9th edn. W B Saunders, Philadelphia, p 389–515

Lebovitz H E 1997 Diabetic ketoacidosis. Medicine 25(7):51–54

Lemley K V, Bayliss C 1997 The renal circulation. In: Jamieson R L, Wilkinson R (eds) Nephrology. Chapman and Hall, London

Levy E M, Viscoli C M, Horwitz R I 1996 The effect of acute renal failure on mortality: a cohort analysis. Journal of the American Medical Association 275:1489–1494

Nolan C R, Adamson R J 1998 Hospital-acquired acute renal failure. Journal of the American Society of Nephrology 1998: 710–718

Orth D N, Kovacs J 1998 The adrenal cortex. In: Wilson J D, Foster D W, Kroenberg H M et al (eds) Williams textbook of endocrinology, 9th edn. W B Saunders, Philadelphia, p 560–565

Roberts I, Alderson P, Bunn F et al 2005 Colloids versus crystalloids for fluid resuscitation in critically ill patients (review). The Cochrane Library (4). Online. Available: http://www.thecochranelibrary.com

Spital A 1988 Clinical assessment of extracellular fluid volume in hyponatraemia. American Journal of Medicine 84:562

Unger R H, Foster D W 1998 Diabetes. In: Wilson J D, Foster D W, Kroenberg H M et al (eds) Williams textbook of endocrinology, 9th edn. W B Saunders, Philadelphia, p 973–1059

Van den Berghe G, Wouters P, Weekers F et al 2001 Intensive insulin therapy in critically ill patients. New England Journal of Medicine 345:1359–1367

References and further reading

Poisoning

Kyee Han

After reading this chapter you should be able to:

- *Follow an airway, breathing and circulation (ABC) approach to the care of the poisoned patient*

- *Use gastric lavage in appropriate cases*

- *Follow treatment algorithms for most common serious poisons*

- *Understand the need for a multidisciplinary approach to the care of a patient following intentional overdose*

CASE 12.1

A 25-year-old housewife is brought by ambulance to your accident and emergency (A&E) department. It is 02.45 and the paramedics were responding to a 999 call made by her partner. She had allegedly taken an overdose of the following drugs: kapake, dothiepin and aminophylline together with cider. On arrival at the house the paramedics found the patient lying on the floor.

Initial prehospital assessment:

Airway	**Patent but nasopharyngeal airway inserted**
Breathing	**Spontaneous at rate of 20/min**
Circulation	**Pulse 100/min regular, blood pressure (BP) 140/80 mmHg, SpO$_2$ 98%**
Disability	**Patient responding to voice.**

Prehospital treatment:

Oxygen 12 L/min using mask with O$_2$ reservoir
Nasopharyngeal airway
ECG monitoring.

En route, the patient's level of consciousness deteriorates to GCS 7 (E2 V2 M3) and she tolerates an oropharyngeal airway:

E2: Eye opening to painful stimuli
V2: Incomprehensible noises
M3: Flexes to painful stimuli.

You are the receiving doctor in the A&E department. How would you proceed?

Answer
After initial assessment, continued administration of high-flow oxygen and venous access to the patient's airway was secured by orotracheal intubation. In view of the tachycardia and ECG findings sodium bicarbonate was given with good effect. The paracetamol level was above the treatment line and acetylcysteine was started in A&E before transfer to the intensive care unit.

The patient was referred to the liaison psychiatry team whilst in hospital.

INTRODUCTION

Poisoning is a leading cause of death in patients less then 40 years of age. It is also the commonest cause of non-traumatic coma in this age group. Self-poisoning with therapeutic or recreational drugs is the main reason for acute medical admissions.

Poisoning may be accidental or intentional. Homicidal poisoning is rare. A 10-year overview of poisoning data in the USA revealed that 78% involved oral ingestion, 13% were by inhalation and 5% were due to parenteral administration. 7% of poisonings involved multiple agents.

Around 15–20% of the workload of medical units and 10% of the work-load of A&E departments in the UK are due to self-poisoning. Alcohol is often taken with the poison(s) and this makes assessment and management more difficult.

Very occasionally industrial accidents and, rarely, warfare, may result in chemical exposure on a larger scale. In such an event, the safety of the staff treating the victims must be considered. Appropriate protective equipment should be worn. Decontamination facilities for the victims must also be provided as close to the scene of the incident as possible, to prevent contamination of the receiving hospital. Although the severity of poisoning has diminished over the past 12 years the total number of deaths from poisoning in the UK remains steady at 4000 per year.

INITIAL ASSESSMENT

A significant number of patients present with an altered level of consciousness and the conventional method of taking a history, examining the patient, investigation, diagnosis and treatment cannot be adhered to. It is important to identify and address the immediate life-threatening factors and address these before moving on with evaluation and treatment of other factors. Only when the airway, breathing and circulation are secure and stable should one take a brief history and plan appropriate investigation and definitive treatment.

Airway

Airway obstruction and respiratory arrest secondary to a decreased consciousness level is a common cause of death.

- Ensure that the airway is clear.
- Test for loss of protective laryngeal reflexes.
- If a Guedel (oropharyngeal) airway is tolerated seek the opinion of an anaesthetist as to whether or not definitive airway protection is necessary.
- Protect the cervical spine if there is any possibility of associated injury.

Breathing

- Assess rate and quality of breathing.
- Remember there may be respiratory depression even if the respiratory rate and arterial oxygen saturation tests are normal.
- Give supplementary oxygen via non-rebreathing mask at a flow rate of 12 L/min.
- Only in the case of possible paraquat poisoning (extremely rare in the UK) should a high concentration of oxygen be withheld as it increases pulmonary injury.

Circulation

- Assess rate and quality of pulse in the carotid and radial artery.
- Observe colour and temperature of hands and assess capillary refill.
- Obtain IV access in the cubital fossa of the arm using a large bore cannula.
- Give fluid bolus if evidence of cardiovascular compromise. Take blood samples at the time of inserting intravenous access.
- Look for injection sites if IV drug abuse is suspected.
- If the patient is fitting, control with IV diazepam 10 mg (child 0.1–0. 3 mg/kg) or lorazepam (0.07 mg/kg).

Disability and decontamination

Assess level of consciousness using the Glasgow Coma Score. If it is 8 or below, seek an anaesthetist for endotracheal intubation and mechanical ventilation.

- Assess the size of pupils and response to light.
- Consider the need for decontamination if toxic chemical exposure is suspected.

Exposure

- Cut the patient's clothes off if necessary for full clinical examination but take measures to avoid hypothermia.
- Connect the patient to a cardiac and vital signs monitor.
- Catheterize the patient to monitor urine output (particularly if the patient is unconscious).

In the event of a cardiorespiratory arrest, follow advanced life support guidelines using the European Resuscitation Council guidelines.

WHEN THE PATIENT IS ADEQUATELY RESUSCITATED

1. Take a brief history from any relative, ambulance personnel or the patient

Enquire for:

What – bottles, packets or tablets (including regularly prescribed or over the counter (OTC) medication)
When – time the relevant agent(s) were taken
How – its route
Why – suicide notes, psychiatric history, morbid ideas.

2. Examine the patient fully with particular reference to other causes of unconsciousness and specific signs of poisoning

Examine particularly for:

- odours
- respiratory rate and quality
- heart rate and rhythm
- blood pressure
- core temperature
- level of consciousness (GCS)
- pupil size and reaction to light
- skin signs – needle tracts, cuts, scars or blisters
- associated signs of injury
- signs of corrosion in the mouth.

3. Investigations

The following tests are recommended on the blood sample taken at the time of obtaining venous access:

- Blood glucose
- Urea and electrolytes
- INR and liver function tests
- Plasma paracetamol and salicylate levels
- Toxicology

- Arterial blood gases
- A 12-lead ECG is essential to detect cardiac arrhythmias.

A sample of urine (50 mL) must be stored in a refrigerator for toxicology screen later.

TREATMENT

If the patient is unconscious and no cause has been found, give:

- 50 mL of 50% glucose solution, intravenously. If there is no response and there are features compatible with opioid poisoning (pinpoint pupils, respiratory depression, absent bowel sounds, injection marks), give: 800 µg (0.8 mg) naloxone intravenously and a further 400 µg (0.4 mg every 2 min) until there is a response or until 2 mg has been given. In children the dose is 0.01 µg/kg.
- If life-threatening tachyarrhythmias occur, cardioversion is indicated except in Torsade de Pointes.

Drug-induced hypotension (systolic < 90 mmHg) is common after self-poisoning. This usually responds to fluid therapy, but occasionally inotropic support is required.

SPECIFIC TREATMENT

There are few specific therapeutic measures for poisons that are useful in the immediate situation. However, if there is a drug for which there is a specific elimination measure or for which a specific antidote or treatment exists, appropriate measures should be undertaken.

METHODS TO PREVENT DRUG ABSORPTION

Three methods have commonly been used with the aim of reducing the absorption of poisons taken by mouth. These are oral-activated charcoal, gastric lavage, and the induction of vomiting using syrup of ipecacuanha. These methods have been greatly overused, considering that:

- there is little evidence that any of these methods reduce drug absorption when used more than 1 h after ingestion of poison, even in the presence of drugs which delay gastric emptying (e.g. salicylates, tricyclic antidepressants, opiates).
- there is very little evidence that they affect clinical outcome. They can, however, cause complications.
- none of these methods are required unless the poison taken carries a significant hazard to the patient.

The European Association of Poisons Centres and Clinical Toxicologists (EAPCCT) and American Association of Clinical Toxicology (AACT) have recently published joint position statements on the use of these methods. The guidance that follows is consistent with these.

Activated charcoal

- This is preferred for the majority of poisons because it is the safest, most convenient method and is as, or more effective than, the other techniques.
- The dose should preferably be *at least* 10 times the quantity of poison taken, as the larger the dose the more pronounced the effect. Doses of 50–100 g (adults) or 25–50 g (children) should be aimed for.
- In patients who vomit or who refuse to swallow the activated charcoal, it can be administered via a nasogastric tube. However, there is always the potential for pulmonary aspiration of activated charcoal if the patient has an impaired (or falling) level of consciousness and in such circumstances it is rarely used.
- If the patient has already been intubated and ventilated for an impaired GCS, the airway is already protected and activated charcoal should be given via nasogastric tube if this is indicated.
- Activated charcoal can be administered in a more palatable form for children by dissolving it in flat cola.
- Repeated doses of activated charcoal are also effective at increasing the elimination of some poisons from the body.
- Activated charcoal is *ineffective* for poisoning with lithium, iron salts, hydrocarbons and some insecticides.

KEY POINT
- Patients with a reduced level of consciousness should not be administered activated charcoal unless the airway is protected, because of the high risk of aspiration pneumonitis, which can be life threatening.

Gastric lavage

- This is only likely to be of benefit if it is used within 1 h of ingestion.
- It carries the risk of gut perforation and aspiration. It may also compromise the patient's airway.
- It should *never* be used to remove hydrocarbons (petrol, diesel, mineral oil, paraffin, turpentine, white spirit), because of the risk of aspiration pneumonitis, or caustic substances (paint stripper, caustic soda, bleach), because of the risk of gut perforation.
- Endotracheal intubation is mandatory in unconscious patients or those with poor gag reflexes.
- For most poisons, activated charcoal is a better option but gastric lavage can be justified for:

– large life-threatening drug overdoses (> 5 g toxin) when there is a significant risk of adverse effects (activated charcoal should also be given via the gastric tube after lavage)
– clinically significant overdoses of drugs not absorbed by activated charcoal such as iron and lithium.

Induced emesis

- Syrup of ipecac is probably ineffective at removing significant amounts of poisons. The vomiting it produces may confuse the clinical picture and prevent the subsequent use of activated charcoal.
- The use of syrup of ipecac is therefore *not justifiable* in adults unless other treatments have been refused.
- Induced emesis may occasionally be justified in children who are at risk of developing symptoms from the poison they have swallowed, will not take activated charcoal, are too small for gastric lavage and present within 1 h. Its use should be discussed in advance with the Poisons Information Service.

> **KEY POINT**
> • **Syrup of ipecac should never be used when activated charcoal is indicated.**

METHODS OF ENHANCING DRUG ELIMINATION

Repeated activated charcoal

According to AACT/EAPCCT guidelines the elimination of the following poisons can be enhanced by repeated doses of oral activated charcoal:

- Carbamazepine
- Dapsone
- Phenobarbital
- Quinine
- Theophylline/aminophylline.

Repeated doses of activated charcoal are best given as follows:

- An initial dose of 50 g oral-activated charcoal *then* 50 g 4 hourly or 25 g oral-activated charcoal every 2 h. Routine use of a laxative (e.g. 20 mL lactulose or 20 mL 40% magnesium sulphate every 2 h, unless the patient already has diarrhoea) is advocated by some but is unproven and often unnecessary.
- Half these doses of activated charcoal may be used in older children.
- Ensure that bowel sounds are present before administering charcoal.
- Intravenous anti-emetics may be required if vomiting is a feature of toxicity (e.g. theophylline poisoning).

- Recent studies indicate that multiple dose activated charcoal improves elimination of some substances but there is no direct evidence of improved outcome.

Haemodialysis or haemoperfusion

Poisons whose elimination can be enhanced by haemodialysis or haemo-perfusion are shown in Table 12.1. If appropriate, consider referring the patient to your local renal unit. Further advice can be obtained from NPIS (National Poisons Information Service), Tel: 0870 600 6266, Website: http://www.spib.axl.co.uk

Altering urinary PH

This affects the tubular reabsorption of weak acids and bases, enhancing the elimination of the poison in the urine (Table 12.2).

For adult symptomatic salicylate poisoning give 1.5 L of 1.26% sodium bicarbonate IV over 3 h with 40 mmoL of KCl.

Forced alkaline diuresis is no longer recommended.

Table 12.1 Poisons for which haemodialysis or haemoperfusion may be considered. *preferred or more effective method

Agent	Haemodialysis	Haemoperfusion
Amphetamines	*	*
Aminophylline		*
Amylobarbitone		*
Carbamazepine		*
Chloral hydrate		*
Ethanol	*	
Ethylene glycol	*	
Lithium	*	
Methanol	*	
Metformin		*
Phenytoin		*
Salicylates	*	*
Sodium valproate	*	
Theophylline		*

Table 12.2 Enhanced elimination depending on acid/alkaline urine

Enhanced elimination depending on acidic/alkaline urine	
Acidic	Alkaline
Weak bases	Weak acids
(pH 7.5–10.5)	(pH 3.0–7.5)
Amphetamines	Salicylate
Phencyclidine	Phenobarbital
	Phenoxyacetate herbicides

Table 12.3 Poisons which may require specific antidotes

Poison	Antidote
Adder bite	Zagreb antivenom
Antimony	Dimercaprol (BAL)
Arsenic	Dimercaprol (BAL)
Benzodiazepines	Flumazenil
Beta-blockers	Glucagon, isoprenaline
Bismuth	Dimercaprol (BAL)
Copper	Penicillamine
Cyanide	Dicobalt edetate (kelocyanor)
Digoxin	Fab antibodies (digibind)
Ethylene glycol	Ethanol or fomepizole
Hydrofluoric acid	Calcium gluconate – topical or IV
Iron	Desferrioxamine
Lead	Sodium calcium edate, dimercaprol
Mercury	Dimercaprol (BAL)
Methanol	Ethanol
Opiates	Naloxone
Organophosphates	Pralidoxime
Paracetamol	Acetylcysteine
Scorpion stings	Specific antivenom
Snakebite	Specific antivenom
Thallium	Dimercaprol (BAL)

ANTIDOTES

Although the emphasis of treatment is on intensive supportive therapy with correction of hypoxia, acid-base and electrolyte disturbances, there are a few

---

Tip

Initial assessment

- A = Airway and cervical spine protection
- B = Breathing
- C = Circulation
- D = Disability and decontamination
- E = Exposure

Resuscitate and stabilize

Take a history	Establish what (including amount), when, how and why
Treat	Generally *supportive*
	Consider methods to prevent drug absorption or enhancing elimination
	Antidotes or specific treatment
Document	Integrated care pathway
Refer	Refer to liaison psychiatry team if poisoning is deliberate self-harm

If patient has a cardiac arrest resuscitate along ERC guidelines
Be prepared for a prolonged resuscitation attempt

---

specific antidotes for poisons that reverse or minimize the adverse effects of the poison (Table 12.3).

ONGOING MANAGEMENT

It is imperative to bear in mind that the condition of the poisoned patient can deteriorate on the ward. Close regular observation is necessary to identify the changes and appropriate action should be taken as required. If the poisoning is an act of deliberate self-harm, a suicide intent score must be calculated and the patient cared for in an appropriate environment.

CASE 12.2

A 20-year-old male student is brought from a club at 02:00 after having had an intravenous injection of heroin in the toilet. His friends noticed him slumped in a corner with minimal breathing effort and rang for an ambulance.

On arrival in A&E, he had pinpoint pupils and was given naloxone 800 μg intravenously. As he woke up and his breathing improved he was admitted to the acute medical ward.

15 min after arrival the nurse on the ward discovers that he has become unrousable with a respiratory rate of 5/min. A cardiac arrest call was put out for the team to attend. How would you proceed?

Answer
With bag valve assisted ventilation the patient started breathing and a further dose of intravenous naloxone 800 μg was given. An infusion of naloxone was immediately set up to prevent further episodes and he was observed in a medical high dependency unit.

The patient was referred to the liaison psychiatry team whilst in hospital.

MANAGEMENT OF COMMON OR IMPORTANT POISONS

Amphetamines and ecstasy

Drugs of misuse continue to present problems, particularly in the inner city areas. Deaths still result from ecstasy poisoning.

The potentially toxic dose is unpredictable as serious effects may occur from ingestion of a single tablet.

The effects are seen over 20 min to 6 h and the half-life is 8 h.

Common effects

- Increased muscle tone/trismus
- Adrenergic features (sweating, dry mouth, anxiety, tachycardia, hypertension, mydriasis)
- Neurological effects (anorexia, insomnia, confusion, ataxia, nystagmus)
- Gastrointestinal effects (nausea, vomiting, abdominal pain, diarrhoea).

Severe effects

- Neurological (delirium, coma, convulsions)
- Cardiovascular system (arrhythmias, acute respiratory distress syndrome (ARDS))
- Hyperpyrexia, rhabdomyolysis, renal failure, acidosis
- Disseminated intravascular coagulation
- Hyponatraemic acidosis
- Hepatocelluler necrosis
- Intracerebral haemorrhage
- ARDS.

Management

- Activated charcoal 50 g if presentation is within 1 h
- Monitor BP, ECG and temperature if signs of toxicology are present
- Correct metabolic acidosis using intravenous sodium bicarbonate.

Severe agitation or fits

- Give diazepam 10 mg (adult) or 0.1–0.03 mg/kg (child) intravenously and repeat if needed (beware respiratory depression)
- *Do not give neuroleptics* for agitation as these may provoke fits and hypotension.

Tachycardia and hypertension

- Control anxiety and agitation as above
- In most cases, persisting tachycardia and hypertension do not require drug treatment
- In extreme cases a beta-blocker may be used (beware paradoxical increases in BP due to unopposed alpha-receptor stimulation, which can be treated with the alpha-blocker phentolamine 2.5 mg IV). Sublingual nifedipine (5–10 mg) can be used for severe hypertension.

Hyperpyrexia, rigidity, rhabdomyolysis

- Give adequate intravenous fluids
- Consider giving dantrolene 1 mg/kg over 15 min, repeated if necessary (maximum 10 mg/kg)

- If this fails, consider using paralysis and mechanical ventilation
- Monitor liver function tests
- Check blood glucose.

Aggressive management and early involvement of the critical care team are appropriate.

Benzodiazepines

Oral benzodiazepines alone rarely cause deep coma. Suspect the synergistic effect of another agent (e.g. alcohol) or a predisposing factor (chronic obstructive pulmonary disease (COPD), old age).

Potentially toxic doses

- Greater than 1–2 mg/kg diazepam or nitrazepam, 2–4 mg/kg temazepam, or 3–6 mg/kg chlordiazepoxide or equivalent
- Lower doses may cause toxicity if taken in combination with other sedatives (e.g. alcohol) in patients with other illnesses (e.g. COPD, muscular weakness), or the elderly.

Establish

- Product taken
- Time taken
- Amount taken
- Other substances/products taken at the same time (e.g. alcohol/paracetamol)
- Other relevant illness (COPD).

Look for

- Drowsiness (Glasgow Coma Score)
- Ataxia
- Hypotension.

Management

If the patient is comatose or there are signs of respiratory disease

- Measure arterial blood gases.

If fewer than 30 tablets have been taken and there is no other poison

- Observe until the patient is awake and walking and talking.

If more than 30 tablets have been taken and it is less than 1 h since ingestion

- Give oral activated charcoal (50 g for an adult, smaller doses in children).

If there is respiratory depression (e.g. PCO_2 above 6 kPa) consider giving flumazenil, particularly in pure benzodiazepine poisoning in the high-risk group, e.g. chronic lung disease, neuromuscular disease.

Flumazenil dose

- Give sufficient amounts to maintain airway and respiration
- 0.5 mg IV, repeated every 30 s up to total dose of 1.5 mg
- Repeat as needed ($T^1/_2 = 1$ hour) every 20 min
- Give no more than 3 mg in 1 h.

  Flumazenil is not advocated in:

- Mixed/identified drug overdose
- Epileptic patients
- It should not be used as a diagnostic test.

Carbon monoxide

Carbon monoxide poisoning is common in patients with smoke inhalation. Such patients may also have cyanide intoxication.

Clinical features

- Mild poisoning – headache, nausea, irritability, dizziness
- Severe poisoning – drowsiness, ataxia, respiratory failure, cerebral oedema, rhabdomyolysis, myocardial infarction, cardiac failure, renal haemorrhages.

Suggested management

- Remove patient from exposure
- Ensure a clear airway
- Ensure the patient is given 100% oxygen to breathe
- Monitor cardiac rhythm and perform an ECG
- Measure oxygen saturation and perform arterial blood gases (oxygen saturation may be reduced even if the PO_2 is normal)
- Confirm ABGs analyzed with co-oximeter and also send blood for carboxyhaemoglobin concentration for laboratory analysis.

If the patient is in coma and ventilation is inadequate

- Seek assistance from the critical care/anaesthesia departments to intubate and commence artificial ventilation with 100% oxygen.

If papilloedema is present

- Give mannitol 0.5–1 g/kg (i.e. 200–400 mL of 20% mannitol for 80 kg patient) over 1 h.

Hyperbaric oxygen therapy may be of value in severe carbon monoxide poisoning although clinical trial evidence is inconclusive. It may be considered under the following circumstances:

- Reduced level of consciousness at presentation, or unconsciousness at any time after exposure
- Focal neurological or psychiatric features (other than mild headache)
- Cardiac dysrhythmias, ischaemia or infarction
- Carboxyhaemoglobin greater than 25% regardless of symptoms
- Pregnancy.

At present, facilities are limited and CO levels are often normal by the time the patient reaches the hyperbaric centre. However, some authorities believe that long-term neuropsychiatric outcome is superior after hyberbaric treatment for severe poisoning (> 25%). Potential benefit must be weighed against transfer risks. Liaise with the critical care team on these risks and call NPIS for advice.

Opiates

Beware of the risk of cross-infection with blood-borne viruses from intravenous drug users.

Opiates and opioids include:

- buprenorphine
- codeine (*sometimes* with paracetamol – treat both)
- dextropropoxyphene (*usually* with paracetamol – treat both)
- diamorphine
- dihydrocodeine
- diphenoxylate (in lomotil which also contains atropine)
- heroin
- morphine (MST)
- pentazocine
- pethidine
- tramadol
- buprenorphine is atypical – naloxone is less effective and only at high doses.

Potentially toxic doses

- > 100 mg morphine/diamorphine or 10–20 co-proxamol tablets/70 kg in an adult may cause serious toxicity
- Higher doses are required to produce serious toxicity from codeine (> 1000 mg/70 kg in an adult) or dihydrocodeine (> 500 mg/70 kg in an adult)
- Toxic effects may be potentiated by co-ingestion of other sedative agents, including alcohol.

Management

- Suspect the diagnosis in any patient with small pupils.

If the patient is unconscious or has respiratory depression

- Ensure clear airway
- Give naloxone 800 µg (0.8 mg) IV and a further 400 µg (0.4 mg) IV every 2 min until the patient improves (respiratory rate, pupil size, consciousness) or 3.2 mg has been given
- In children the dose is 0.01 mg/kg
- In A&E departments it is accepted practice to give 800 µg IM at the time of the IV dose, as there is the danger that the patient might walk out of the department before further IV doses are administered.

If the patient responds to IV naloxone, remember

- Relapse is likely after about 20 min
- Paracetamol (co-codamol, co-dydramol, co-proxamol) may also have been taken in significant amounts
- Opiates delay gastric emptying and some are slow release; effects may therefore be prolonged.

If relapse occurs

- Repeat IV naloxone 400 µg (0.4 mg) IV every 2 min until patient improves or 2 mg has been given.

If a large dose has been taken, or relapse has occurred

- Set up an infusion (5 × 400 µg ampoules naloxone = 2 mg in 500 mL 5% dextrose) at a rate that equals two-thirds of the dose needed to wake the patient up per hour
- Mechanical ventilation may be indicated in selected cases
- Acute withdrawal reactions may be precipitated in addicts.

Paracetamol

KEY POINT
- Check aspirin and paracetamol levels in all patients suspected of overdose as these are common drugs taken as part of multidrug overdoses; these may be life threatening and require specific treatment.

Potentially toxic doses

Normal-risk patients

- At least 12 g paracetamol is usually required to produce serious toxicity in adults, unless the patient is at high risk (see below).
- Children are comparatively resistant to paracetamol toxicity. Doses of less than 150 mg/kg are very unlikely to have toxic effects.

High-risk patients

- Lower doses might produce toxicity, e.g. > 7.5 g (adults) or > 100 mg/kg (children). The following put patients at higher risk of paracetamol-induced toxicity:
  - Malnutrition/cachexia (e.g. eating disorders, cystic fibrosis, AIDS), chronic high alcohol consumption
  - Hepatic enzyme-inducing drugs, e.g. phenytoin, barbiturates, primidone, rifampicin, carbamazepine, St John's Wort.

Establish

- Product and amount taken
- Time taken
- Other poisons taken at the same time (e.g. co-analgesics containing opiates)
- Presence of factors which put the patient at a higher risk (see above).

For the early management of paracetamol overdose and the use of activated charcoal, gastric lavage and acetylcysteine, *follow the clinical algorithms*

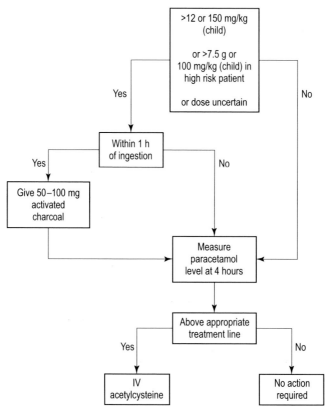

Figure 12.1 Algorithm for the management of paracetamol overdose within 4 h of ingestion.

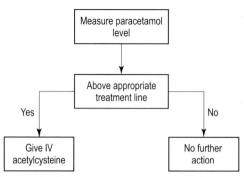

Figure 12.2 Algorithm for the management of paracetamol overdose between 4 and 7 h after ingestion.

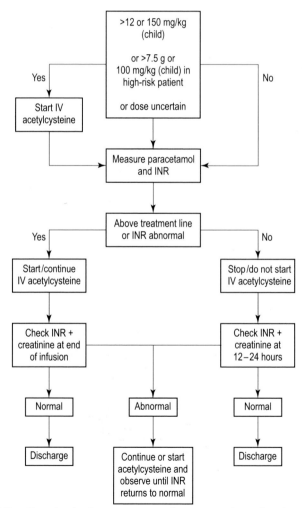

Figure 12.3 Algorithm for the management of paracetamol overdose between 7 and 24 h after ingestion.

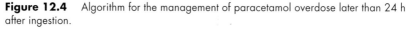

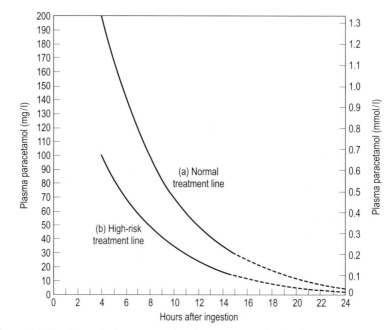

Adverse symptoms and signs
Drowsiness, nausea or vomiting, liver pain, encephalopathy

Figure 12.4 Algorithm for the management of paracetamol overdose later than 24 h after ingestion.

Figure 12.5 Nomogram treatment chart for paracetamol poisoning.

corresponding to the time after ingestion. When the time of overdose is uncertain, use the earliest time that it may have occurred. For staggered overdoses, use the time that the first paracetamol overdose was taken. If in doubt treat with acetylcysteine. See Figures 12.1–12.5.

Laboratory tests

Urgent
All patients:

- Paracetamol concentration immediately and at least 4 h after overdose (if time of overdose known).

Patients with severe poisoning (potentially toxic dose (see above) and/or paracetamol concentration above nomogram treatment line):

- Test urine for blood and protein
- Blood glucose
- Urea, creatinine
- Electrolytes
- Prothrombin time or INR
- Blood gases
- Daily urine output.

Routine

- Liver function tests.

These tests should be repeated at least every day until recovery.

Management

Activated charcoal
This should be given in a dose of 50 g if:

- the patient has taken the overdose within the previous hour, and
- a potentially toxic amount has been taken (see above).

N-acetylcysteine

- Acetylcysteine should be used in patients with a paracetamol level above the appropriate (high or low risk) treatment line between 4 and 24 h after overdose. *If in doubt treat with N-acetylcysteine* (e.g. when the interval between the overdose and the blood sample is uncertain). Treatment should not be started until the plasma paracetamol level is known unless:
  – a potentially serious amount has been taken (see above) *and*
  – the result of the paracetamol level will not be known until 8 h or more has elapsed (or the interval between overdose and presentation is uncertain). This is because acetylcysteine is almost completely effective up to 8 h after overdose, but becomes progressively less effective after 8 h.
- An urticarial reaction may occur in up to 10% of patients – give chlorpheniramine (chlorphenamine) for itch and continue acetylcysteine, reducing the infusion rate if symptoms do not resolve immediately.
- Pregnancy is not a contraindication to acetylcysteine.

Acetylcysteine
Acetylcysteine should be given as an intravenous infusion as follows:

- 150 mg/kg in 200 mL 5% dextrose over 15 min

- 50 mg/kg in 500 mL 5% dextrose over 4 h
- 100 mg/kg in 1000 mL 5% dextrose over 16 h.

If the PTR is > 2.0 (or PT > 30 s)

- Give oral lactulose 20 mL every 2 h until diarrhoea occurs, and IV vitamin K 10 mg once only.

If the blood glucose is < 4.0 mmol/L

- Give an infusion of 10% glucose starting at a rate of 100 mL/h and adjust to keep blood glucose levels between 5 and 10 mmol/L.

Criteria for specialist advice

- PTR/INR > 2.0 or PT > 25 s and rising
- Renal failure (creatinine > 200 µmol/L and rising, or oliguria)
- Metabolic acidosis (pH < 7.3)
- Reduced level of consciousness
- Hepatic tenderness
- Hepatic failure (liver flap, encephalopathy, jaundice)
- Hypotension (systolic BP < 100 *or* mean BP < 60 following volume resuscitation)
- Abnormal bleeding
- Hypoglycaemia
- Late presentation of a potentially serious overdose
- Timing of overdose is uncertain.

Seek advice from your local liver unit or nearest centre of the NPIS (National Poisons Information Service).

SSRI and related antidepressants

These notes cover the management of overdose with selective serotonin reuptake inhibitor (SSRI) antidepressants. The newer antidepressants, nefazodone and venlafaxine (serotonin and noradrenaline reuptake inhibitor, SNRI), have similar toxicity but less data is available. Mirtazapine (tetracyclic SNRI) and reboxetine (noradrenaline reuptake inhibitor) have different patterns of toxicity. For these newer agents you are advised to use TOXBASE or contact the NPIS for the most up-to-date information.

SSRI antidepressants

SSRI antidepressants include:

- citalopram
- fluoxetine
- fluvoxamine
- paroxetine
- sertraline.

Potentially toxic doses (acute overdose)

- SSRIs are of low toxicity in overdose. Toxic effects are unlikely at doses less than:
  - 1.5 g (adult) or 3.6 mg/kg (child) for fluoxetine
  - 3 g (adults) or 6 mg/kg (child) for fluvoxamine
  - 3.6 g (adult) or 8 mg/kg (child) for sertraline
  - 1.2 g (adult) or 2.5 mg/kg (child) for paroxetine
- Citalopram and venlafaxine may be more toxic since QT prolongation and ventricular arrhythmias have been reported
- Toxic effects are more likely if alcohol or other drugs have been co-ingested.

Establish

- Time taken
- Presence if there are symptoms/signs.

Neurological

Common: agitation, insomnia, tremor, drowsiness
Uncommon: nystagmus, hyperventilation, convulsions

Cardiovascular

Common: sinus tachycardia, bradycardia, hypertension, prolonged QT
Uncommon: junctional rhythm

Others
Common: nausea, vomiting

Laboratory tests

- Electrolytes, urea and creatinine
- ECG
- Cardiac monitor (for citalopram and venlafaxine overdose).

Immediate management

- Give a single dose of oral activated charcoal (50 g for an adult, smaller doses in children) if the patient has taken a potentially serious overdose within the previous hour
- Control prolonged convulsion with intravenous diazepam 10 mg (child 0.1–0.3 mg/kg) given slowly and repeated if necessary (beware respiratory depression)
- Give supportive treatment for complications.

Tricyclic and related antidepressants

These include:

- amitriptyline
- lofepramine
- clomipramine
- maprotiline
- desipramine
- mianserin

- dothiepin (dosulepin)
- nortiptyline
- doxepin
- trazodone
- imipramine
- trimipramine.

Potentially toxic doses

- More than 500 mg (adult) or 7.5 mg/kg (child) may cause serious toxicity, especially overdoses involving dothiepin or amitriptyline
- Lofepramine is less toxic – doses of less than 3.5 g (adult) are unlikely to produce symptoms.

Immediate management

- Ensure airway, breathing and circulation
- Control fits using intravenous diazepam 10 mg (child 0.1–0.3 mg/kg) given slowly and repeated if necessary (beware respiratory depression).

Establish

- The product taken
- The amount taken
- The time from ingestion
- Symptoms of anxiety, restlessness, dry mouth, urinary retention, palpitation, blurred vision.

Examine for

- Hot, dry skin
- Pupillary dilation
- Tachycardia
- Urinary retention (palpable bladder)
- Hypertonia and hyperreflexia
- Agitation, delirium, fits and coma.

Estimate

- Urea, electrolytes and blood glucose
- ECG, in particular the QRS duration. If this is greater than 0.16 s (160 ms, 4 small squares) the patient is at *high risk of arrythmias and fits* and needs *urgent treatment.*

If there are symptoms or signs, or if a potentially toxic dose has been taken

- Monitor the electrocardiogram
- Measure the blood gases
- Correct any metabolic acidosis immediately using sodium bicarbonate. Start with 50 mL 8.4% sodium bicarbonate given over 20 min (reduce quantity for children)
- Give activated charcoal 50 g (adults) or 10 times the ingested dose of tricyclic antidepressant (children) if within 1 h of the overdose.

If there are fits and these are prolonged

- Give IV diazepam 10 mg (child 0.1–0.3 mg/kg) and repeat if necessary. Beware respiratory depression.

If there are any arrhythmias or the QRS duration is > 160 ms

- *Immediately* start IV infusion of 50 mL 8.4% sodium bicarbonate over 20 min, even if the patient is not acidotic (dose for children < 10 kg = 5 mL/kg). Recheck arterial pH and repeat as necessary until ECG is normal and no longer acidotic
- Consider prophylactic insertion of a pacing wire or DC cardioversion for arrhythmias
- *Do not use anti-arrhythmic drugs in this context.*

If cardiac arrest occurs

Do not stop cardiac massage. Patients may survive after several hours of resuscitation. Consider using mechanical CPR device.

Toxicology advice

Advice on treatment of poison could be obtained from TOXBASE, a computerized database of the UK poisons information service online: http://www/spib.axl.co.uk.

Further expert advice can be obtained by telephoning the UK NPIS, Tel: 0870 600 6266. Alternatively one can contact the regional poisons service.

CASE 12.3

A 32-year-old man is being brought by ambulance to your A&E department. It is 02:31 in the morning and the paramedics responded to a 999 call. He had allegedly taken alcohol and antiepileptics in the presence of his partner at 01:50. A suicide note had been written.

Initial pre-hospital assessment:

Airway   **Clear**

Breathing   **Spontaneous at 16/min**

Circulation   **Pulse 80/min and regular, BP not taken, SpO_2 96%**

Disability   **Patient fully conscious, GCS 15/15**

   Pre-hospital treatment: none in transit.

You are the receiving doctor in the A&E department. How would you proceed?

Answer

After continued high-flow oxygen and gaining venous access the patient was to be admitted to an acute medical ward awaiting the results of blood levels of phenytoin. Whilst waiting for a bed on the ward, however, he became incontinent, his level of consciousness dropped to a GCS of 9 and he developed myoclonic movements. With continued observation his GCS dropped further to 7 and he was therefore intubated and ventilated by the critical care team. Inotropes were also used for the hypotension he developed. Phenytoin levels were significantly raised at 900 mg/L and the patient was dialysed by the renal team on the intensive care unit.

The patient was referred to the drug misuse centre on discharge from the ward.

POISONING AS AN ACT OF DELIBERATE SELF-HARM

A high proportion of deliberate self-harm patients self-poison and usually present to local A&E departments. It is important to identify the motive in taking the poison. A comprehensive assessment by the liaison psychiatric team should start immediately after the acute physical care of the patient. Evaluation of the suicide intent score and mental assessment must be carried out and management individualized on the basis of assessment. A multi-disciplinary team approach is integral to the successful overall management.

KEY POINTS

- Poisoning may be accidental or intentional.
- It comprises a significant workload for A&E departments and acute medical wards.
- The ABCD approach can be appropriately used in the initial management of poisoned patients.
- Treatment is generally supportive but specific therapeutic measures and antidotes are indicated with certain agents.
- Advice and help is always available after the initial resuscitation.
- The patient should be observed closely on the ward after good initial response to treatment.
- A multidisciplinary approach is required for successful management of deliberate self-harm patients.

DOCUMENTATION

Accurate and comprehensive documentation can be ensured by locally produced Deliberate Self Harm Integrated Care Pathways between A&E, acute medicine and liaison psychiatry teams.

FURTHER READING

Andrzejowski J C, Myint Y 1998 The management of acute poisoning. British Journal of Intensive Care 97:102

Isacsson G, Rich C L 2000 Regular review – management of patients who deliberately harm themselves. BMJ 322:213–215

Jones A L 2002 Poisoning. In: Haslett C, Chilvers E R, Boon N et al (eds) Davidson's principles and practice of medicine, 19th edn. Churchill Livingstone, Edinburgh, p 165–184

Jones A L, Volans G 1999 Recent advances - management of self poisoning. BMJ 319:1414–1417

NHS Northern and Yorkshire Regional Drug and Therapeutics Centre National Poisons Information Service 1999 Management of poisoning, 4th edn. Wolfson Unit of Clinical Pharmacology, Newcastle Upon Tyne

Nolan J, Baskett P, Garbott D et al (eds) 2000 Advanced life support manual, 4th edn Resuscitation Council (UK), London

Practical procedures

13

Kaye Cantlay

OBJECTIVES

After reading this chapter you should have an understanding of:

- *Three of the more commonly performed emergency medical practical procedures:*
  - *central venous catheterization*
  - *chest drain insertion*
  - *lumbar puncture*

- *How these procedures can be performed more easily and with fewer complications*

- *The indications, contraindications, techniques, and complications for each of the procedures*

A few points pertinent to all procedures are presented below:

- All practical procedures carry potential risks. These must be considered carefully and weighed up against the potential benefits before undertaking the procedure. If you are in any doubt, consult a senior colleague.
- Never undertake a procedure you are unfamiliar with without appropriate senior supervision or assistance.
- Assemble all necessary equipment prior to starting the procedure.
- Ideally at least two suitably qualified people should be available to assist you. One to help you with the actual procedure and a second to look after the patient.
- Explain to the patient and any relatives what you intend to do and why. Mention any possible complications. If possible, obtain their verbal consent and document the discussion clearly in the patient's notes.
- Similarly, document in detail the procedure undertaken, including any difficulties encountered.

- Always bear in mind the potential complications of any procedure and be prepared to observe your patient for these over an appropriate time period.

CENTRAL VENOUS CATHETERIZATION

Central venous catheterization refers to the placement of an intravenous catheter within one of the large central veins, such that the tip usually lies within the superior or inferior vena cava. It must be remembered that, except in unusual cases such as the insertion of a temporary pacing wire, the placement of the line is not in itself a therapeutic procedure! This is a procedure with many possible complications, and so the relative risks and benefits must always be weighed up carefully in each individual.

Indications

The most common indications for central venous catheterization in the emergency setting include:

- central venous pressure (CVP) monitoring
- administration of potent drugs such as inotropes
- venous access where peripheral access is very poor.

Other indications include venous access for renal replacement therapy, total parenteral nutrition, temporary pacing wires, pulmonary artery catheters, and longer-term tunnelled line placement for chemotherapy or protracted antibiotic therapy.

Contraindications

These depend to an extent on the planned site of insertion, but include the following:

- Overlying *infection.*
- *Coagulopathy or low platelets:* This is a relative contraindication as critically ill patients frequently display clotting abnormalities. The subclavian site should be avoided as it is difficult to apply pressure on an inadvertently punctured artery at this site.
- *Carotid artery disease:* Avoid the internal jugular in case of inadvertent carotid arterial puncture and the risk of dislodging an embolus.
- *Raised intracranial pressure:* The internal jugular vein should be avoided as this may impair venous drainage from the head on that side.

Equipment

- Hat, mask, sterile gloves and gown
- Sterile pack
- Cleaning fluid for the skin

- Gauze or sponges to apply cleaning fluid
- Large drapes
- Selection of syringes and needles
- Local anaesthetic
- Central line kit
- Scalpel and blade
- Ultrasound machine if available
- Saline to flush the line
- Three-way taps or bungs
- Suture
- Dressing.

Types of central line

Various different types of central venous catheters exist. Some differences include the following:

- *Number of lumens:* Lines generally have between 1 and 5 lumens. Greater numbers of lumens may be associated with an increased incidence of catheter-related infection, possibly due to increased line handling. A line with the smallest number of lumens necessary should therefore be chosen.
- *Gauge of lumens:* Lumens are generally of the order of 16 to 18G, which is the same as many commonly-used peripheral cannulae. However, as most lines are considerably longer than peripheral cannulae, the rate of infusion through them is relatively slow. This makes them unsuitable for the rapid infusion of large volumes of fluid. Central lines with much wider bore lumens are manufactured for purposes such as renal replacement therapy. These lines allow much more rapid flow.
- *Catheter material:* The most frequently used materials are silicone, polyurethane, polyvinylchloride, polypropylene and Teflon. Lines impregnated with antiseptics such as chlorhexidine or silver sulfadiazine, and antibiotics such as rifampicin or minocycline exist. These are expensive but may be associated with a lower incidence of infection.
- *Tunnelled lines:* These may be associated with a lower rate of line infection where a long indwelling time is expected. Examples include Hickman lines placed for chemotherapy.

Sites of insertion

The internal jugular vein

- *Advantages:* It may be easily visualized using ultrasound. There is less risk of pneumothorax compared with subclavian lines.
- *Disadvantages:* There is a risk of carotid puncture. It may impede cerebral venous drainage resulting in a rise in intracranial pressure. It is uncomfortable for the patient.

The subclavian vein

- *Advantages:* It is more comfortable for the patient. It has the lowest risk of infection and thrombosis.
- *Disadvantages:* It has the highest risk of mechanical complications, in particular pneumothorax. This site should not be used where there is an abnormal bleeding tendency as it is not possible to apply direct pressure to the artery in the event of inadvertent puncture.

The femoral vein

- *Advantages:* It is the easiest to access in an emergency. There is no risk of a pneumothorax. The patient does not need to be tilted head-down.
- *Disadvantages:* It has the highest risk of infection and thrombosis. It does not give accurate CVP readings as the tip will not lie within the thorax.

The antecubital fossa

- A 'long-line' may be inserted via a vein in the antecubital fossa to reach the subclavian vein or superior vena cava. This does not risk a pneumothorax and may be performed in the presence of deranged clotting. They may be tricky to thread all the way into the thorax and sometimes do not give very reliable central venous pressure readings. They are single lumen and therefore cannot be used for CVP monitoring and inotropes together and, although often useful for CVP monitoring in the perioperative phase, they will not be discussed further.

Landmarks and positioning

The internal jugular vein (Figs 13.1 and 13.2)

- The right internal jugular vein is easier to find than the left, particularly by a right-handed operator.
- Remove the patient's pillow and turn the head away from the side to be cannulated.
- Tilt the bed head-down into the Trendelenburg position. This is done both to distend the vein, and also to reduce the risk of air embolism through the needle when the syringe is removed.
- There are a number of described approaches to the internal jugular vein. Two of the more common are as follows:
  1. Palpate the carotid artery with the fingertips of the non-dominant hand. The internal jugular vein will be found superficial, lateral, and parallel to the carotid artery.
  2. For a higher approach, the needle should be inserted just lateral to the carotid artery pulsation at approximately the level of the thyroid cartilage at 45 degrees to the skin.
- A lower approach is also possible, but carries a higher risk of pneumothorax. The needle should be inserted at the apex of the triangle formed by the two heads of the sternocleidomastoid muscle and the clavicle (Fig. 13.2).

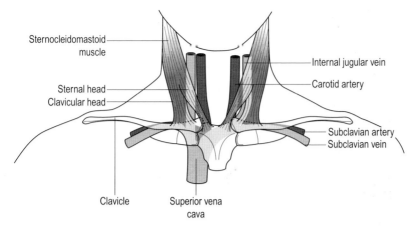

Figure 13.1 Anatomy of the internal jugular and subclavian veins.

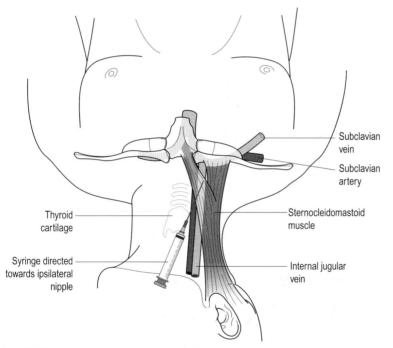

Figure 13.2 Approach to the internal jugular vein.

- The needle should be advanced whilst aspirating gently, in the direction of the ipsilateral nipple.
- If the vein is not hit in this plane, the needle is withdrawn to skin and then advanced in a slightly more medial direction until the vein is found.

The subclavian vein (Figs 13.1 and 13.3)

- The patient lies with their head on a pillow in the neutral position.
- The bed should be tilted head-down.

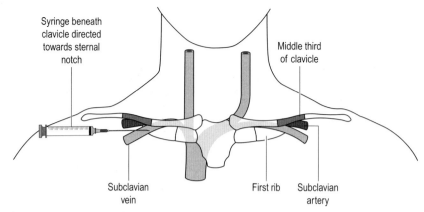

Figure 13.3 Approach to the subclavian vein.

- Several approaches to the vein have been described but the following is commonly used.
- Locate the junction of the middle and medial thirds of the clavicle.
- The needle is inserted approximately 1 cm below this junction.
- The needle should be advanced in the horizontal plane towards the clavicle until bone is hit.
- The needle is then 'walked' under the clavicle.
- Once under the clavicle the needle is then swung round to point towards the suprasternal notch.
- The needle is then advanced towards the notch taking great care to keep it within the horizontal plane.
- If the vein is not encountered, the needle should be withdrawn and the process repeated, this time aiming slightly more cranially.

The femoral vein (Fig. 13.4)

- The patient lies flat with the corresponding leg slightly abducted and externally rotated.
- The pulse of the femoral artery is located with the fingers of the non-dominant hand.
- The vein lies medial and parallel to this pulsation.
- The needle is inserted 1 cm medial to the arterial pulsation at 30 degrees to the skin, and in a direction that is parallel to the artery.

Ultrasound guidance

Two-dimensional ultrasound (Fig. 13.5) may be used to identify the precise position of veins such as the internal jugular and the femoral. It may allow distinction from the adjacent artery by demonstrating compressibility of the vein, and changes in its diameter with postural adjustment, coughing or the Valsalva manoeuvre. Anatomical variants may be detected, as may thrombi within the vein.

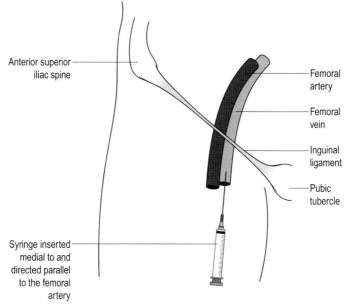

Figure 13.4 Anatomy and approach to the femoral vein.

Pooled data from a number of trials have shown that using real-time ultrasound guidance to facilitate needle placement in internal jugular catheterization can reduce the incidence of complications such as arterial puncture or multiple unsuccessful attempts. There is also some evidence to support its use in catheter placement at other sites. This has led the National Institute of Clinical Excellence (NICE) to issue guidance in 2002 recommending ultrasound over traditional landmark-based methods for vein location during internal jugular catheterization. Training is necessary to achieve competence in ultrasound-guided venous access and so NICE have

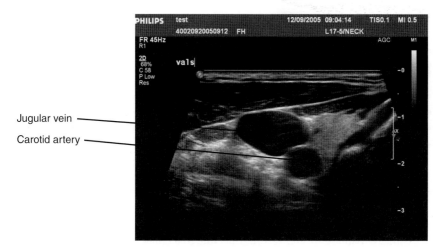

Figure 13.5 Ultrasound of internal jugular vein.

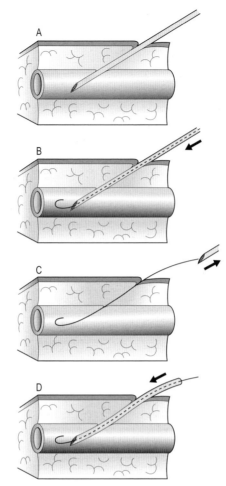

Figure 13.6   The Seldinger technique.

also issued a recommendation that individuals practising central line placement be trained in its use.

The Seldinger technique (Fig. 13.6)

- Choose the most appropriate site for insertion.
- Position the patient as described above.
- Put on a mask and hat, scrub hands, and put on sterile gown and gloves.
- Draw up your local anaesthetic, flush all the lumens of your line with saline and apply three-way taps or bungs to all except that through which your guidewire will emerge.
- Clean a wide area of skin around the site of insertion with antiseptic solution.
- Apply large drapes to all sides leaving a small area of cleaned skin visible. If you are inserting a jugular line in a conscious patient, avoid completely covering their head with the drapes; this may be extremely

distressing in an already frightened and sick individual. Place your drapes such that your patient is still able to see out, and have a second helper sitting where they can see them to help to reassure them during the procedure.

- Establish the location of the vein either using ultrasound guidance or by the landmark technique.
- Apply local anaesthetic to your intended site of puncture, first to the skin using a 25G needle, and then to the subcutaneous tissues using an 18G needle. Always aspirate prior to injecting anaesthetic to avoid inadvertent intravascular injection.
- Take your central line needle and attach a 5 or 10 mL syringe. Puncture the skin and then advance the needle slowly in the appropriate direction for the chosen site as described above. Aspirate continuously whilst advancing. When the vein is entered, blood will be aspirated. Check that a free flow of blood into the syringe is present. It should be noted that even in the obese patient the jugular vein is a relatively superficial structure. It should therefore be accessible using a standard 2.5 cm 18G needle. It is good practice to establish the location of the jugular vein using a small 'seeker' needle first before moving onto the large central line needle. This is not usually an option for the more deeply situated subclavian and femoral veins.
- Gently remove the syringe from your central line needle taking care not to dislodge the position of the needle within the vein. Unless the patient is extremely hypovolaemic, venous blood should be seen to flow from the needle hub. Very red or obviously pulsatile blood flow is suggestive of arterial puncture. If this is observed, remove the needle and apply pressure for a number of minutes to prevent haematoma formation. Note that in the hypotensive and hypoxic patient, arterial blood may in fact appear to be venous.
- Thread your guidewire through the needle lumen. This should pass without resistance. Never force the guidewire if resistance is felt. If the wire will not pass, then remove the needle and wire together and start again. Do not remove the wire through the needle as this risks shearing off the tip of the guidewire inside the patient. Pass the guidewire to around 20 cm or so watching the patient's ECG monitor. Do not be tempted to pass the entire guidewire through the needle as it will pass into the right cardiac chambers resulting in the risk of arrhythmias. If ectopics are seen on the ECG during guidewire passage then withdraw the wire until they disappear.
- Now remove the needle leaving only the guidewire in the vein.
- Make a small nick in the skin using a scalpel blade at the site the guidewire emerges.
- Pass the dilator over the guidewire: use your non-dominant hand to stabilize and slightly stretch the adjacent skin. Pass the dilator in a slight twisting motion to a depth of around 1 to 2 inches. The purpose of the dilator is to stretch up the skin and subcutaneous tissues. It does not need to be inserted to the hilt as this may causes considerable damage to the underlying vein.

- Remove the dilator leaving the guidewire in situ.
- Railroad the central line over the guidewire and into the vein to a depth of around 15 cm at the skin in the average adult. Always ensure that the guidewire protrudes from the end of the line before the line tip disappears through the skin.
- Withdraw the guidewire.
- Check that it is possible to freely aspirate venous blood from all lumens of the line and flush each with saline so that residual blood is not visible.
- Secure the line carefully with sutures. More local anaesthetic will be necessary at the site of each suture.
- Apply a dressing.
- For subclavian and jugular lines request a chest X-ray to view line placement and exclude a pneumothorax. The line should be seen to pass from the point of insertion along the anatomical path of the vein and into the superior vena cava (SVC). The tip of the central line should be seen to lie in the SVC approximately at the level of the carina (see Fig.13.7). If the tip is lower than this there is a risk of it lying within the atrium or even the ventricle which will put the patient at risk of arrhythmias, and the line should be withdrawn by an appropriate amount and resutured.
- Where doubt exists as to the position of the line tip, connection to a pressure transducer and waveform monitor may help. The normal central venous pressure in an unventilated patient will be around 3–8 mmHg with a waveform similar to that described for the jugular venous pulse. Similar numbers and waveform will be seen for placement in both the distal SVC and the atrium. A line tip in the ventricle will display much higher pressures and a 'taller' pressure wave (15–20 mmHg systolic and 0–10 mmHg diastolic). If the line has been placed in the arterial system the mean pressure will be seen to approximate the mean arterial blood pressure, and an arterial waveform will be seen. A blood gas sample

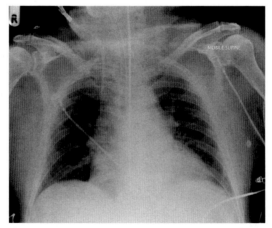

Figure 13.7 This patient is a critically ill patient who is intubated and ventilated. The patient has a wide bore dialysis line inserted into the right internal jugular vein. The tip lies just above the carina. Note also the presence of an oesophageal doppler probe and ECG leads.

taken from the line may also differentiate between arterial and venous placement.

Troubleshooting

Failure to locate the vein

- Withdraw the needle slowly aspirating as you go – you may have transected the vessel, especially in the hypovolaemic patient, and may find it during needle withdrawal.
- Try again angling your needle slightly more laterally/medially, or cranially depending on the site chosen.
- Check your landmarks are correct.
- Use ultrasound guidance for the femoral or jugular if you were previously relying on the landmark technique.
- Do not persist as the risk of mechanical complications will significantly increase. Consider another site or seek senior help. Do not be tempted to try siting a line on the opposite side of the chest as you risk causing bilateral pneumothoraces.

Unable to pass guidewire

- This is usually due to the needle tip not being well within the vein, or being dislodged during removal of the syringe.
- Always ensure blood can be freely aspirated before attempting to pass a guidewire and never force the guidewire. Rotating the bevel of the needle slightly may facilitate free aspiration of blood.
- Occasionally the obstruction to guidewire passage may be anatomical, e.g. due to a stricture within the vessel. *Gently* rotating the guidewire may manipulate it past such an obstruction.

Aspiration of air

- You have almost certainly caused a pneumothorax. If the patient remains stable and well oxygenated you may complete line placement and confirm the pneumothorax on the post-procedure chest X-ray. If the confirmed pneumothorax is large, the patient dyspnoeic, or if the patient is ventilated, a chest drain will be required.

Arterial puncture

- Withdraw the needle and apply pressure for several minutes.

Ectopics or arrhythmias during guidewire insertion

- The guidewire is in too far. Withdrawing it will usually be sufficient to terminate the problem.

Possible complications of central line insertion

Possible immediate or early complications are numerous and include the following:

- Failure to locate vein
- Failure to pass guidewire
- Haematoma
- Arterial puncture
- Arterial laceration
- Pneumothorax (subclavian > internal jugular)
- Aberrant venous placement, e.g. jugular line passing down subclavian vein instead of into the superior vena cava
- Haemothorax
- Cardiac tamponade due to perforation of the vessel wall below the pericardial refection or a cardiac chamber
- Air embolism
- Arterial line placement
- Nerve damage
- Thoracic duct damage
- Arrhythmias – care particularly in high-risk patients, e.g. tricyclic overdose.

The most common later complications include:

- infection
- thrombosis.

KEY POINTS
- Central line insertion per se is rarely therapeutic. It is what is done with the line that matters!
- There are numerous possible complications, particularly with inexperienced operators so consider carefully the risks to your patient.
- Always use ultrasound guidance to locate the jugular vein if it is available.

CHEST DRAIN INSERTION

Indications

The principal indications for chest drain insertion include the following:

- Pneumothorax:
  - in any ventilated patient
  - tension pneumothorax after needle thoracocentesis
  - persistent or recurrent pneumothorax after simple aspiration
- Pleural effusion:
  - traumatic haemothorax
  - empyema
  - malignant pleural effusion.

Contraindications

- Coagulopathy or low platelets. These should be corrected if possible prior to drain placement.
- Lung densely adherent to the chest wall throughout the hemithorax.

Equipment

- Hat, mask, sterile gloves and gown
- Sterile pack
- Gauze or sponges, and cleaning fluid for the skin
- Large sterile drapes
- A selection of syringes and needles
- Local anaesthetic
- Blade and scalpel
- Forceps for blunt dissection if a large bore drain is to be placed
- Seldinger kit if a small bore tube is to be placed
- Chest drain
- Sutures
- Connecting tubing
- Underwater seal bottle and sterile water, or drainage bag
- Dressing.

Positioning and landmarks

The patient is usually best positioned semirecumbent in bed. The arm on the ipsilateral side is abducted, externally rotated, with the elbow flexed and the hand behind the patient's head. An alternative is to have the patient sitting up and leaning forward onto a table in front of them. The drain should be sited within what is termed the 'safe triangle' bordered by the anterior border of latissimus dorsi, the lateral border of pectoralis major, and a horizontal line superior to the level of the nipple (Fig. 13.8).

In the case of small or loculated collections of fluid, alternative insertion sites may be used as determined, e.g. by ultrasound guidance. If the drain is not placed at the time of the ultrasound, and the site has been marked by the ultrasonographer, always remember to position the patient as they were positioned at the time of ultrasound.

Drain size and type

Small drains of the order of 10 to 14 F are more comfortable for the patient and are probably adequate for the majority of patients. These are often supplied in kits for insertion by the Seldinger technique.

Larger drains may be necessary for large air leaks, viscous pleural collections, and for traumatic haemothorax. For the latter it has been recommended that a drain of at least 28 to 30 F be used to facilitate drainage of the thoracic cavity and to assess ongoing blood losses. Larger drains are more commonly sited following blunt dissection through the chest wall.

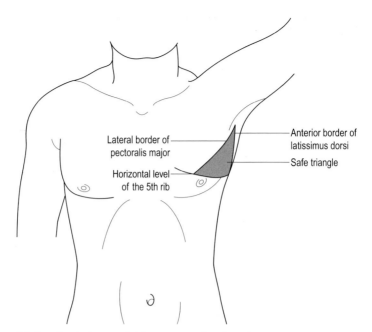

Figure 13.8   The 'safe triangle' for insertion of a chest drain.

Seldinger drains are often easier, quicker and less painful to insert than conventional drains. However, Seldinger drains should only be used where there is a definite collection of fluid or air between the underlying lung and chest wall, e.g. a pleural effusion confirmed and marked with ultrasound. If there is a possibility that underlying lung may be apposed to the chest wall, there is a risk of causing lung perforation with this technique. In such a situation, blunt dissection would be preferable.

Technique

- Confirm the need for and appropriate side for the chest drain both clinically and radiologically.
- Position the patient as above.
- Put on a hat and mask, scrub hands, and put on a sterile gown and gloves (see Box 13.1).
- Clean a wide area of skin with antiseptic solution.
- Apply ideally a single large drape with a hole over the 'safe triangle'.
- Identify a rib space within this triangle. You will be inserting the drain over the superior border of the rib below, in order to avoid damaging the corresponding neurovascular bundle which runs beneath the lower border of the rib (Fig. 13.9).
- Draw up your local anaesthetic (see Box 13.2).
- Apply local anaesthetic first to the skin using a fine 25G needle. Then infiltrate the subcutaneous tissues, intercostal muscles, pleura, and adjacent periosteum using an 18G needle. Use plenty of local anaesthetic,

Box 13.1   Aseptic technique

- In all of the procedures described in the text there is a real risk of introducing infection to the patient with potentially devastating consequences.
- It is therefore imperative that strict asepsis is observed.
- Long hair should be tied back.
- Ideally a hat and face mask should be worn. These may be obtained from the operating theatre suite if not readily available on your ward.
- Hands should be thoroughly scrubbed and a sterile gown and gloves worn.
- A wide area of skin should be cleaned with an antiseptic solution such as 1% povidone iodine or 0.5% chlorhexidine in alcohol. The latter may be associated with a lower risk of infection in the case of central line insertion. It must, however, be remembered that it should be allowed to dry before it becomes effective. Particular care should be taken to ensure the entire area of skin is covered when using a colourless antiseptic solution.
- Apply three or four large drapes to the sides of the area such that only a triangle or square of skin remains visible. All of this visible area should have been cleaned as described above. A single large drape with a hole in the centre is a useful alternative if available.
- Anatomical landmarks such as the iliac spines may be felt through these drapes.
- Be scrupulously careful not to touch anything other than the drapes, the cleaned area of skin, and your sterile instruments and tray.

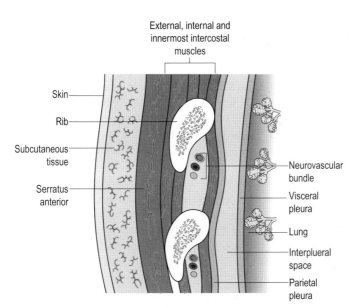

Figure 13.9   Layers of the chest wall.

without exceeding the safe limit for your patient (Box 13.2). Chest drain insertion is a painful procedure.

- For the insertion of a *Seldinger drain*, take your needle and attach a syringe. Point the bevel upwards for a pneumothorax, and downwards for an effusion. Pass your needle perpendicularly through the skin and

Box 13.2   Local anaesthesia

- The most commonly used anaesthetic is lidocaine
- This is usually provided as a 1% solution which contains 10 mg/mL. 0.5% and 2% lidocaine formulations are also available, as are preparations containing adrenaline (epinephrine). Always check the label carefully.
- Plain 1% lidocaine is the most suitable for the procedures discussed in this chapter.
- Always aspirate with your syringe before injecting local anaesthetic to ensure the tip of your needle is not in a blood vessel
- Remember to allow at least 1 or 2 min for it to take effect.
- The maximum safe dose of plain lidocaine that may be administered at one time is 3mg/kg. In an average 70 kg male this equates to 21 mL of the 1% solution, or just 10.5mL of 2% solution. Clearly, however, the safe limit will vary with the size of your patient and should be calculated beforehand, particularly for small patients.
- In overdose, or following intravascular injection, signs of toxicity may develop including perioral paraesthesia, tinnitus, fitting, or even cardiac arrest.

over the top of the rib, aspirating as you go. On entering the pleural cavity you will aspirate air or fluid depending on the indication for the drain. Pass your guidewire through the needle. It should pass easily without resistance. Remove your needle. Make a small nick in the skin where the guidewire exits using a blade. Now dilate up the track by passing the dilator or dilators provided over the guidewire. Finally pass the drain over the guidewire into the pleural cavity. Ensure that it is inserted to such a depth that all of the side holes at the drain tip are within the pleural cavity.

- For a *conventional drain*, a skin incision is made using a blade just above the top of the rib below the chosen intercostal space. The incision should follow the direction of the rib and should approximate in size to the diameter of the drain to be inserted. Before proceeding, insert a single horizontal mattress suture to close the wound with following drain removal (Fig. 13.10A). For a larger wound a mattress suture either side of the drain may be necessary (Fig. 13.10B). Purse-string sutures used in the past tended to cause unsightly scarring and are no longer recommended. You must now use forceps such as Spencer-Wells to bluntly dissect down to and through the pleura. The track is created by applying pressure with the tip of the closed forceps, then opening up the forceps in order to spread apart the muscle fibres. Once the pleura has been breached, it should be possible to slide the drain *without force* into the pleural cavity. Do not use the trochar to assist pushing the drain in. In the case of a wide bore drain, a finger should first be inserted through the track into the pleural cavity, and a 'finger sweep' performed to ensure there are no underlying organs which may be damaged by the passage of the drain. Direct the drain apically for a pneumothorax, and basally for an effusion.
- Connect the drain to the appropriate drainage system. An underwater seal drainage bottle is most commonly used as this allows only one-way flow and enables ready inspection of the respiratory swing, bubbling, and

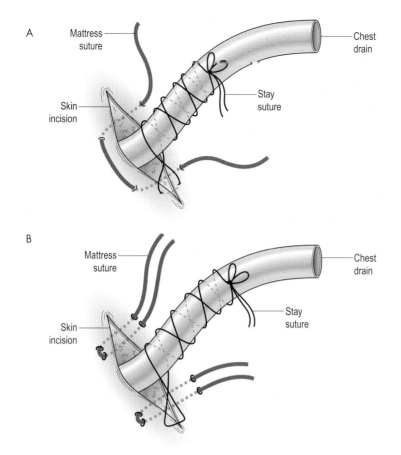

Figure 13.10 (A) Securing a chest drain. (B) Double mattress suture for a larger incision and drain.

drainage (Fig. 13.11). Occasionally a drainage bag is used for a small effusion.
- Secure the drain with a stay suture.
- Apply a dressing.
- Request a chest X-ray.

Troubleshooting

The drain will not pass easily into the pleural cavity

- Do not use force. Remove the drain and use further dissection to widen the track.

The patient develops subcutaneous emphysema

- It is likely that all of the drainage holes are not within the pleural cavity. Remove the drain and site a new one at a different site. Do not push the non-sterile external tube into the chest as this risks introducing infection.

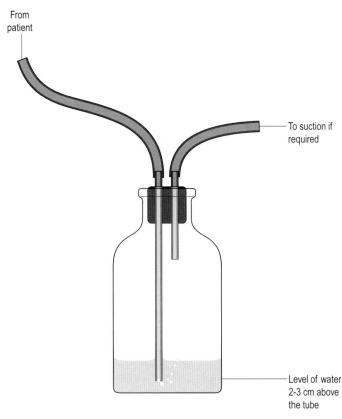

From
patient

To suction if
required

Level of water
2-3 cm above
the tube

Figure 13.11   An underwater seal drainage system.

The drain stops swinging

- It may have been pulled out of the pleural cavity. Check the drain and resite a new one if one is still required.
- It may be kinked either within the chest or at the exit site. Check the dressing and ensure the problem does not reside here. If the drain is in a long way, withdrawing may help as long as the drainage holes remain within the chest. Otherwise resite if necessary.
- The tube may be blocked with thick secretions or clots. Occasionally these may be cautiously 'milked' down the tubing. Alternatively a wider bore tube may be necessary.

A pneumothorax fails to re-expand

- The tube may be blocked in which case it will not be bubbling or swinging. Refer to the above.
- If it continues to bubble there may be a persistent bronchopleural fistula. Suction may be applied to the underwater seal drain and may help to expand the lung. Occasionally a cardiothoracic opinion must be sought.

An effusion fails to drain

- The tube may be blocked as above and therefore not swinging.
- The drain may be directed apically and failing to drain basal fluid.
- The fluid may be loculated. Consider another drain insertion with radiological guidance.

Possible complications of chest drain insertion

- *Intercostal vessel* damage resulting in bleeding
- *Intercostal nerve* damage
- *Splenic, hepatic,* or *cardiac* damage if the appropriate landmarks are not adhered to, or a trochar is used to apply force during insertion
- *Subcutaneous emphysema* if all of the drainage holes are not within the pleural cavity
- *Failure to drain* an effusion or pneumothorax due to a blocked or kinked tube
- *Re-expansion pulmonary oedema* if an effusion is drained too rapidly. Do not drain more than 1 L at one time
- *Empyema* due to introduction of infection. Always remove a drain as soon as air or fluid has stopped draining.

KEY POINTS
- Always ensure you are inserting a drain on the correct side.
- Remove the trochar before inserting a chest drain.
- Never use force to insert the drain into the pleural cavity.
- A drain should rarely be clamped and never if it is bubbling.
- Do not rapidly drain a large pleural effusion.

LUMBAR PUNCTURE

A lumbar puncture is a simple means of obtaining cerebrospinal fluid (CSF). The first person to remove CSF by this method for analysis was Quinke in 1891. He also measured CSF pressure using a manometer and introduced the use of a stylet which forms the basis of the instruments we use today.

Indications

A lumbar puncture is almost always done to provide *diagnostic* information. Occasionally, however, the procedure may be performed *therapeutically* either to remove CSF, or to introduce drugs into the CSF.

The most common indications in the *emergency* setting are as follows:

- Suspected *meningitis*
- Suspected *subarachnoid haemorrhage*
- Suspected *Guillain-Barré syndrome*.

Lumbar puncture

Less common indications include the evaluation of suspected demyelinating disease or other neurological disorders, diagnosis and treatment of benign intracranial hypertension, administration of intrathecal chemotherapy, and spinal anaesthesia.

Contraindications

- *Local infection* in the region of the puncture site. This is an absolute contraindication as there is clearly a risk of introducing infection into the CSF.
- *Raised intracranial pressure.* Clinical signs suggestive of this include a reduced consciousness level, focal signs such as a hemiplegia, cranial nerve palsies, in particular the third and sixth cranial nerves, papilloedema, and the Cushing reflex resulting in hypertension and bradycardia. Lumbar puncture in the presence of raised intracranial pressure risks the patient coning. If there is any doubt, a CT scan of the head should be performed prior to attempting the procedure.
- *Coagulopathy or low platelets.* This may be apparent from the patient's blood tests or drug history, but the presence of a non-blanching petechial rash in a case of suspected meningitis is highly suggestive of a coagulopathy secondary to meningococcal septicaemia. A lumbar puncture should not be performed under such circumstances.

Equipment

- A sterile pack such as a dressing pack
- A hat and mask
- Sterile gown and gloves
- Fluid to clean the skin
- Gauze or sponges to clean the skin
- A large drape with a hole in the centre or several large plain drapes
- Local anaesthetic (see Box 13.2)
- A syringe, 25G and 18G needles for the local anaesthetic
- Appropriate selection of spinal needles (see below)
- A manometer set for pressure measurement
- At least three sterile containers and a fluoride-oxalate tube to collect specimens.

Spinal needles

These are manufactured in a range of sizes and designs. All are essentially hollow needles containing an inner removable stylet. The stylet prevents tissue from entering and blocking the needle during insertion.

Variable features of these needles are as follows:
- *Length.* The standard needle is 10 cm long. 5-cm needles exist for paediatric use and 15-cm needles for obese patients.
- *Diameter.* Needles range from a large 18G to very fine 29G. Larger needles are easier to insert but are associated with an unacceptably high incidence

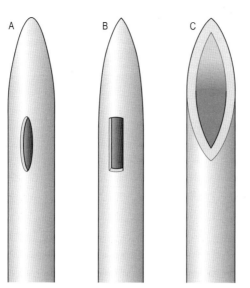

Figure 13.12   Spinal needle tips: (A) Sprotte (B) Whittaker (C) Quinke.

of post-dural puncture headache following the procedure. Finer needles have a tendency to bend during insertion and may require an introducer needle to stabilize them at the skin. The flow of CSF is also slower but the incidence of headache is far less. In general a needle no larger than 22G should be used for lumbar puncture.

- *Tip.* Needles such as the Yale or Quinke have a sharp, cutting tip. Sprotte and Whittaker needles have more blunt 'pencil-point' tips with a side-port (see Fig. 13.12). The latter are thought to divide tissue planes rather than cutting through them and are associated with a lower incidence of headache.

Positioning

This is possibly the single most important part of the procedure and can make the difference between success and failure, so spend time getting it right (Fig. 13.13). Patients are usually positioned in the left lateral position if you are right-handed, and right lateral if you are left-handed. Occasionally the sitting position may be useful if the patient is very obese as this makes the midline easier to identify. Ensure that the patient is lying on a firm mattress or surface. They should be lying in the 'fetal position' with the thoracolumbar spine as flexed as possible. Excessive neck flexion is both unimportant and uncomfortable. The lumbar region should be vertical at the edge of the bed. Place a pillow beneath the patient's head, and a second between the knees to improve comfort, reduce torsion of the spine, and prevent the patient from tilting forwards. A second helper is invaluable and should be in front of and facing the patient. This will reduce the tendency of the patient to turn in response to your voice from behind the patient.

Lumbar puncture

13

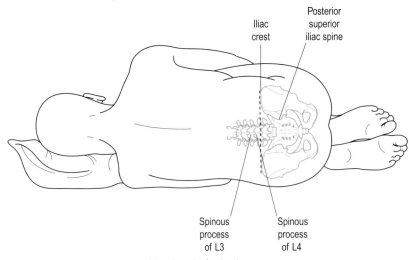

Figure 13.13   Positioning and landmarks for lumbar puncture.

Landmarks

In adults the spinal cord ends at the level of approximately L1/2 (Fig. 13.14). This however is variable and may occur at L2/3 in some individuals. It is therefore unwise to use an interspace higher than L3/4. An imaginary line joining the patient's iliac crests will cross the vertebral column at about L4

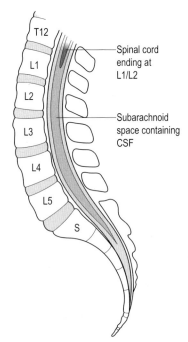

Figure 13.14   Relationship of the spinal cord to the vertebral column.

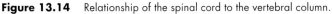

(Fig. 13.13). The spaces immediately above (L3/4) or below this spinous process (L4/5) will be suitable. Use whichever feels most accessible to the palpating fingers.

Technique

- Position the patient carefully as above.
- Put on the hat and mask, scrub hands, and put on the gown and gloves.
- Draw up your local anaesthetic and put together the manometer set ensuring the three-way tap turns freely.
- Clean the patient's skin and place the drapes.
- Establish landmarks.
- Place the tips of the middle and index fingers of your non-dominant hand on the spinous processes either side of the interspace to be punctured. Use these fingers to slightly stretch the skin overlying the space.
- Inject local anaesthetic to the skin at a point midway between the spinous processes using a 25G needle. Use an 18G needle to inject slightly deeper to this.
- Take your spinal needle with bevel facing upwards. Pass it through the anaesthetized skin in a plane parallel to the floor in the direction of the patient's umbilicus.
- Slight resistance will be felt as the needle passes through the interspinous ligament, and then again as it passes through the tougher ligamentum flavum. A characteristic 'give' will be appreciated as the needle passes beyond this ligament. Move the needle a further 1 to 2 mm. A second 'give' will usually be felt as the needle punctures the dura to enter the subarachnoid space (Fig. 13.15).
- Withdraw the stylet. If the needle is in the subarachnoid space then CSF will appear in the hub of the needle. If there is no CSF, rotate the needle slightly in case it is lying against a nerve root. Failing this, reinsert the stylet and move the needle forward another 1 mm and repeat the process.
- Measure CSF pressure using the manometer set.
- Collect the CSF from the manometer tubing into one of your sterile containers.
- Remove the manometer and allow further CSF to drop into your other containers. Around 10 drops per container is sufficient. Remember also to collect around 6 drops into a fluoride-oxalate blood tube for glucose analysis.
- Remove the needle, clean the patient's skin and apply a simple dressing to the puncture site.
- Samples should be inspected for colour, and sent to the appropriate labs for analysis of cell count, Gram stain, protein, glucose, and any other tests considered necessary according to the patient's history. Always remember to simultaneously send a blood sample for a glucose level for comparison with CSF.
- The patient should lie flat following the procedure for around an hour.

Lumbar puncture

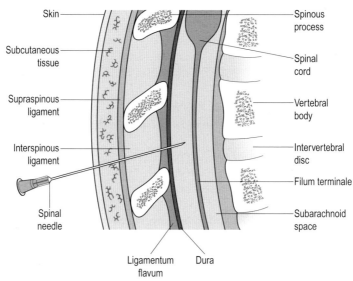

Skin — Spinous process

Subcutaneous tissue — Spinal cord

Supraspinous ligament — Vertebral body

Interspinous ligament — Intervertebral disc

Filum terminale

Spinal needle — Subarachnoid space

Ligamentum flavum   Dura

Figure 13.15 Layers and ligaments of the back.

Troubleshooting

Failure to find the space

- This is most commonly due to poor positioning of the patient so reassess this.
- Ensure your needle is in the horizontal plane, and that the puncture site is midway between spinous processes.
- Try angling the path of the needle slightly more cranially or caudally.
- If you are still unsuccessful, call for more experienced help.

Bloody tap

- If frank blood oozes slowly from the needle then it is likely that an epidural vein has been entered. Remove the needle and flush it. Try a space above or below.
- If blood stained CSF is observed, this will usually appear to clear in successive samples. Three samples should be sent for cell counts to demonstrate a fall in red cell count in consecutive samples.
- If the samples do not appear to clear with time, this may be due to the genuine presence of red cells within the subarachnoid space as in subarachnoid haemorrhage. Serial cell counts will show consistent numbers of red cells.

Paraesthesia

- If the patient experiences a shooting pain or paraesthesia this may be due to the needle encountering a nerve root or even spinal cord. Do not advance the needle. Remove the needle and ascertain your landmarks, in particular the level of the space you are puncturing.

Complications

- *Post-dural puncture headache* is the most common complication and is due to ongoing leak of CSF from the dural sac through the hole made in the dura. The risk may be reduced by appropriate needle selection as described above. The headache is characteristically frontal and made worse by sitting up. Conservative management with simple analgesia and good hydration is usually sufficient, but occasionally a blood patch may be required to terminate the CSF leak.
- *Nerve or cord damage*. This is rare and would usually be characterized by shooting pain or paraesthesia experienced during the passage of the spinal needle.
- *Epidural haematoma*. This is rare. It is characterized by severe back pain and signs of cord compression such as leg weakness, altered sensation, and sphincter disturbance. The diagnosis may be confirmed by MRI and an urgent neurosurgical opinion sought.
- *Epidural abscess*. With strict attention to asepsis this is also extremely rare. Presentation is similar to an epidural haematoma but with the addition of pyrexia and other signs of infection.
- *Coning*. Coning of the brainstem may occur if a lumbar puncture is performed on a patient with critically elevated intracranial pressure. This will be identified when you measure the CSF pressure with your manometer. Following the procedure the patient's level of consciousness may drop, they may become bradycardic and hypertensive, and the pupils may become dilated and unreactive to light. This is an emergency with extremely high mortality. Mannitol should be given and urgent intubation and ventilation instituted.

KEY POINTS
- Never perform a lumber puncture if you suspect raised intracranial pressure.
- Never perform a lumbar puncture in the presence of deranged clotting.
- Always position your patient meticulously.
- Always try to use a needle that is 22G or smaller.

REFERENCES AND FURTHER READING

Laws D, Neville E, Duffy J et al 2003 BTS guidelines for the insertion of a chest drain. Thorax 58(suppl II):ii53–ii59

National Institute for Clinical Excellence 2002 Guidance on the use of ultrasound locating devices for placing central venous catheters. Technology Appraisal Guidance No. 49. National Institute for Health and Clinical Excellence. Online. Available: http://www.nice.org.uk

Polderman K H, Girbes A R 2002 Central venous catheter use. Part 1: Mechanical complications. Intensive Care Medicine 28:1–17

Polderman K H, Girbes A R 2002 Central venous catheter use. Part 2: Infectious complications. Intensive Care Medicine 28:18–28

Turnbull D K, Shepherd D B 2003 Post-dural puncture headache: pathogenesis, prevention, and treatment. British Journal of Anaesthesia 91(5):718–279

Tracheostomy management

Nicky Cree, Stephen Bonner

OBJECTIVES

After reading this chapter you should:

- *Understand the indications for insertion of a tracheostomy and other surgical airways*

- *Understand the relevant anatomy of surgical airway devices*

- *Recognize the importance of tracheostomy care on the ward including endotracheal suctioning and inner tube changes*

- *Be familiar with the variety of tracheostomy tubes available and understand their different characteristics*

- *Be able to identify when a tracheostomy change is required and how to change the tubes*

- *Understand aids to weaning and speaking*

- *Be able to perform appropriate resuscitation in a patient with a tracheostomy tube in situ*

INTRODUCTION

Care of a tracheostomy is a basic ward skill, but unfamiliarity with tracheostomies and the simple rules governing their care often leads to poor management, which can result in life-threatening complications. This is increasingly important as the current trend is for more tracheostomies to be performed in critically ill patients, resulting in more patients discharged to wards with tracheostomies in situ. These patients will usually be continuing to wean with the intention to remove the tracheostomy when this is possible. There has been an increase in the number of tracheostomies on the wards for many reasons. Increasing numbers of intensive care admissions and an older critical care unit population, together with a vogue for early tracheostomy tube insertion facilitated by percutaneous bedside insertion techniques in the critical care unit, mean that more tracheostomies are performed in the critical care unit. In addition, more radical head and neck cancer surgery is being performed and developments such as invasive home ventilation for patients with neuromuscular disorders, such as motor neuron disease, who previously would have received terminal care, are increasingly available and demanded by patients.

Tracheostomy care on the ward, therefore, remains a core skill for all hospital doctors and nurses and is likely to be increasingly important. A carer's unfamiliarity with tracheostomy tubes can lead to a great deal of anxiety for both the carer and the patient. Failure to care for these patients appropriately may result in the development of largely preventable complications which can have an impact on the patient's recovery, discharge from hospital and ultimate outcome.

This chapter aims to provide an overview of how to manage a patient in the ward setting who has a tracheostomy tube in situ.

WHAT IS A TRACHEOSTOMY?

Definitions

Tracheostomy: This is an artificial opening into the trachea through the neck, kept patent with a tracheostomy tube. The tube allows air to flow directly into the lungs via the trachea, bypassing the nose, pharynx and larynx. However, during weaning, air is slowly directed again via the larynx.

Stoma: This is the passage left by the tracheostomy when the tracheostomy tube has been removed.

Minitracheostomy: This is a small tube inserted into the trachea through the cricothyroid membrane.

Laryngectomy: This is the surgical removal of the larynx. The anatomy of a patient having undergone a laryngectomy is permanently changed with the trachea sutured in position on to the anterior surface of the neck. This forms a permanent stoma and the patient is no longer able to breathe through their upper airway. A tracheostomy tube in this circumstance maintains the patency of the stoma and if this is blocked the patient will be unable to breathe.

History of the tracheostomy

Tracheostomies have been performed since ancient times and in many different cultures including the Romans, Egyptians and in ancient India. The oldest reference probably relates to a pictogram on an Egyptian wooden tablet dating to around 3000 BC in the reign of King Aha. Interestingly the depiction of this tracheostomy has the image of the Ankh above both operator and subject, appropriately thought to represent the gift of life from one to the other (Pahor 1992). The practice of tracheostomy fell out of favour in the Middle Ages, probably because of poor surgical technique and lack of understanding of the indications leading to poor outcome. However, a gradual return to the technique included the first documented percutaneous tracheostomy by Sanctorius Sanctorius in Padua around 1600 using a trochar. The technique gained popularity in the 18th century for relief of life-threatening upper airway obstruction, such as diphtheria. By 1909 the tracheostomy had been standardized by Chevalier Jackson who quoted:

There is no other justifiable life-saving operation whose reign of usefulness has not been extended by modern methods.

Tracheostomy became the accepted technique of securing the airway and administering intermittent positive pressure ventilation (IPPV) for long periods of time during the polio epidemics in Europe in the 1950s, but it was not until 1982 that Larsen and Engstrom introduced the tracheostomy and IPPV for respiratory insufficiency due to under-ventilation (Whittet & Waldmann 1995). Tracheostomy is now a frequently indicated treatment for critically ill patients on the intensive care unit although the indications, timing and method of insertion remain issues for debate. The TracMan study aims to be the definitive trial of tracheostomy timing and outcome in the critically ill and this is currently in progress. Tracheostomy is also indicated in the management of many other longer-term medical and surgical conditions such as bulbar palsy associated with motor neuron disease and head and neck malignancy.

Indications for tracheostomy tube insertion

Although tracheostomy insertion was originally developed for the relief of acute upper airway obstruction, current indications for insertion include:

- To facilitate weaning from positive pressure ventilation in patients with respiratory failure on the critical care unit
- Prophylactic or therapeutic relief of actual or anticipated upper airway obstruction
- To allow tracheal suctioning and removal of bronchial secretions, e.g. in patients with respiratory failure or weak cough
- To protect the tracheobronchial tree from aspiration of substances when pharyngeal and laryngeal reflexes are obtunded, e.g. neuromuscular disease, impaired consciousness (e.g. head injury)
- To obtain a patent airway in patients with injuries to or following surgery to the head and neck
- To facilitate long-term invasive ventilation, e.g. high spinal injury with respiratory failure or motor neuron disease.

The advantages of a tracheostomy over an endotracheal tube in the critical care patient include:

- Reduced airway resistance leading to decreased work of breathing and theoretically easier weaning from ventilation
- Decreased need for sedation
- Increased patient comfort

- Improved oral hygiene
- Easier communication through oral movement and possible vocalization
- Easier mobilization of the patient, even if the patient is still ventilated artificially
- Intake of oral nutrition
- Reduced physical erosive damage and infection to the larynx, mouth or nose from prolonged endotracheal intubation.

A tracheostomy tube is usually a temporary measure with the majority of patients having normal respiration through the larynx and restoration of speech upon removal of the tracheostomy. However, in some cases the tracheostomy is permanent, e.g. prior to laryngectomy, upper airway tumours, permanent bilateral vocal cord palsy or in those patients requiring permanent assisted ventilation. Before considering tracheostomy change or removal, the operator must be aware of the reasons for insertion and the nature of the upper airway above the tracheostomy.

> **KEY INDICATIONS FOR TRACHEOSTOMY**
> - Weaning from IPPV
> - Upper airway obstruction
> - Sputum retention
> - Protection from aspiration
> - Long-term ventilation

Anatomy of the trachea

The adult trachea is approximately 10 cm long and 2 cm wide. It descends from the lower border of the cricoid cartilage at the level of C6 through the neck and thorax to end at its bifurcation into the left and right main bronchi. This occurs at the sternal angle level with the 4th thoracic vertebra. The tracheal walls are formed from fibrous tissue reinforced by 15–20 U-shaped cartilaginous rings. These are deficient posteriorly and united behind by fibrous tissue and smooth muscle. Internally the trachea is lined by ciliated respiratory epithelium.

In the neck the trachea lies in the midline, anterior to the oesophagus and with the recurrent laryngeal nerve in the groove between them. It is crossed by the isthmus of the thyroid gland anteriorly (over the 2nd to 4th tracheal rings) and the lobes lie laterally (Fig. 14.1). Also in front of the trachea lie the cervical fascia, infrahyoid muscles and the jugular venous arch. The carotid sheath and inferior thyroid artery lie laterally. Although the anterior neck over the trachea is often assumed to be relatively avascular, this is often not the case. There is significant variation in the presence of both arteries and veins, the large anterior jugular veins often being encountered even during percutaneous tracheostomy, and the thyroidea ima artery lies in the midline supplying the thyroid isthmus in 3% of cases. The operator must be vigilant for vessels during the procedure and be aware that haemorrhage may occur as a delayed reaction to tracheostomy or during the first tracheostomy change.

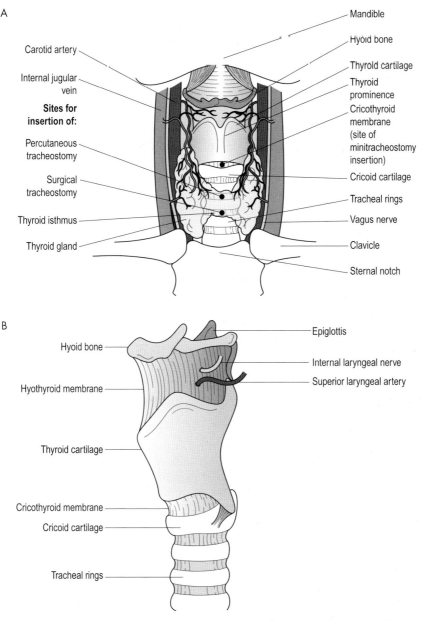

A

Mandible

Carotid artery

Hyoid bone

Internal jugular vein

Thyroid cartilage

Thyroid prominence

Sites for insertion of:

Cricothyroid membrane (site of minitracheostomy insertion)

Percutaneous tracheostomy

Surgical tracheostomy

Cricoid cartilage

Tracheal rings

Thyroid isthmus

Vagus nerve

Thyroid gland

Clavicle

Sternal notch

B

Epiglottis

Hyoid bone

Internal laryngeal nerve

Superior laryngeal artery

Hyothyroid membrane

Thyroid cartilage

Cricothyroid membrane

Cricoid cartilage

Tracheal rings

Figure 14.1   (A) Anterior view of the larynx showing different sites of insertion of tracheostomy tubes and some surrounding structures. (B) Lateral view of the larynx.

Whilst it is superficial at the level of the cricoid, as the trachea descends into the thoracic cavity it progressively moves posteriorly, sometimes at a steep angle, particularly in the elderly, becoming much deeper and less easily accessible.

KEY POINTS
- Trachea 10 cm long
- Runs from C6–T4
- 15–20 U-shaped cartilaginous rings
- Lined by ciliated epithelium
- Crossed by isthmus of thyroid gland and jugular venous arch in the neck

Sites for insertion of tracheostomy tubes (Figs 14.1 and 14.2)

Minitracheostomy

A minitracheostomy tube is inserted through the avascular cricothyroid membrane. This passes from the thyroid cartilage above to the cricoid cartilage below. The minitracheostomy tube and technique for cricothyroid puncture in an emergency are described later in this chapter.

Percutaneous tracheostomy

Percutaneous tracheostomies are now the most commonly performed type of tracheostomy in the critically ill. They are performed at the bedside in a critical care unit with the patient sedated. The tube is placed between the first and second or second and third tracheal rings. A variety of techniques exist, the commonest being the Ciàglià technique where a guide wire is inserted through a horizontal incision made over the anterior neck and a dilator forms a track to pass the tracheostomy tube through.

Surgical tracheostomy

The surgical tracheostomy is performed in the operating theatre, usually under general anaesthesia, but if upper airway obstruction is present, this is occasionally performed under local anaesthesia. A larger skin incision

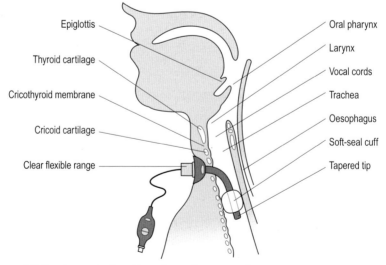

Epiglottis

Thyroid cartilage

Cricothyroid membrane

Cricoid cartilage

Clear flexible range

Oral pharynx

Larynx

Vocal cords

Trachea

Oesophagus

Soft-seal cuff

Tapered tip

Figure 14.2 Anatomical position of a tracheostomy tube.

compared to the percutaneous technique is made over the second and third tracheal rings. The surrounding anatomical structures are clearly identified. A slit or square opening is created in the trachea and the tube placed under direct vision. The wound usually requires sutures, which can be removed after approximately 7 days.

Figure 14.2 shows the anatomical position of a tracheostomy tube in situ from the lateral aspect.

Physiological changes associated with a tracheostomy

A tracheostomy bypasses the upper airway. This reduces the upper airway anatomical dead space (volume of inspired air that takes no part in gas exchange) by up to 150 mL or 30–50% of the total. The benefit of this to the patient is to reduce the work of breathing by decreasing airway resistance and increasing alveolar ventilation when compared to ventilation via a standard endotracheal tube. For example:

$$\text{alveolar ventilation (Va)} = \text{respiratory rate (RR)} \times [\text{tidal volume (Vt)} - \text{dead space volume (Vd)}]$$

Without a tracheostomy:
Vt = 400 mL
RR = 20/min
Vd = 150 mL
Va = 20 × (400–150) mL/min
 = 20 × 250 mL/min
 = **5.0 L/min**

With a tracheostomy:
Vt = 400 mL
RR = 20/min
Vd = 75 mL
Va = 20 × (400–75) mL/min
 = 20 × 325 ml/min
 = **6.5 L/min**

The use of a tracheostomy therefore increases alveolar ventilation (minute ventilation involved in gas exchange) in this example from 5 L to 6.5 L without necessarily increasing the work of breathing. This is a significant advantage over a patient trying to breathe with an endotracheal tube in place where airway resistance will be higher than with a tracheostomy. However, airway resistance with a tracheostomy in situ will be higher than in a patient breathing through their mouth and therefore patients are often given a trial of extubation and, if this fails, a tracheostomy is considered. The actual impact on the work of breathing through a tracheostomy also depends on the size and type, and in particular, internal diameter of the tracheostomy

KEY POINTS
A tracheostomy:
- Reduces upper airway anatomical dead space
  - increases alveolar ventilation
  - reduces airway resistance c.f. endotracheal tube
- Warming, humidification and filtering of air does not occur and must be provided if gases are administered via the tracheostomy

Table 14.1 Example of differences between internal and external diameter in mm with some common tracheostomy tubes

Size	Portex Blueline		Tracoe comfort		Shiley		Mallinckrodt Tracheosoft		Rusch 502	
	OD	ID	OD	ID	OD	ID	OD	ID	OD	ID
7	10.5	5.5	10.5	7			9.6	7	10.4	7
8	11.9	6.5	11.3	8	12.2	7.6	11.0	8	11.4	8
9	13.3	7.5	12.6	9			12.0	9	12.4	9

tube used. The number of the tracheostomy indicates the internal diameter, but there are significant differences between internal and external diameters. If swapping between different types of tubes do not try and insert a tracheostomy of larger external diameter than the one in situ (Table 14.1).

COMPLICATIONS OF A TRACHEOSTOMY

In the critical care setting, tracheostomy insertion for weaning from IPPV was historically considered after a period of 2–3 weeks of artificial ventilation due to the complication rates associated with tracheostomies. Before the late 1980s, all these tracheostomies were open surgical tracheostomies. With the advent of the bedside percutaneous tracheostomy with fibre-optic confirmation of correct placement, which appears to be associated with fewer complications than surgical tracheostomy (Dulguerov 1999), increasing numbers of tracheostomies are performed to aid weaning in critical care. However, although widely used to aid weaning in critical care, there is little evidence from randomized studies on improved outcome or the correct timing of tracheostomy, with preliminary studies suggesting a shorter critical care unit stay but no improved mortality from earlier tracheostomy (Griffiths et al 2005). This question may be answered by the TracMan study which is a UK-based multicentre trial comparing tracheostomy insertion within four days of admission to the critical care unit to insertion after 10 days, if still required at that stage. This study hopes to recruit 1200 patients and report findings by 2007 (http://www.tracman.org.uk).

Complications can be divided into those that occur immediately (i.e. related to insertion), are delayed or are late. Immediate complications are usually obvious, e.g. bleeding, pneumothorax (Fikkers et al 2004) or misplacement. However, later complications may be more insidious in nature and should be actively sought in patients on the ward who have had a tracheostomy.

Any patient with a tracheostomy who complains of breathlessness without an obvious respiratory cause, or in whom a suction catheter cannot be passed through the tracheostomy, may have an occluded tracheostomy. This often occurs with blood or secretions, particularly if non-humidified oxygen has been used and the secretions have dried in the tracheostomy. Alternatively the tracheostomy may no longer be sitting entirely within the trachea, leading to obstruction. Most tracheostomies have an inner lumen and this should be removed and cleaned at least once a day. Despite this, it still may block if the patient has profuse secretions. The inner lumen should be immediately removed and replaced. If this does not immediately cure the breathlessness, it is possible that the tracheostomy may have migrated out of the trachea. To replace this blindly is only safe it there is a smooth well-formed stoma, and it is usually safer in these circumstances to confirm the position of the lumen with a fibre-optic scope and if necessary the tracheostomy can be railroaded over a scope under direct vision to sit in a central position in the trachea. This should only be performed by a skilled operator. Tracheostomy malpositioning usually only occurs with tracheostomies that have been recently performed and it may also be noticeable that the tracheostomy is standing proud of the skin.

Tracheostomies allow better physiotherapy to the chest and removal of infected sputum. However, as a foreign body they can act as a nidus of infection themselves. For this reason, as well as to avoid tube blockage and to ensure a smooth stoma, they should be regularly replaced. Little evidence exists on the required interval between tracheostomy changes, but every 30 days is often quoted for an inner lumen tube. This period may be more frequent if secretions are copious and infection exists, or the tube may be left for much longer if there are no secretions and the stoma is well formed and smooth. A recently inserted single lumen tracheostomy tube should be changed every 7–10 days. If left longer it may block with secretions and may become stuck in situ.

Late bleeding can occur, although it is rare more than 10 days after a tracheostomy. It is usually due to the tracheostomy tube eroding through adjacent vessels and if it does not settle with pressure or infiltration with adrenaline (epinephrine) solutions, it will require surgical exploration. Very rarely it may be due to the cuff or the tip of the tube eroding through the trachea and intrathoracic vessels leading to massive haemorrhage, which may be fatal. Other indications for surgical referral include the inability of a patient to speak or breathe through their mouth when the cuff is deflated. This may indicate the presence of granulation tissue around the larynx, which may be diagnosed by indirect laryngoscopy, and which necessitates surgical removal.

Other rare, but serious complications include tracheal rupture or tracheo-oesophageal fistula, either from erosion of the tracheal wall or secondary to the operative procedure. These are life threatening and require urgent surgical referral. Another complication, which is probably underdiagnosed is tracheal stenosis. This may produce breathlessness which starts weeks or months after the tracheostomy is removed. Studies of asymptomatic post-tracheostomy patients report significant tracheal stenosis in as many as 10% of patients (Law et al 1997). Patients often do not report breathlessness until the tracheal lumen has been narrowed by more than 75% and such patients will demonstrate fixed obstruction spirometry and need CT scanning of the trachea and urgent referral to specialist surgeons for consideration of tracheal reconstruction. Tracheal stenosis may occur either at the site of the tracheostomy as the trachea heals with scar tissue which contracts, or at the site of the cuff, possibly due to high cuff pressures from overinflation

Complications of a tracheostomy

causing necrosis of the tracheal wall with subsequent scar formation. Although the risk of tracheal wall necrosis also depends partly on the type of cuff, it is good practice to measure the cuff pressure daily on any cuffed tracheostomy tube and deflate the cuff until the pressure is in the range of 20–25 mmHg. However, pressures of less than 18 mmHg may not protect against the risk of aspiration (Stewart et al 2003). Higher pressure should only be required in patients being ventilated at airway pressures higher than this.

Potential complications of tracheostomy

Immediate

- Haemorrhage – minor to life threatening
- Misplacement – pretracheal tissues or main bronchus
- Pneumothorax
- Tube occlusion – secretions, compression by the cuff, occlusion against the carina
- Subcutaneous emphysema.

Delayed

- Tube occlusion with secretions
- Infection – stoma site, tracheitis, pneumonia
- Tracheal ulceration and necrosis from high cuff pressures, asymmetrical inflation of the cuff or tube migration
- Suboptimal tube position and ventilation in obese or fatigued patients who have difficulty extending their neck
- Tracheo-oesophageal fistula formation
- Tracheal erosion into surrounding blood vessels.

Late

- Tracheal stenosis
- Tracheal dilation
- Granulomata of the trachea leading to respiratory difficulty on tube removal
- Persistent sinus at tracheostomy site
- Scar formation requiring surgical revision.

KEY POINTS

Main complications of tracheostomy include:

- haemorrhage
- tube occlusion
- misplacement
- infection
- fistula formation
- tracheal stenosis

TYPES OF TRACHEOSTOMY TUBE

Tracheostomy tubes can be plastic or metal, cuffed or uncuffed, fenestrated or non-fenestrated. Common features of all tubes include:

- Wings attached to the proximal part of the tube for securing it in place with ribbon or sutures
- The proximal end has a standard 15 mm connector (connects to an Ambu bag)
- The tip of the tube is cut horizontally so as to reduce the chance of obstruction by lying against the tracheal wall.

Each is described in more detail below.

Cuffed tracheostomy tubes

Cuffed tracheostomy tubes (Fig. 14.3) are the most common tubes encountered on the intensive care unit and postoperatively. These plastic tubes have *low pressure, high volume* cuffs which are inflated with air from a syringe via a pilot balloon. (Note that some more unusual tracheostomy tubes may have a self-inflating balloon, e.g. the Bivona Fome-cuf has a special syringe for removal of air for tracheostomy insertion and, on removal of the syringe, the cuff self-inflates to a preset pressure.)

These tubes are used to:

1. Allow intermittent positive pressure ventilation (IPPV) or maintain continuous positive airway pressure (CPAP). By inflating the cuff until a

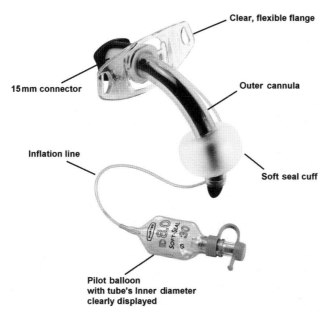

Clear, flexible flange

15mm connector

Outer cannula

Inflation line

Soft seal cuff

Pilot balloon
with tube's inner diameter
clearly displayed

Figure 14.3 Portex cuffed tracheostomy tube.

leak is no longer heard around the tracheostomy site the air/oxygen mix being delivered to the patient is prevented from escaping. This allows accurate delivery of a required percentage of oxygen and maintains the desired level of positive end expiratory pressure (PEEP) or CPAP. These modes of ventilatory support are not routinely encountered outside the critical care unit.

2. Decrease the risk of any aspirate reaching the lungs. The cuff effectively creates a mechanical barrier and so reduces the likelihood of aspiration in a patient with impaired swallowing. However, the cuff can interfere with the swallowing mechanism itself and when patients are able to take an oral diet, the cuff should ideally be deflated when eating if they have been assessed as not being at risk of aspiration.

Disadvantages of cuffed tracheostomy tubes are:

1. The cuff acts as a foreign body occluding the trachea, i.e. if the lumen of the tube becomes blocked with secretions, or the lumen is occluded by a decannulation cap with the cuff still inflated, this prevents any passage of air/oxygen past the tube and leads to total airway obstruction. *Unless the cuff is deflated or the tracheostomy tube removed a respiratory arrest will occur.*
2. Pressure trauma. The pressure exerted by the cuff on the tracheal wall reduces the perfusion of the tracheal mucosa. This will eventually lead to tracheal erosion, ulceration, dilation and stenosis.
3. The patient will be unable to speak or swallow with comfort.

Cuff inflation and prevention of pressure trauma

• High volume low pressure cuffs reduce the risk of trauma by dissipating the pressure exerted over a wider surface area.

> pressure = force/area

• Air is gradually inserted into the cuff via the pilot balloon at 0.2–0.5 mL increments with a 10 mL syringe. Stop inflating when an air leak is no longer audible and document the volume of air in the medical notes.
• The cuff pressure must also be measured using a hand pressure manometer. This is attached to the pilot balloon via a luer lock and the pressure on the dial is read. Care must be taken not to allow deflation of the cuff during the procedure. *Cuff pressure must not exceed 25 mmHg.*

Tracheostomy tubes with inner cannulae

Tracheostomy tubes with inner cannulae were introduced to minimize the frequency with which a normal tube required changing. Initially the recommendations were to replace a tube (without an inner cannula) every 7–10 days to minimize the risk of the tube lumen becoming narrowed or occluded by secretions. Patient discomfort and potential trauma to the stoma site were two disadvantages of this guideline. A tracheostomy tube with an inner cannula, however, can be left in situ for up to 30 days. The inner cannula can be changed frequently to reduce the risk of occlusion and this may also reduce the risk of infection.

It must be noted that the inner cannula for a tracheostomy tube reduces the internal diameter of the lumen by 1–1.5 mm and can increase the effort it takes for the patient to breathe. However, when the fenestrations are open (vide infra) this then reduces airways resistance.

Airflow is proportional to the radius of the tube to the power of four:

$$Q \propto r^4$$

Inner cannulae are designed to fit a specific size of tracheostomy tube. The correct diameter and length of cannula must be used. The inner cannula should be removed and cleaned at least once per day and as frequently as four hourly if secretions are profuse and tenacious. This must be performed using universal precautions and the cannula then discarded if disposable, or cleaned with normal saline if reusable. A twist lock action system is usual for most tubes where the tube is stabilized and the inner tube twisted in an anticlockwise direction to unlock it. The cannula can then be gently pulled out. The reverse is done when replacing it, ensuring that the arrows are lined up on the connector.

KEY POINT
- When the inner tube is removed from the tracheostomy tube the 15 mm connector is also removed. An adaptor or spare cannula must be available should hand ventilation be necessary in an emergency.

Uncuffed tracheostomy tubes (Fig. 14.4)

An uncuffed tracheostomy tube is indicated in a patient who no longer requires IPPV or CPAP, or protection of the airway from aspiration. These

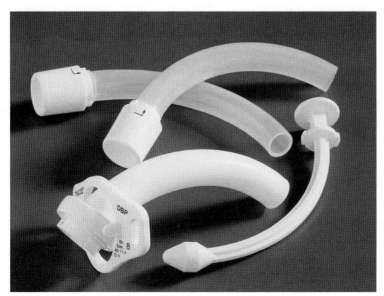

Figure 14.4   Uncuffed, non-fenestrated tracheostomy tube.

patients are usually those who have been discharged to the ward following a prolonged stay on the critical care unit but still require tracheal suctioning and physiotherapy. The uncuffed tubes are easier to replace, do not necessarily require inner tubes, are suitable for long-term use and allow the patient to speak. They also do not lead to total airway obstruction if the lumen of the tube becomes blocked. A fenestrated tube will further reduce the work of breathing and aid speech.

KEY POINT
- If manual ventilation is required with this type of tube most of the air will be forced upwards through the mouth and the tube should be changed for a cuffed variety.

Fenestrated tracheostomy tubes (Fig. 14.5)

Note that there are two inner tubes, one unfenestrated for tracheal suction and one fenestrated to facilitate speech. The internal diameter is marked on the flange as 8 mm and the external diameter as 11.4 mm. This varies between different makes of tube.

Fenestrated tracheostomy tubes have either a single window or multiple holes in the greater curvature of the tube. The two benefits of the fenestrated tube are:

1. Air is channelled to the vocal cords through the fenestrations allowing the patient to speak.
2. The work of breathing is reduced when the cuff is deflated as air can flow around the cuff and also through the fenestrations in addition to entry via the stoma. This can assist weaning of the spontaneously breathing patient from the tracheostomy.

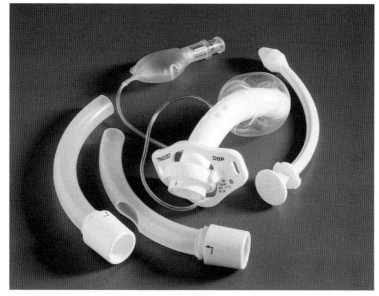

Figure 14.5 Fenestrated cuffed tracheostomy tube.

Tracheostomy tubes with a variable flange

Variable flange (i.e. length) tracheostomy tubes have been designed for patients who have 'deep set tracheas'. Morbidly obese patients and patients with pretracheal oedema or inflammation come into this category. The adjustable flange allows the tube to be set at the desired length and altered to the ideal position as the clinical situation dictates. Positioning of the end of the tube at the optimal position in the trachea may be performed using a CXR or fibre-optic bronchoscopy. Most variable flange tubes have a numbered scale to show the length of tube at the skin and this should be recorded in the notes to ensure that if the tube slowly migrates out of the neck, it may be reinserted to the appropriate length.

Tip
Routine adjustment of variable flange tracheostomies is not recommended due to the risk of tube displacement.

Metal tracheostomy tubes

These tubes are used for patients requiring long-term tracheostomy. They are coated with silver which is non-irritant and bactericidal. They are uncuffed and some have a reusable inner tube. They do not have a 15 mm connector and if a patient with a silver tube requires ventilatory support, i.e. at cardiac arrest, then it should be changed for a cuffed tube to allow ventilation; however, if a cuffed tube is not at hand some ventilation may be provided using a 15 mm connector from an endotracheal tube of an appropriate size to fit into the end of the tracheostomy tube. Alternatively if the patient has a patent upper airway, the tube may be removed and the patient intubated through the larynx.

CARE OF THE PATIENT WITH A TRACHEOSTOMY

Postoperative care

The majority of patients undergoing a surgical tracheostomy will return to a high dependency or intensive care area. Some surgical specialities will have a ward area able to provide a higher level of care.

The following guidelines refer to the immediate care of a patient having undergone a surgical tracheostomy.

- Essential equipment must be with the patient at all times, at the bed space and at times of transfer:
  - tracheostomy tube – same size plus one size smaller
  - Ambu bag
  - 10 mL syringe
  - suction unit, suction catheters and gloves
  - Spencer Wells forceps
  - access to resuscitation equipment.
- The patient must be under direct supervision during the initial postoperative period. Observations must include:
  - respiratory rate
  - effort and sound of breathing
  - patient colour
  - oxygen saturations
  - regular inspection of stoma site for bleeding or haematoma formation.
- A portable chest X-ray (CXR) is usually performed when the patient returns from theatre. The position of the tracheostomy must be at least 2–3 cm above the carina and should be positioned vertically in line with the trachea (see the CXR in Fig. 14.6). The CXR also helps to exclude a pneumothorax, surgical emphysema or segmental collapse due to blood clots or sputum retention.
- Check cuff pressure with a hand-held portable manometer (estimated techniques, such as feeling the tension of the pilot balloon, are

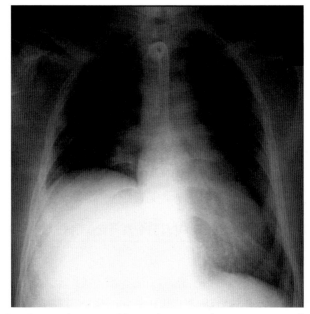

Figure 14.6 Correct placement of the tracheostomy tube, pointing vertically down the trachea ending 3–4 cm above carina. Note this patient also has an elevated right hemidiaphragm due to unilateral phrenic nerve paralysis.

unreliable!). Ensure the pressure is less than 25 mmHg in a spontaneously breathing patient.

- Check that the ties used to secure the tracheostomy tube in situ are reasonably tight when the neck is in the flexed position (surgery is usually performed with the neck extended where the circumference measurement is maximal).

> **KEY POINT**
> - Do not change the tracheostomy tube for at least 72 h unless absolutely required. Ideally leave the first change until 7–10 days when a track has formed. Prior to this time the stoma will close and the track may be lost.

Delivery of oxygen and humidification

The upper respiratory tract is normally responsible for the filtering, warming and humidification of inspired gases. In a patient with a tracheostomy this protective mechanism is bypassed. Inhalation of dried air or unhumidified oxygen may cause drying of the respiratory mucosa and reduced ciliary activity, keratinization and ulceration, increased tenacity of mucus and sputum retention, atelectasis and impaired gas exchange. With time the mucosa adapts to the drier, cooler air, but patients with a new tracheostomy are at high risk of the above complications. It is important to increase the moisture content of inspired gases by means of a humidification device.

Ventilated patients or patients on a CPAP circuit

A heat-moisture exchanger (HME) can be placed into the breathing system. This efficient device not only heats and humidifies the inspired gases but acts as a filter and supplemental oxygen may be delivered through the HME. It can be used in the short term provided secretions are not too tenacious (occlusion can occur).

Self-ventilating patient with oxygen

Place a tracheostomy mask over the tracheostomy tube site and connect to a humidifier system and oxygen by elephant tubing (Fig. 14.7). Alternatively a T-piece may be used and connected in the same way to the system. Inspired gas is usually bubbled through cold sterile water. Despite being relatively inefficient at humidification and not warming the gases, it is a cost-effective method with a low complication profile. The water used must be changed every 24 h to reduce the risk of pseudomonas colonization and subsequent infection.

Self-ventilating patient on air

An HME device can be directly attached to the tracheostomy tube, e.g. 'Thermovent T'. This must be checked every 4 h and replaced if soiled.

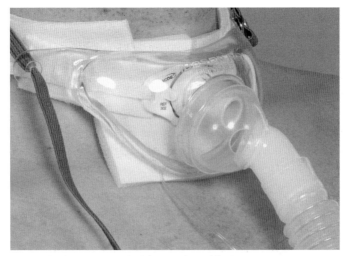

Figure 14.7 Tracheostomy mask delivering humidified oxygen.

This will humidify gases and may also be used to deliver supplemental oxygen (Fig. 14.8).

Nebulized 0.9% saline can also be used as a form of humidification and to loosen secretions. A nebulizer is attached to the tracheostomy mask as to a normal facemask and connected to a gas source with a flow rate of 6–8 L/min.

Suctioning

Suctioning via the tracheostomy tube is performed to clear bronchial secretions. It is a very traumatic procedure for the patient as there may be an inability to

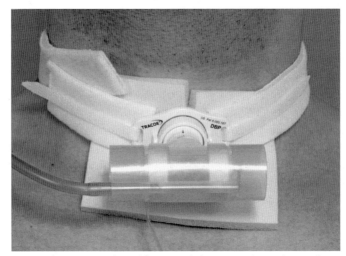

Figure 14.8 'Thermovent T' humidifier ('Swedish nose') with supplemental oxygen delivery.

inspire during suctioning itself. Other consequences include hypoxia, bradycardia (particularly in patients with autonomic dysfunction such as spinal injuries), tracheal mucosal damage and bleeding, and introduction of infection. Each patient needs recurrent individual assessment to ascertain the frequency with which suctioning is required and, where possible, patients should be encouraged to cough up their own secretions (Buglass 1999). The procedure is as follows:

- Suctioning should be done using an aseptic technique.
- The sterile suction catheter should have a diameter no greater than half that of the tracheostomy tube:

> Suction catheter size (Fg) = 2 × (size of tracheostomy tube − 2)
> For example: 8.0 mm ID tube: 2 × (8 − 2) = 12 Fg

- The lowest possible vacuum pressure should be used: = 100–120 mmHg (13–16 kPa).
- Hyperoxygenate the patient for at least 3 min prior to suctioning.
- Insert the suction catheter approximately 10–15 cm into the tube before applying suction and slowly withdrawing the catheter.
- Suction should be applied for a maximum of 10 s.

Suctioning can be performed either with single-use sterile suction catheters or with closed system multiple-use suction units. The closed system units are commonly used in patients who are ventilator-dependent or who have copious infected secretions. There is no strong evidence to recommend either form of suctioning over the other with respect to infection risk (Branson 2005). Patients who are at risk of developing hypoxaemia may require pulse oximetry monitoring during suctioning.

Changing tracheostomy tubes

- Tracheostomy tubes without an inner cannula are generally changed every 7–14 days until the patient is free of pulmonary secretions and has a well-formed clean stoma, when tube changes may become less frequent.
- Inner lumen tracheostomy tubes may remain in situ for approximately 30 days before requiring a tube change.
- The first tracheostomy tube change:
  - should not be performed within 72 h following a surgical tracheostomy and not before 3–5 days after a percutaneous tracheostomy to allow the stoma to become established. Opinions vary but it is the author's practice to leave the first change until after 7 days
  - the decision to change the tube must be made by a medical practitioner competent in the care of tracheostomies
  - must be carried out by a medical practitioner with appropriate, advanced airway skills.
- Subsequent changes can be made by experienced personnel trained in tracheostomy tube changes. Many hospitals now have specialist tracheostomy nurses.

Care of the patient with a tracheostomy

A standard procedure for changing a tracheostomy tube is described below. Two skilled practitioners should be present when changing the tube, e.g. a doctor and nurse, and resuscitation equipment must be readily available (Minza & Cameron 2001).

If a patient has a smooth long-term stoma and has regular tracheostomy changes, the new tube may usually be inserted using the tracheostomy introducer. If this is the first change, or difficulty with changing the tube is anticipated due to abnormal anatomy, it may be more appropriate to change the tube over an airway exchange device such as a bougie. Both the Frova and Cook Airway Exchange Catheter™ have the advantage of allowing oxygenation by insufflation of oxygen whilst changing the tube. In these circumstances, this should only be performed by someone with the appropriate advanced airway skills.

There is a risk of paratracheal tube placement with any blind technique and some institutions recommend exchange and confirmation of tube placement with a fibre-optic bronchoscope.

Procedure for changing a tracheostomy tube

1. Equipment:
   – dressing pack and 0.9% saline sachet
   – tracheostomy tubes – same size plus one size smaller
   – 10 mL syringe if the tracheostomy tube is cuffed
   – lubricant
   – tracheostomy dressing
   – sterile gloves and protective eyewear
   – suction – suction catheters and yankeur sucker
   – tracheostomy exchange device – gum elastic bougie.
2. Explain the procedure to the patient – verbal consent should be obtained if appropriate.
3. Ensure the patient has been nil by mouth for a minimum of 4 h and that the nasogastric tube is aspirated if present.
4. Place the patient in the semi-recumbent position.
5. Administer 100% oxygen for at least 5 min prior to the change if the patient is oxygen-dependent and monitor oxygen saturations in all patients.
6. If the new tracheostomy tube is cuffed, inflate the cuff with air to ensure there is no leak. Deflate the cuff fully before insertion.
7. Lubricate the new tracheostomy tube.
8. Remove the old tracheostomy dressing and clean around the stoma with the 0.9% saline.
9. Suction the back of the patient's mouth to clear any secretions and suction via the tracheostomy.
10. Slowly deflate the tracheostomy cuff.
11. If using an airway exchange device, pass this down the tracheostomy once the patient has stopped coughing to a depth equal to that of the tube. The tube is then removed leaving the exchange catheter in place,

over which the new tracheostomy may be railroaded insufflating oxygen down the airway exchange device if required.

12. If inserting the new tracheostomy tube using the introducer, remove the old tube and reinsert the new tube into the stoma with the introducer inserted, ensuring that the first movement is vertically down and then gently rotate to allow passage into the trachea.
13. The new tracheostomy tube is usually inserted during exhalation. Once the tracheostomy tube is in position, remove the bougie and inflate the cuff and re-administer oxygen.
14. Observe the patient's respiration and assess chest movement, air entry and pulse oximetry.

Care of the stoma

The tracheostomy site must be kept clean and dry to prevent infection and irritation occurring. It should be inspected daily and cleansed with 0.9% saline. A slim, absorbent dressing is appropriate to use and the tape or tube holder should be assessed at least every 24 h.

OTHER ASPECTS OF CARE OF THE TRACHEOSTOMY

Speech and tracheostomy tubes

A patient with a cuffed, non-fenestrated tracheostomy tube will not be able to vocalize as air is unable to pass through the vocal cords. This problem can be overcome by the following methods:

- Cuff deflation or uncuffed smaller tracheostomy tubes
- Fenestrated tracheostomy tubes
- Intermittent finger occlusion by the patient or one-way speaking valves with a fenestrated tube.

Speaking valves

One-way speaking valves allow air to be entrained during inhalation but not when exhaling, thus airflow is redirected either through fenestrations in the tracheostomy tube or back down the tube, up into the larynx and out through the vocal cords.

Swallowing

Each patient with a tracheostomy must be individually assessed before allowing oral intake by either a speech and language therapist or by a trained medical practitioner.

> **KEY POINT**
> - Speaking valves must not be used with a non-fenestrated tube with the cuff inflated because exhalation will not be possible.

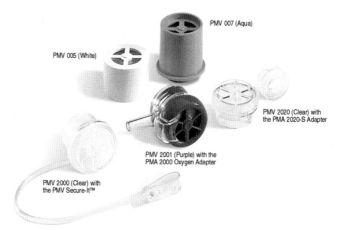

A **Passy-Muir Tracheostomy and Ventilator Speaking Valves**

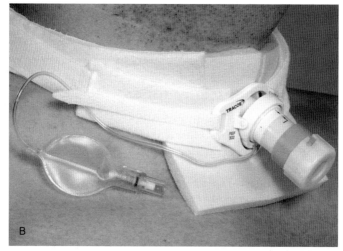

B

Figure 14.9 (A) A selection of 'speaking' valves, some for use with artificial ventilation or administration of oxygen. (B) The 'speaking valve' in place; note that the fenestrated inner tube is in place and the cuff deflated, encouraging air to escape past the vocal cords allowing speech.

Patients find it easier to eat and drink with the cuff of the tracheostomy tube deflated. This prevents the cuff compressing the oesophagus, making swallowing difficult and increasing the risk of aspiration. Sips of sterile water are initially given and if tolerated without coughing, desaturation, fatigue or signs of aspiration on tracheal suctioning, thickened fluids may be introduced followed by a soft diet. Additional coloured dye tests may be

KEY POINT
- Cuff deflation is safe in patients receiving CPAP (< 10 cm) with only a slight fall in pressure support and continued respiratory stability (Conway & Mackie 2004).

appropriate to assess risks of aspiration, but are not very sensitive and occasionally endoscopic evaluation of laryngeal function may be required.

Weaning and decannulation

Weaning from ventilatory support and dependence on a tracheostomy tube can be a prolonged process depending on the individual patient and their illness. Most patients will return to the ward breathing spontaneously on a tracheostomy mask from a critical care area. Depending on the clinical condition of the patient, the intention is usually to wean and remove the tracheostomy before discharge.

Certain criteria must be met before weaning can commence:

- The condition necessitating the insertion of a tracheostomy has resolved.
- Lung function remains stable and oxygen requirements are less than 40%.
- The patient is able to swallow, and has a good cough and a gag reflex.
- Nutritional status is adequate.
- The patient is comfortable with the cuff deflated.

If the patient meets these criteria, weaning can begin with lengthening periods of time with the cuff deflated. Begin with 5–15 min periods with at least a 30-min rest interval until the patient can manage 4 h at a time. This gradually increases respiratory muscle strength. Once this stage has been reached the process is repeated with the tracheostomy tube capped off, initially with a one way 'speaking valve' then onto an occlusion cap, with the cuff deflated and the inner lumen fenestrated tube in place. This effectively allows the patient to breathe solely through the upper airway but maintains access to the airway if there is any deterioration in the patient's condition. Speech should be restored at this stage. If it is not, an ENT opinion should be considered before decannulation as patients can develop granulation tissue above the tracheostomy that may require surgical resection.

Once this stage has been reached and the patient can tolerate having the tracheostomy tube capped off, removal of the tracheostomy tube should be considered. The optimal time for this is early morning when the patient has been rested overnight and there is time to observe their condition over the day.

To remove the tube, ensure the patient is sitting upright and is comfortable. Suction the oropharynx and down the tracheotomy tube. Fully deflate the cuff if present and gently but firmly withdraw the tube during

---

KEY POINTS
- Have the criteria for weaning been met?
- Begin with 5–15 min periods of respiration with the cuff deflated.
- Rest for at least 30 min between intervals of cuff deflation.
- Extend periods by 15–30 min up to 4 h.
- Repeat this sequence with the tracheostomy tube capped off, initially with a speaking valve, then occlusive cap.
- If tolerated for 4 h or overnight, consider decannulation.

exhalation with an outward and downward movement. Apply a dry dressing to the stoma site and cover with an occlusive dressing to provide an effective seal. Closely monitor the patient's respiratory status following the procedure.

EMERGENCY ALGORITHMS

Tracheostomy tube occlusion

Tracheostomy tube occlusion is a potentially life-threatening situation and must be recognized and dealt with promptly. The protocol in Figure 14.10 is designed for use in the general ward setting.

Tracheostomy tube change failure

Failure to reinsert a tracheostomy tube after removal is fortunately a rare occurrence but can have serious consequences including those of losing the airway completely, culminating in respiratory arrest and the complications of tube misplacement. The protocol in Figure 14.11 has again been developed for use outside the critical care area.

Cardiorespiratory arrest

Establishing a patent airway is the first priority in any arrest situation. In this group of patients it is important to identify early if the cardiorespiratory arrest is directly related to a problem with the tracheostomy tube itself (Fig. 14.12).

MINITRACHEOSTOMY AND CRICOTHYROID PUNCTURE

The minitracheostomy

The minitracheostomy tube is a plastic tube up to 10 cm long with an internal diameter usually greater than 4 mm (Fig. 14.13). The proximal end allows a 15-mm connector to be attached, or newer versions have an integral 15-mm connector in common with other airway devices allowing attachment to a breathing system (Fig. 14.14). It also has wings to secure the tube in place. It is inserted under local anaesthesia through the cricothyroid membrane.

The main indication for using a minitracheostomy tube is for the management of sputum retention both on the ward and in critical care. The advantage of this technique is to allow tracheal suctioning whilst preserving glottic function. In some cases tracheostomy can be avoided by their use.

It can also be used in the emergency situation as a temporary airway in cases of acute upper airway obstruction. The minitracheostomy set enables easy cricothyroidotomy and provides a means to deliver oxygen.

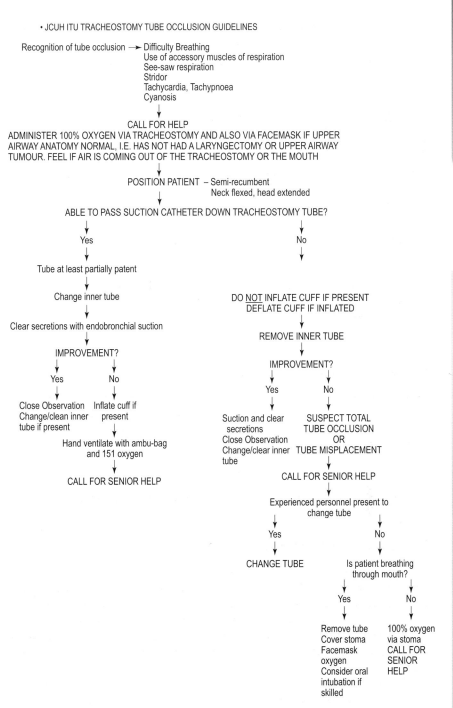

• JCUH ITU TRACHEOSTOMY TUBE OCCLUSION GUIDELINES

Recognition of tube occlusion → Difficulty Breathing
Use of accessory muscles of respiration
See-saw respiration
Stridor
Tachycardia, Tachypnoea
Cyanosis

CALL FOR HELP
ADMINISTER 100% OXYGEN VIA TRACHEOSTOMY AND ALSO VIA FACEMASK IF UPPER
AIRWAY ANATOMY NORMAL, I.E. HAS NOT HAD A LARYNGECTOMY OR UPPER AIRWAY
TUMOUR. FEEL IF AIR IS COMING OUT OF THE TRACHEOSTOMY OR THE MOUTH

POSITION PATIENT – Semi-recumbent
Neck flexed, head extended

ABLE TO PASS SUCTION CATHETER DOWN TRACHEOSTOMY TUBE?

Yes

Tube at least partially patent

Change inner tube

Clear secretions with endobronchial suction

IMPROVEMENT?

Yes   No

Close Observation   Inflate cuff if
Change/clean inner   present
tube if present

Hand ventilate with ambu-bag
and 15l oxygen

CALL FOR SENIOR HELP

No

DO NOT INFLATE CUFF IF PRESENT
DEFLATE CUFF IF INFLATED

REMOVE INNER TUBE

IMPROVEMENT?

Yes   No

Suction and clear   SUSPECT TOTAL
secretions   TUBE OCCLUSION
Close Observation   OR
Change/clear inner   TUBE MISPLACEMENT
tube

CALL FOR SENIOR HELP

Experienced personnel present to
change tube

Yes   No

CHANGE TUBE   Is patient breathing
through mouth?

Yes   No

Remove tube   100% oxygen
Cover stoma   via stoma
Facemask   CALL FOR
oxygen   SENIOR
Consider oral   HELP
intubation if
skilled

NB: Fibreoptic confirmation of tube patency and position is very useful in this situation if skilled endoscopist available

Figure 14.10   Protocol for dealing with tracheostomy tube occlusion.

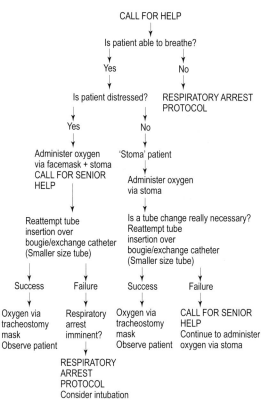

Figure 14.11 Protocol for dealing with tracheostomy tube failure.

Cricothyroid puncture

A cricothyroid puncture may only be performed in the emergency setting if all other methods of oxygenating the patient have failed. The person performing the procedure must be aware of the anatomy involved, the equipment required and the complications they may face. It is a holding measure prior to a definitive airway being obtained, particularly as oxygenation may be maintained, but CO_2 will progressively rise over the ensuing 20–30 min. A Sanders injector may also be used to deliver oxygen under high pressure but with an increased risk of barotrauma in unskilled hands. If upper airway obstruction exists, a second cannula may need to be inserted to allow expiration. Ventilation via cricothyrotomy has significant associated risks and should only be performed by experienced personnel.

The technique for insertion of a minitracheostomy tube and performance of a cricothyroid puncture are described below.

• CARDIORESPIRATORY ARREST PROTOCOL IN TRACHEOSTOMY PATIENT

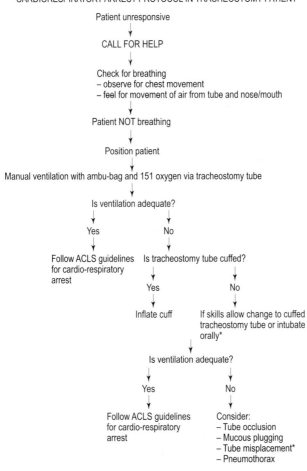

*If unable to replace tube and ventilation inadequate, consider removing tracheostomy tube, occluding stoma and performing bag and face mask ventilation until senior help arrives. If unable to ventilate, the tube may be malpositioned in the anterior neck, this is a dangerous situation as a tension pneumomediastinum can be created, beware particularly if surgical emphysema develops on controlled ventilation. Do not vigorously ventilate if in doubt and consider removing tracheostomy and intubating through the larynx.

Figure 14.12   Protocol for dealing with cardiorespiratory arrest.

Minitracheostomy and cricothyroid puncture

Elective

1. Position patient with sandbag under shoulders +/− a headring support
2. Identify cricoid and thyroid cartilages – the cricothyroid membrane lies between them
3. Local infiltration of 1% lidocaine + 1:200 000 adrenaline (epinephrine)
4. Puncture membrane with 16G short bevelled needle:
   - this should be attached to a 5 mL syringe containing 2 mL 0.9% saline
   - insert in midline, in slight caudad direction, with bevel of needle facing down
   - aspirate until air → in trachea

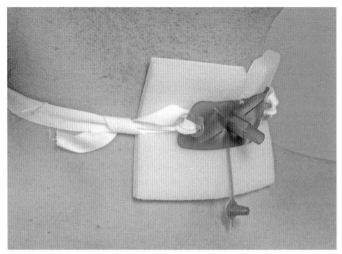

Figure 14.13 Minitracheostomy in situ. Note the position higher in the neck at the level of the cricothyroid membrane.

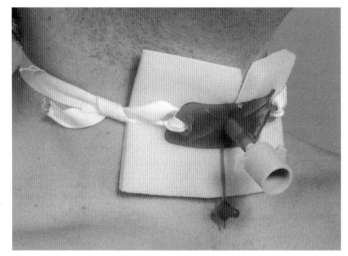

Figure 14.14 Minitracheostomy with 15-mm connector attached, allowing emergency attachment to breathing circuits, e.g. Ambu bag. Note: due to the small diameter of the airway, artificial ventilation will not be possible for long with a minitracheostomy (see text). Newer devices are available for emergency subglottic airway control which allow more prolonged ventilation, but require experience for their insertion and management.

5. Feed guide wire down the needle then remove the needle over the wire
6. Pass small dilator over the wire
7. Replace dilator with minitracheostomy tube – apply firm pressure to insert with a downwards and backwards movement
8. Secure in place with neck tie
9. Connect to standard 15-mm connector.

Emergency

1. Position patient as above
2. Identify cricothyroid membrane
3. Puncture membrane with 14G vascular access cannula or cricothyroid cannula
4. Remove syringe and ensure that it is possible to aspirate air from cannula
5. Secure in place to avoid kinking of plastic cannula
6. Connect to 3.5 mm tracheal tube connector with:
   - 2 mL syringe with plunger removed + 8 mm tracheal tube connector inserted into open end
   - injector device connected to needle hub
   - oxygen tubing with hole in side of tubing.

SUPPORT SERVICES

Various support services may be available in hospital to medical and nursing staff caring for patients with a tracheostomy tube. These include:

- a dedicated tracheostomy care nurse
- critical care medical and nursing staff
- 'outreach' team
- local, trust wide and national guidelines.

Recent studies have shown that with the introduction of specialist tracheostomy services, tracheostomy tubes remain in situ for shorter periods of time and fewer patients suffer from tracheostomy-related complications (Norwood et al 2004). It is important to be aware of services offered by the particular hospital you are working in and to make appropriate use of them.

CASE 14.1

An obese 48-year-old man develops myasthenia gravis and is ventilated in the critical care unit. A tracheostomy is performed using a variable flange (long) tracheostomy tube and he returns to the neurology ward where he develops respiratory distress and is in peri-arrest when you are asked to review him. Describe the CXR (Fig. 14.15), the underlying problem and outline your plan of treatment.

Answer
The CXR shows malpositioning of the tracheostomy tube which is straight and does not appear to proceed down the trachea. It is clearly lying in the trachea horizontally and partially blocking the tracheal lumen. The first course of action is to let the cuff down as the inflated cuff will be blocking the trachea. This was carried out and the patient subsequently improved considerably and was able to breathe through his mouth. The tracheostomy needs repositioning either in theatre or using the flexible fibre-optic bronchoscope as a guide to railroad the tracheostomy into the

14

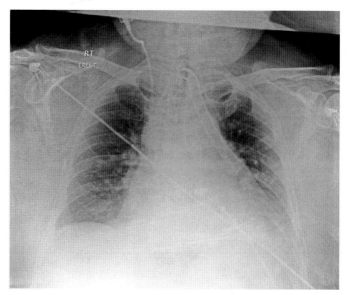

Figure 14.15 CXR.

trachea. If this man had arrested, it would have been better to have removed the tracheostomy completely and intubate him through the larynx under direct vision, as from this CXR you cannot be sure that the tracheostomy is in the trachea at all.

CASE 14.2

A 66-year-old man has a tracheostomy performed to facilitate weaning from ventilation on the critical care unit and returns to the ward. The tracheostomy becomes dislodged and the nursing

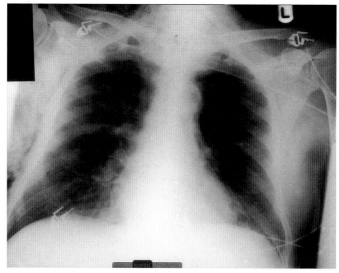

Figure 14.16 Emergency CXR.

staff are unable to replace it. He develops central chest pain and shortness of breath. His CXR is shown (Fig. 14.16). What is the diagnosis? Outline a plan of treatment.

Answer

The tracheostomy has been pushed back to create a false passage allowing air to enter the mediastinum, creating a pneumomediastinum. Note the double border to the heart and extensive surgical emphysema in the soft tissues.

This can be a life-threatening emergency and experienced help should be called immediately. The first priority is to ensure oxygenation. If he is breathing through his mouth administer high-flow oxygen over both his mouth and tracheostomy stoma. He may settle with conservative management, particularly as the cause of the false passage has now been removed. If the tracheostomy needs to be replaced this may require placement under direct vision using a fibre-optic bronchoscope and an experienced operator. Rarely a pneumomediastinum may develop into a tension pneumomediastinum which may require decompression with chest drain insertion and cardiothoracic referral. Massive surgical emphysema may also develop if the leak is ongoing and this may be relieved with subcutaneous incisions over the upper chest wall.

Acknowledgements

Thanks to Smiths Medical PLC and Kapitex Healthcare for the provision of diagrams and pictures, which have been adapted for this chapter.

REFERENCES AND FURTHER READING

Al-Shaikh B, Stacy S 2001 Essentials of anaesthetic equipment, 2nd edn. Churchill Livingstone, London

Branson R D 2005 The ventilator circuit and ventilator-associated pneumonia. Respiratory Care 50(6):774–785; discussion 785–787

Buglass E 1999 Tracheostomy care: tracheal suctioning and humidification. British Journal of Nursing 8(8):500–504

Conway D H, Mackie C 2004 The effects of tracheostomy cuff deflation during CPAP. Anaesthesia 59(7):652–657

Dulguerov P 1999 Percutaneous or surgical tracheostomy; a meta analysis. Critical Care Medicine 27:1617–1625

Fikkers B G, van Veen J A, Kooloos J G et al 2004 Emphysema and pneumothorax after percutaneous tracheostomy: case report and anatomic study. Chest 125:1805–1814

Griffiths J, Barber V S, Morgan L et al 2005 Systematic review and meta-analysis of studies of the timing of tracheostomy in adult patients undergoing artifical ventilation. BMJ 330:1243–1246

Law R C, Carney S, Manara A R 1997 Long term outcome after percutaneous dilational tracheostomy. Endoscopic and spirometry findings. Anaesthesia 52:51–56

Lewarski J S 2005 Long-term care of the patient with a tracheostomy. Respiratory Care 50(4):534-537

Minza S, Cameron D S 2001 The tracheostomy tube change: a review of technique. Hospital Medicine 62(3):158–163

Norwood M G, Spiers P, Bailiss J et al 2004 Evaluation of the role of specialist tracheostomy services. From critical care to outreach and beyond. Postgraduate Medical Journal 80(946):478–480

Pahor A L 1992 Ear, nose and throat in Ancient Egypt. Journal of Laryngology and Otology 106:773–779

Paw H G W, Bodenham A R 2004 Percutaneous tracheostomy; a practical handbook. Greenwich Medical Media, Cambridge

St George's Healthcare NHS Trust 2001 Guidelines for the care of patients with tracheostomy tubes. St George's Hospital, London

Stewart S L, Secrest J A, Norwood B R et al 2003 A comparison of endotracheal tube cuff pressures using estimation techniques and direct intracuff measurement. AANA Journal 71(6):443–447

Whittet H, Waldmann C 1995 Review article: percutaneous tracheostomy. Care of the Critically Ill 11(5):198–202

Ethical issues in critical care

Stephen Bonner, Nick Pace

15

OBJECTIVES

After reading this chapter you should be able to:

● *Understand the ethical principles upon which medical decision-making is based*

● *Translate these principles into clinical decision-making in critically ill patients*

INTRODUCTION

Ethics is the philosophical study of the moral value of human conduct and of the rules and principles that ought to govern it. From the medical profession's perspective, it defines the code of behaviour considered to be correct. This is frequently related to a particular culture and time. It is based on moral philosophy, morality and value judgements, mostly related to doing good or harm. What is thought of as ethical may be thought of as no more or less than what is moral. Morality in any society is based on prevailing religious principles and influenced by society's values and must therefore always be interpreted in a specific cultural setting.

In everyday practical terms, specific ethical principles may be narrowly interpreted according to a 'list' of concepts and values applicable to a particular culture, or may be more broadly interpreted as value judgements made for another person and with their best interests at heart.

All such judgements are subject to the rule of law, which is also based on religious principles and influenced by prevailing values in society. Many legal principles cross national boundaries. For example, all countries in the European Union are now subject to the European Convention on Human Rights. English common law is based on case law, where preceding judgements in a particular situation form legal principles which then act to guide future judgements. Such a framework responds to new developments in society, such as advances in medical technology, by holding test cases where a ruling is laid down which then acts as guidance for future cases. Such cases may be brought before the courts with the specific intent of generating a ruling where no case law exists, thereby generating legal precedent. It should also be remembered that Scotland has a separate legal system and when this differs significantly from English law it will be highlighted.

The emphasis of medical ethics changes with time according to influences from society. Recently there has been a dramatic shift away from paternalism and ethics founded on religious principles towards humanistic ethics, autonomy, the rights of the individual and some would say 'the patient as consumer'. Although case law gives reassurance in ethical dilemmas where a particular situation has already arisen, it may be difficult to decide on the correct course of action in the shifting sands of society's values if no such judgement is available.

This makes it even more important to ensure that actions must be guided by a set of ethical principles and justified according to an established ethical and legal framework.

This chapter discusses some of the basic ethical principles needed to guide doctors through such decisions as well as reviewing some more recent influences of society. Firstly it is important to understand some of the background in the development of these ethical principles.

HISTORY

There are three well-described streams of development of Judeo-Christian medical ethics. Hippocrates (460–377 BC) exhorted physicians to do no harm to the patient, but only to do good, and to accept that there were limits to one's skill. This guidance is in the ancient Greek tradition of craftsmanship: to step beyond the limit of one's craft is to be guilty of pride (*hubris*). True beneficence, as in doing good, even to one's own detriment, is thought to stem from the Samaritan tradition of medicine. St Luke was a physician. It is also thought that the Good Samaritan in the gospel of St Luke was a physician who administered a mixture of oil and wine to the man fallen by the wayside. This medical ethos was further developed in the third tradition during the Crusades by the Knights Hospitallers, who founded hospitals to care for sick pilgrims on the road to the Holy Land and subsequently cared for the wounded during the Crusades. This Order came from noble families and established a tradition of 'gentlemen physicians' and has been blamed for the paternalistic tradition of western medicine, much criticized in recent years.

These traditions of medical ethics have, in modern times, come into conflict with social changes. The rise of patients' rights groups and the concept of the patient as a healthcare 'consumer' do not sit easily with the need to ration healthcare resources. The right of the patient to decide, autonomy, has always been central in the practice of Western medicine but has recently become of overwhelming importance throughout all aspects of healthcare. This is now also being extended to the families of patients, as seen in the recent scandal surrounding the retention of organs. These changes have been driven from outside the profession, which in turn can be criticized for failing to keep with the wishes and desires of society. However, it is important to stress that these changes still follow basic medical ethical principles, the difference being which one is given prominence.

BASIC PRINCIPLES

The four basic underlying principles that have guided Western medicine for more than 2000 years are:

- autonomy
- beneficence
- non-maleficence
- distributive justice.

All medical treatment should be given with these principles in mind and actions may be subsequently judged according to them. Patient autonomy is currently given the highest priority. If a patient is competent, they have an absolute right to be involved in the decision-making process. Thus they need to be given sufficient information to enable them to make an informed choice and appreciate the consequences of that choice. Before surgery, this would require disclosure of complication rates, while in the critical care setting this should include a discussion of the risks, such as the potential for distress and the realistic chances of recovery, of intensive care or cardiopulmonary resuscitation. Patients may thus refuse the treatment offered, even if in the mind of the doctor such treatment is essential for the well-being of the patient.

Beneficence means that all treatment given to, or withheld from, a patient should be in their best interests. This is to be judged by the medical and nursing staff and discussed with the patient and/or relatives. The principle of non-maleficence states that no harm should be deliberately done to a patient, although it is understood that there are risks associated with all treatment. The concept of distributive justice means that the greatest good should be done for the greatest number of patients within the available resources. Furthermore, resources should be distributed equitably.

There are clearly many occasions, particularly in critical care, when not all of these principles sit happily together. For example, when moving a critical care unit patient to another unit to make room for another critically ill patient, there is a conflict between the various ethical principles. It is clearly not in the interests of the patient being moved out, yet any risks of harm to this patient should be minimal in relation to a less stable acutely ill patient. An alternate and more controversial ethical view would be that the acutely ill patient is the one in need of resources and should be transferred to where those resources exist. In practice it should be demonstrated that all options have been explored, that the patient being moved has been stabilized and being transferred to an appropriate place and the reasons for this choice of patient are documented.

The recent case of Mr Leslie Burke (R v GMC 2004) highlights the conflict between autonomy and distributive justice. Mr Burke suffers from cerebellar ataxia. He challenged guidelines produced by the General Medical Council

(GMC) on withholding and withdrawing life-prolonging treatment. He feared that when he lost the power to swallow and communicate doctors might decide to stop providing artificial nutrition and hydration. In July 2004 a High Court judge ruled that the guidance placed too much emphasis on the right of the patient to refuse treatment and not enough on the patient's right to require treatment. It was for patients and not doctors to decide what was in their best interests. Therefore Mr Burke had the right to decide for himself whether he should receive artificial nutrition and hydration. The GMC have successfully appealed this decision claiming that doctors would have to provide treatment that the patient demanded despite the doctor considering it clinically inappropriate. It is possible that this case will be further referred to the House of Lords.

This brief review intends to explore some of these basic concepts to allow application of these principles to manage ethically difficult situations. It is only by understanding these concepts that doctors can perform their duties responsibly and even question those duties if the needs of a particular patient or situation warrant it.

> **KEY POINTS**
> - Always act in a way that you feel is in the best interests of the patient at the time.
> - Difficult decisions can be reviewed later in light of new information.

Autonomy and consent

The existence of the patient's right to make his own decisions may be seen as a basic human right protected by the common law. (Lord Scarman 1985) (Sidaway v BRH 1985)

Obtaining consent for treatment serves two purposes. Firstly, and from a clinical perspective, obtaining the patient's cooperation and trust is a major factor contributing to the proposed treatment's success. The second serves a legal purpose and is quite different. There is no law, per se, of consent. However, obtaining consent provides a defence to a charge of assault or battery. Any treatment given, surgery performed or intimate physical contact made without the patient's consent may be interpreted legally as assault. In a well-documented and discussed case an anaesthetist was found guilty of assault when, without her consent, he inserted an analgesic suppository into an unconscious female patient undergoing dental treatment. Consent is informed when it is based on full knowledge of the facts. The issue of informed consent was an important feature in the investigation into paediatric cardiac surgery services in Bristol where relatives claimed that they were never told the risks of surgery. In response to several high profile cases the Department of Health has recently summarized 12 key points on issues of consent (DoH 2001a). Some of these are summarized and annotated here:

- Consent should always be obtained for any medical examination, treatment, surgery or research. Usually patients presenting themselves for treatment are assumed to have offered a degree of consent. For example, if a patient is asked to roll up his sleeve to have his blood pressure checked, consent is implied when he does so. If a patient is not capable of giving consent, for example an unconscious patient in A&E, consent to urgent treatment is assumed until they are deemed able to consent/refuse treatment themselves. Patients may change their mind and withdraw their consent to a treatment at any stage. The person providing the treatment should 'obtain' consent.

- Consent may be written or verbal. Written consent should be obtained for complex treatments and where the risk of harm is significant. In such situations, patient understanding requires explanation, discussion and confirmation of acceptance.
- Children below the age of 16 years may give their own consent to treatment but this should be on an individual basis. 'Gillick' competence relates to previous case law where a teenage girl was receiving the oral contraceptive pill without parental consent (Gillick v West Norfolk & Wisbech Area Health Authority 1985). The House of Lords ruled that a mature child capable of understanding the implications, issues and risks of that treatment could give their own consent. It is recommended that parents and guardians should be involved (while paying due regard to issues of confidentiality) but if a child is deemed competent (by healthcare professionals), and consents to treatment, then their decision cannot be over-ruled by their parents/guardian.
- It is not quite as straightforward if a child below the age of 16 refuses treatment. Discussion of these issues in any detail is beyond the scope of this chapter and in such situations it is strongly recommended that legal advice is sought. It appears that legally a parent can consent to treatment for a competent child who refuses, but this should be a rare event. In a noted recent case, a child of 15 years refused heart transplantation but the court ruled that it should be carried out against her wishes since her parents and medical staff were in agreement. She was subsequently grateful and admitted to refusing because she was understandably scared. It is important to note that the law in Scotland pertaining to children has been interpreted as slightly more liberal. Expert advice is usually required in such cases on both sides of the border.
- Patients between the ages of 16 and 18 years, although not yet adults in the full face of the law, are assumed to be competent to give their own consent.
- If a child is under the age of 18 years and deemed to be incompetent, the parents/guardians will need to give consent for treatment.
- Any competent adult has the right to refuse treatment, even when this puts their life at risk, the only exception being if the patient is detained under the Mental Health Act 1983. A competent pregnant woman has the right to refuse treatment even when this puts the life of her baby at risk.
- In England, no one can give consent on behalf of an incompetent adult (including those unconscious through critical illness or sedation in the critical care unit). Thus, the treatment offered must be based on the best interests of the patient, including religious beliefs, current state of health

and the premorbid wishes of the patient, if known. The legal principal of necessity covers this. Relatives and friends should act to inform professionals on these factors. The situation in Scotland is very different following the enactment of the Adults with Incapacity (Scotland) Act 2000. This makes provision for legally valid proxies to consent on behalf of incapable adults. In addition, authority to treat is given if a registered medical practitioner completes a prescribed form. If no proxy exists, this authority has legal standing.

- If a competent adult has signed an advanced directive, this holds weight in law and usually should be obeyed when that patient is not competent to express their views. This only relates to specifics mentioned in that directive and can be difficult to interpret.
- Consent should be voluntary and not influenced by professionals, family or friends. However, it is not inappropriate for professionals to offer advice and even to attempt to persuade patients about the correct action to take. For example, if a patient wanted a hazardous treatment, such as refusing to stop warfarin before a routine liver biopsy, it would only be proper for the doctor to express concern. The doctor may also refrain from undertaking what in his mind is inappropriate treatment and refer the patient to a colleague.

The GMC has described informed consent as a five-stage process. The stages are:

- *Competence* (to understand the information)
- *Information disclosure* (the risks/benefits of proposed treatment and any alternatives)
- *Patient comprehension* (ask them to repeat their understanding if necessary)
- *Voluntary decision making* (no outside influences affecting their decision making)
- *Authorisation* (allowing treatment to proceed).

Necessity

In England, the common law principle of necessity states that an unconscious patient should be treated with their best interests in mind, since their consent cannot be sought. This should protect the doctor from a charge of assault. However, the doctor should have made an effort to determine the wishes of the patient, if expressed or documented whilst competent. This may necessitate speaking to family, friends or the GP. Furthermore, treatment in such situations should only be for saving 'life or limb'. In addition, what is in the best interests of the patient involves considering whether the doctor's skill had been applied in accordance with accepted medical practice and whether the decision to proceed would be accepted by a responsible body of medical opinion, the so called 'Bolam test'.

There is a potential problem when treating an attempted suicide in that the patient could later claim to have been assaulted, particularly if survival was accompanied by a diminished quality of life. A court would need to consider whether the wish to end a life was always indicative of an unsound mind. Furthermore, the court would also need to consider whether erring on the side of life was paramount. Any defence would be based on the principle of necessity. Reassuringly, such an action has never yet been brought.

Beneficence and non-maleficence

All treatment should be in the best interests of the patient and deliberate harm should not be done to the patient. These principles acknowledge that there is risk associated with all treatment but there is an expectation that the physician will perform a reasoned and well-judged assessment of risk. In the critical care setting this is most important when considering limitation of treatment decisions, where stopping or limiting treatment may be considered as doing the patient harm as it may result in death. However, if further treatment is regarded as futile, then continuing treatment may not be in the best interests of the patient and will only serve to produce further suffering and indignity, i.e. doing harm without the expectation of doing good.

English law expects the doctor to act in the best interests of the patient. This needs to be considered in slightly more detail. For example, it is obviously in the best interests of a patient with a severe intracranial bleed to be admitted to the critical care unit for further treatment. However, this could be inappropriate if death is certain and admission is solely for the purpose of consideration for organ donation. In such a situation, admission is arguably not in the patient's best interests but potentially in the best interests of another. Such elective ventilation is controversial and probably illegal, particularly since some patients may survive with gross neurological impairment and thus directly against their best interests. Relatives cannot give consent for this action, since the patient is still alive and, under English law, an adult cannot give consent for another, even when incompetent. However, in certain situations the patient may give consent. For example, if the patient had a brain tumour and consented to admission to the critical care unit as part of postoperative treatment for this and agreed that if he died organ donation could be carried out, this would be appropriate provided such resources were being used appropriately and not denying other patients potential access to that critical care unit bed.

Distributive justice and rationing health care resources

Undoubtedly, patients and their families are demanding more from healthcare and wish to see every possible medical intervention or treatment being undertaken. Doctors are regularly asked whether a critically ill patient with a failing heart can have a heart transplant, regardless of age or comorbidity, yet this is an extremely limited resource and some form of prioritization of treatment must be undertaken. The concept of utility argues that the greatest good should be done for the largest number within the resources available, but how does this concept fit into everyday clinical practice? Fortunately, such issues rarely need to be considered at an individual level in routine everyday practice. However, on a national scale such issues do arise, particularly in the use of expensive drugs, e.g. β interferon in multiple sclerosis, drugs in the treatment of Alzheimer's disease and the treatment of relapsing haematological malignancies.

Within the critical care unit setting, more money is spent on patients who die there than on those who survive. Patients who die tend to spend longer periods of time there than those who are admitted, improve rapidly and are then discharged. Equally, patients who survive the critical care unit after long-term ventilation subsequently have a poorer quality of life, mostly resulting from neurological disability or poor physiological reserve, than those who are ventilated for shorter periods of time.

The utilitarian approach requires health improvement to be maximized within available resources. The National Institute for Health and Clinical Excellence (previously known as NICE) was originally set up to de-politicize rationing decisions. Eventually, however, much of its guidance concerned the promotion of good practice which, paradoxically, led to extra resources being consumed. There are further problems in that its economic evaluation depends on evidence of clinical effectiveness. One of the problems of evidence-based medicine is that the research on which it is based produces a complex mixture of substantial benefits for some, little benefit for many and harmful effects for a few. In addition, there are technical limitations regarding what criteria it uses in its cost-effectiveness analysis and many of the limits chosen are arbitrary. In an effort to highlight the importance of social value judgements, a Citizens Council has been set up, representing a cross-section of the population, in order to try to legitimize the decision-making process.

Thus the role of the National Institute for Health and Clinical Excellence may be to give guidance on some of these national issues. In individual cases, doctors need to demonstrate that any decisions have taken into account all factors including the patient's wishes, prognosis, suffering associated with treatment and local availability of resources. There is, however, limited scope for an individual doctor in an individual case to be influenced by concern over distributive justice. It may therefore be appropriate for doctors to use clinical discretion regarding the interpretation of such guidance. However, this still leaves the problem of how and to whom individual doctors should be accountable if they exercise their discretion.

There is therefore no current magic formula or technical analysis that can solve the problem of how best to allocate health resources. It is also essential that both the medical profession and the general public accept any decision-making process. Such decisions need to reflect the values of society and to be taken in ways that are seen to be transparent. Even if all this can be achieved and accepted, there still remains the problem of how macrodecisions about rationing can be used at the delivery end of healthcare, i.e. how to translate an explicit rationing decision into an implicit one that affects an individual patient.

For example, although often discussed, illness severity scoring systems such as APACHE are of little use in predicting the outcome of an individual patient. They really only become useful when comparing critically ill populations, and then mainly for research purposes. Dynamic scoring systems are an improvement because they measure changes in sickness over time, thereby reflecting the response to treatment, and are thus a more predictable measure of survival. Progressive three organ systems failure despite five days of treatment usually results in mortality rates in excess of 90%. However, even these systems are rarely used to decide about individual cases.

What has been suggested as useful to enable rationing decisions to be made on a national scale are measures such as quality adjusted life years (QALYs). The concept of QALYs was introduced in 1979 in an attempt to quantify the success and the attendant economic implications of different forms of medical treatment (Table 15.1). It could therefore be used to define health service priorities. The virtue of such a measure is that it is explicit, and consequently the debate about the allocation of resources is about objective problems such as the measurement of quality of life, its duration and cost rather than subjective and about the political power of doctors competing for scarce resources.

However, although concepts such as QALYs may help society to judge the value of different treatments and ration any such treatment accordingly, they should not be used for decision making at an individual patient level. This is partly because it is notoriously difficult to judge another individual's quality of life or predict outcome in individual cases. This relates particularly to the appropriateness of admission to intensive care. Furthermore, the whole concept of QALYs can be severely criticized on other grounds. The selection criteria on which QALYs are composed are arbitrary and selected for reasons of economy rather than human equality. The definition of health used in the calculation is open to interpretation. It is also assumed that all cases, by and large, are governed by the same few factors. The greatest injustice, however, is that they must necessarily discriminate against the elderly. The older person's life expectancy is bound to be less than a younger person's. The life years gained will be fewer and the quality of those gained often lower. QALYs may therefore be used to legitimize discrimination between people.

Table 15.1 Cost per QALY ranking (after Ridley & Plenderleith 1994)

Treatment	Cost per QALY (£)
Pacemaker implantation	830
Hip replacement	890
CABG	1 580
Kidney transplant	3 560
Respiratory critical illness	7 500
Haemodialysis at home	13 000
Haemodialysis in hospital	16 000

TREATMENT WITHDRAWAL AND END OF LIFE DECISIONS

Withdrawal of treatment

Society's rising expectations and evolving medical technology are offering, at some financial and human cost, greater improvements in outcome. Paradoxically, the withdrawal of active treatment from patients in intensive care has increased in recent years, accounting for up to 90% of deaths on the critical care unit in some series (Turner et al 1996, Prendergast & Luce 1997). There are well-established ethical, moral and legal frameworks for the withdrawal of treatment, even in circumstances where it might be life-saving. In seeking moral support for the withdrawal of life-sustaining treatment, Pope Pius XII acceded that there are circumstances of profound unconsciousness from which artificial ventilation may be withdrawn. The Linacre Centre, a respected Roman Catholic institution, has given quite specific advice confirming the appropriateness of withdrawing inotropes or ventilation in circumstances of medical futility. Recently there has been a re-evaluation of intensive care in terms of the quality of life of the survivors. It is in these terms that the distinction drawn by Rachels (Rachels 1986) of 'having a life' and 'being alive' is vital. 'Being alive is relatively unimportant. One's life by contrast is immensely important. It is the sum of one's aspirations, decisions, activities, projects and human relationships'.

A recent example of this is the case of Miss B. This unfortunate lady was tetraplegic and ventilator-dependent and regarded her quality of life as so poor that she wanted treatment to be withdrawn. Her doctors disagreed, but as she was judged to be competent the courts upheld her views. As a competent adult she had the right to agree to or refuse any treatment and thus the court sanctioned withdrawal of ventilation (Ms B v An NHS Hospital Trust [2002]).

By contrast, when dealing with treatment withdrawal/limitation in children, the recent case of Glass v UK emphasized that the courts should be involved in such decisions if the views of the medical profession and the parents differed in the appropriateness of future medical care.

Ordinary and extraordinary treatment

Withdrawal of medical treatment in cases of futility is ethical, but what is medical treatment and what may be withdrawn? To aid this determination, the distinction between ordinary and extraordinary care was developed in the 16th century. Ordinary treatment is simple and effective, offering benefit without undue expense, pain, or suffering. It carries a reasonable hope of benefit. Extraordinary treatment, on the other hand, may involve pain, expense and suffering whilst offering marginal benefit. The claimed distinction is that ordinary treatment does not produce suffering and is morally obligatory. Forms of medical treatment that fall into this category include hydration, nutrition and oxygen. Extraordinary treatment, on the other hand, involves treatment such as artificial ventilation, with the associated intubation or tracheostomy, or haemodialysis, involving repeated central venous access. These produce suffering, pain and indignity and are expensive. It is claimed that such treatment is not morally obligatory.

The distinction appears to offer doctors a reasonable and straightforward basis of assessing what is obligatory treatment. However, this distinction is imprecise, is likely to change over time and treatments that may be burdensome to one patient will not be to another. Furthermore, the terms 'benefit' and 'burden' are open to interpretation.

Nutrition and hydration

In studies, patients do not see any difference between nutrition, ventilation and cardiopulmonary rescuscitation (CPR), but to some moralists there are significant differences. To them, the provision of nutrition (usually naso-gastric or percutaneous endoscopic gastrostomy (PEG) feeding) is considered ordinary, and therefore morally obligatory treatment. Some argue that to withhold nutrition may be regarded in theory as contrary to the European Human Rights Act. However, the withdrawal of nutrition and hydration is accepted in law. In 1993, permission was granted to withdraw nutrition from Tony Bland, who had spent two years in a persistent vegetative state (PVS) following a severe head injury sustained in the Hillsborough disaster, on the premise that nutrition, when given by a pump through a nasogastric tube, constituted medical treatment. At the time, the courts emphasized that the withdrawal of nutrition remained controversial and such decisions in cases of PVS should always be ratified in advance by the courts (Airedale NHS Trust v Bland 1993). There have, however, now been so many cases where the courts have sanctioned withdrawal of nutrition in PVS patients that there have been recent calls for this to no longer require legal sanctioning. Indeed it is now accepted practice in many hospitals in the USA that nasogastric tube feeding in patients with dementia is not mandatory, if there are concerns that more distress is being caused than relieved. This remains controversial since the distress experienced by hunger and thirst may involve more suffering than the side effects of nasogastric tube or PEG feeding. The rationale is that feeding may produce more distress than starvation due to increased pulmonary aspiration and the discomfort associated with PEG insertion, replacing nasogastric tubes, etc. The BMA have also called for this not to require legal sanction in individual cases, but it remains controversial, despite being ratified in law.

Interestingly, English law forbids the force-feeding of hunger strikers, not on a right to commit suicide premise, but on the principle of respect for autonomy and self-determination. To force-feed a patient of sound mind without consent would constitute a tort (a civil wrong) and leave one open to a charge of assault. Psychiatric patients may be force-fed under the Mental Health Act 1983, but this is not a uniform ruling. In 1993 the English Court of Appeal overruled an earlier ruling to force-feed a girl with anorexia nervosa. In conclusion, the duty to feed is not absolute but must be considered carefully, and currently, legal sanction of its withdrawal is recommended.

Acts and omissions

The acts and omissions doctrine argues that an action which results in an undesirable consequence is morally worse than an inaction which results in the same outcome. This is quite an attractive doctrine as people do not feel as morally responsible for their omissions as they do for their actions. For example, the central argument in the 'Arthur' case, in which a neonate with Down's syndrome was allowed to die by not being given nourishment (R v Arthur 1981), was that although it was not permissible for doctors to kill their patients, sometimes it is morally permissible to allow the patient to die. In other words, there is a distinction between 'killing' and 'letting die'.

This distinction, however, has often produced concern that a patient dying as a result of having treatment actively withdrawn might be regarded, from an ethical or legal perspective, as worse than dying without treatment having been started in the first place. This doctrine makes little sense and has been heavily criticized when applied to healthcare. Thus there can be no legal or moral justification for giving a doctor the right to withhold treatment such as connecting a patient to a ventilator and yet to refuse him the right to withdraw treatment already started. The BMA and the Department of Health agree that there is no necessary difference between treatment withdrawal and not starting treatment in the first place, and that it is the outcome that matters. This has been ratified in case law. However, if one had a duty to act and did not, one must be morally responsible for the consequences arising out of that omission. This moral fact lies at the basis of the legal concept of culpable negligence: the failure to perform an act which, morally speaking, one was duty bound to do. In other words, there is no necessary difference between an act and an omission if the motives, intentions and other background factors are held constant.

Another distinction that needs to be addressed is whether there is a difference between 'allowing' something to happen and 'making' it happen. If death occurs as a direct result of one's actions when no other outcome is possible, then this could be interpreted as causing death to happen, which could lead to a charge of manslaughter. However, if by these actions alternative outcomes are possible, then merely letting die has occurred and the underlying pathological process has caused the death. For example, if ventilation has been withdrawn from a patient who subsequently dies, it is the pathological process that killed them (letting die), since if they were not critically ill they would breathe. If, however, all possibility of breathing has been taken away, for example the patient is paralysed with a muscle relaxant and then taken off a ventilator, then the only possible outcome is death and 'making die' has occurred. This leads to a discussion on the principle of double effect (Buttigieg & Pace 2004).

Double effect

Doctors are frequently faced with the dilemma of wishing to undertake a course of action or administer treatment that has two possible effects, a good and morally desirable one and a bad one. For example, potent pain relieving and sedating drugs may be used in dying patients to prevent distress but they may also shorten life. Assuming that shortening life is an undesirable effect, the use of these drugs is seen to have both good and bad effects and thus the doctors concerned appear to face a dilemma. An even starker problem is highlighted by the use or presence of neuromuscular blocking agents while wishing to withdraw ventilatory support. Such drugs may be useful in aiding ventilation and they are also commonly used during managed withdrawal of life-sustaining treatment in paediatric intensive care units as they help mask any possible signs of terminal distress from the child's parents.

Thus there are situations in which it is impossible to avoid all moral harms. The principle of double effect allows justification of an action that has both a good and a bad effect provided that four criteria can be satisfied. Firstly, the action itself is not inherently immoral. Secondly, the intention is to achieve the good effect, even though the bad effect may be foreseen and inevitable. In other words, there is a moral distinction between intending an effect and not intending, although foreseeing, an effect. Thirdly, the good effect must be a direct result of the action and not secondary to the bad effect. Fourthly, there must be a favourable balance between the good effects and the bad effects.

If all four conditions are satisfied, then the principle argues that it is morally acceptable to undertake the action, even if a harmful effect, such as death, was also to result. Thus, dying patients who are in pain should be given appropriate doses of opiates to relieve their distress, even though the dying process may be hastened. In law, the principle of double effect was accepted in the case of R v Adams [1957]. In this case the judge stated that if the treatment was designed to promote comfort and it was the right and proper treatment, the fact that it shortened life did not convict the doctor of murder.

It should be pointed out, however, that the nature and dose of drugs administered should be considered appropriate and tailored to relieve distress of the patient. Thus, it is acceptable to infuse diamorphine to a dying cancer patient to relieve distress although death may be hastened. This, however, would be unacceptable if the same drugs and doses are given to a patient who is neither distressed nor suffering an imminently terminal condition.

With respect to the use of neuromuscular agents, however, the situation is much less clear. The action of stopping ventilation in a patient unable to breathe as a result of neuromuscular blockade could theoretically be interpreted in law as an intentional killing. Furthermore, even if the drug infusion is stopped, the failure to reverse the effects could be interpreted as an ethically inappropriate act of omission, especially as the intention, the death of the patient, is the same. Even though arguments have been used to justify the use of neuromuscular agents in these circumstances, including the requirement to relieve terminal distress and dyspnoea, there is no evidence for this. Indeed, it is possible that distress may be greater, especially as awareness is always of concern when using these drugs.

Treatment withdrawal and end of life decisions

Although the principle can be useful to clarify the proper course of action pertaining to certain dilemmas such as the use of strong analgesics at the end of life, its main criticism is that it is dependent on the concept of intentionality, i.e. a clear distinction can be made between what a person intends and what is foreseen but unintended. In this respect, it depends heavily on the integrity of the person applying it, as it is easy for anyone to say that a particular result was unintended.

The unconscious patient

It is well recognized that withdrawal of consent may be made at any stage during treatment by a fully informed competent patient. Treatment may also be withdrawn from the incompetent/unconscious patient. Life-sustaining treatment may be withdrawn when, in the opinion of the medical staff, it is futile, i.e. the patient will die despite treatment, since no one is under obligation to provide treatment that will not do good and may do harm. Such a decision may be made in the critical care unit even when a possibility of survival remains, but where the treatment given may produce significant distress, e.g. repeated tracheal suction. It also applies when the quality of life of the survivor will be profoundly impaired in relation to the pain and suffering necessary to ensure survival, e.g. surviving the critical care unit with major neurological disability. Treatment should also be withdrawn where it may be clearly demonstrated that it had been expressly forbidden by the patient whilst competent, either in the form of a legally-produced advance directive (e.g. Jehovah's Witnesses) or it had been clearly and unequivocally expressed to friends and relatives.

KEY POINTS
- Seek experienced advice with difficult decisions.
- If the patient is incapacitated, inform the family about all decisions.
- Ask about advance directives.
- Remember sources of ethical and legal support, and advice.

Advance directives

A competent patient has an absolute right to refuse any and all treatment, even if it is life-enhancing or life-preserving. For example, a physician in the US who administered a blood transfusion to save a patient's life, despite being aware that she carried a card refusing blood transfusion under any circumstances, was successfully sued when she survived. His argument had been that as she was unconscious she could neither confirm that this had been her intent nor that her intent remained the same.

In order to indicate patients' wishes should they become incompetent or unable to express them, the use of advance directives has been widely recommended in the USA. This resulted in the Patient Self Determination Act, passed by congress in 1990, which required all Medicare hospitals to ask all patients on admission whether they had made a living will and inform them of their rights to make one. The validity of advance directives in the expression of patient autonomy has been accepted by both the BMA and the Standing Committee of Doctors in the EU on Living Wills/Advance Directives. The Medical Treatment (Advance Directives) Bill was passed by the House of Lords in the 1992/3 session to clarify that no criminal offence would be committed by a doctor who complied with an advance directive and the Law Commission stated that refusal of treatment made in advance should carry as much weight as a refusal from a currently competent individual. The BMA's statement approved legislation to clarify the non-liability of a doctor who acted in accordance with such a directive. However, like its counterparts in the European Union, it agreed that in appropriate circumstances doctors were not bound irrevocably by advance directives but should endeavor to follow the spirit of an advanced directive. In incapacity, this may involve discussion with family members and GPs, etc., to gain an understanding of what the patient might have wanted.

Despite the widespread acceptance of advance directives, take-up has been low in both the UK and the USA. In surveys, most people would still wish their doctor to make decisions for them in collaboration with a proxy (in the UK this is the next of kin). This is in many ways a more logical situation since many people cannot reasonably make an advance decision about intensive care treatment or resuscitation status when they do not understand either what this entails or the specific circumstances at the time that such treatment is required. This is not informed consent and may only serve to confuse. It would be pointless and a waste of valuable critical care unit resources to ventilate a patient if the doctor was not also allowed to dialyse their potentially reversible renal failure. Similarly if a patient did not want a tracheostomy and yet could not be weaned from ventilation, are doctors committed to long-term ventilation with repeated failed trials of extubation? This would be an intolerable situation to put a patient through simply because they might not have understood either what a particular treatment actually entailed or that the alternatives were worse. Such directives do however hold weight in law and any actions contrary to them may need to be justified. In such situations it would be appropriate to seek colleagues' and legal advice.

Do Not Rescuscitate (DNR) orders

Do Not Resuscitate (DNR) orders detail the care to be given in the specific circumstances of a cardiac arrest. They should always be made with the consent of the competent patient. Because of the inappropriate use of DNR orders when competent patients were unaware that these had been issued, the Department of Health has issued guidelines on their use. This has manifested itself as a document requiring the signature of a senior doctor outlining reasons for the order being given and the nature of the discussions that have taken place with the patient and/or family.

This is a good example of how medical practice changes according to shifting values in society and the move away from 'paternalism' in medicine to 'consumerism'. However, it is important to realize that basic medical ethical values have not changed. A fully conscious patient has the right to decide and be involved in decisions on future treatment. If incompetent, e.g. an unconscious patient, then the relatives are informed of the medical decision not to perform CPR and this is documented. Note that the relatives are not asked for their permission not to perform CPR, since under English law an adult cannot give consent for the medical treatment of another. It would, however, be unusual to disagree sufficiently with the relatives that diametrically opposite views were taken. It should also be noted that a DNR order does not necessarily mean that other treatment, such as dialysis, is inappropriate or should be withdrawn.

On the other hand, if a patient suffers a cardiorespiratory arrest and CPR is performed, this does not imply that further treatment is necessarily appropriate, e.g. critical care unit care, since this is a separate decision made on different grounds using other criteria, such as chances of survival, quality of life, distressing treatment required, etc.

Can relatives force doctors to perform CPR?

It is well recognized that patients have rights. Medical professionals also have rights. One of these is that a doctor cannot be forced into providing treatment that he/she thinks is not in the best interests of that patient. This right is currently well established after multiple legal rulings. For example, in October 2004 Mr Justice Hedley ruled that Charlotte Wyatt should not be revived if she stopped breathing again. Charlotte had chronic respiratory and kidney problems and had severe brain damage that had left her blind, deaf and incapable of voluntary movements or response. The judge agreed with the views of Charlotte's doctors as to what was in her best interests and did not accept her parents' submissions (Portsmouth NHS Trust v Wyatt [2004], Dyer 2005). In another case, Dame Butler-Sloss, President of the Family Division of the High Court, presided over the case of Luke Winston-Jones, who suffered from Edwards's syndrome. This is linked to heart defects and respiratory problems. She gave permission to the doctors caring for him to withhold mechanical ventilation if his condition deteriorated. Following Luke's death, his mother made a formal complaint to the police that procedures that could have prolonged her son's life were withheld (Royal Liverpool Children's NHS Trust and North West Wales v Luke Winston-Jones and Rith Winston-Jones 2004, Dyer 2004). Recently the coroner recorded a verdict of death by natural causes and that the doctors concerned could not have done anything more to help the terminally ill child. These cases show that it can be extremely difficult to apply legal principles to individual cases and these are likely to be strongly disputed by the various interested parties.

To return to the issue of DNR orders, the Department of Health's guidelines on CPR clearly state that 'nobody can insist on having treatment that will not work'. In cases of potential conflict, doctors are duty bound to get a second opinion or refer the patient to another appropriate medical practitioner. In practice it should be rare for such a conflict to arise and usually does so because of poor communication, but rising patients' expectations occasionally produce unrealistic demands. Rarely one may need to resort to a legal ruling in contentious cases. Judging potential outcome and quality of life is difficult, but essential when making rational decisions about the appropriateness of further treatment in critical care.

Admission to the critical care unit

Intensive care is a scarce and expensive resource, which also inevitably inflicts suffering in the hope of enabling patients to survive critical illness. Admission to the critical care unit is only justified when support is required for an acute treatable pathology, i.e. there has not simply been an inexorable deterioration in the patient's underlying condition. There must be a hope that the quality of life of the survivor will be acceptable. This may be difficult to judge and valued differently. Some people may see existing in a handicapped and dependent state as being worthwhile whilst others would not. Interestingly when assessing the quality of life of survivors from the critical care unit, young trauma victims describe their deterioration in quality of life as being the greatest. This is due to having a very good premorbid quality of life and therefore any subsequent restriction is seen as a significant handicap. Each case must be judged on its own merits. To admit someone to the critical care unit with no prospect of recovery would be to subject them to suffering and indignity. It has even been suggested that this could amount to torture under the European Convention on Human Rights, by taking away their autonomy, and subjecting them to degrading behaviour, e.g. repeated bodily exposure and sleep deprivation.

European Convention on Human Rights

The UK is a signatory to the European Convention on Human Rights and this may have a significant impact on the future practice of medicine. The articles encapsulate a series of basic human rights from the 'right to life' to liberty and freedom from torture or degrading treatment. Many procedures in hospital and particularly in critical care may be described as degrading and it is important that any potentially degrading treatment is medically justified and patient comfort is optimized. Difficult ethical problems may be taken to clinical ethics committees, which meet regularly in many hospitals and give guidance on difficult dilemmas. It is also important to remember that round the clock legal support is available, including access to a judge for emergency legal rulings.

ORGAN DONATION

Both tissues (e.g. heart valves, corneas, skin) as well as organs (e.g. heart, lungs, liver, kidneys, pancreas, small bowel) may be donated after death has

KEY POINTS
In difficult ethical cases you may need to seek guidance from:
- experienced senior colleagues
- hospital clinical ethics committees
- British Medical Association Ethics Department
- medical defence organizations
- hospital lawyers/judicial rulings, i.e. emergency wards of court.

Organ donation

been diagnosed. This usually follows certification of death by confirmation of brainstem death. Brainstem death was first described in 1959. As the patient is apnoeic and irreversibly comatose, this was ratified by the Royal Colleges of the UK as equating to death certified by cardiorespiratory criteria, and therefore allowing organ donation (Conference of Medical Royal Colleges 1976, 1979). Curiously, whereas death certified by brainstem death criteria has been ratified in case law, death certified by cardiorespiratory criteria has never been ratified in UK law and indeed, whereas national guidelines exist for the diagnosis of the former, there are currently no national guidelines for the 'conventional' diagnosis of death. This situation is currently under review, and guidance for the diagnosis of death is imminently expected from the Department of Health.

By definition, brainstem dead patients will be apnoeic and therefore ventilated on the critical care unit. However, organ donation may also be performed under some circumstances after asystole and subsequent certification of death and this is called non-heart beating organ donation (NHBOD). This usually follows withdrawal of active treatment in the critical care unit, but may occasionally occur in less controlled settings, such as in A&E and occasionally on a medical ward, usually following a fatal and untreatable head injury or stroke or a failed attempt at CPR. In NHBOD, organs are at risk of significant damage from ischaemia and the warm ischaemia time should be minimized. Steps must be taken rapidly to preserve organs (usually kidneys, liver and rarely lungs), usually within 20 min following asystole and this necessitates consent from a family member, or the patient to be registered as an organ donor on the Organ Donor Register, which should be quickly checked (Tel: 0845 60 60 400). Donor renal function following NHBOD is similar to that following kidneys donated from heart beating brainstem dead donors (Gok et al 2002) and the number of kidneys donated from this source has steadily risen in the UK in the past few years with 140 kidneys being successfully transplanted in the year to April 2005. National UK guidelines for organ donation, including the addition of NHBOD were revised in 2004 by the Intensive Care Society (http://www.ics.ac.uk). Any potential patients suitable for donation should be discussed with the transplant coordinator, ideally before this possibility is offered to the family, as the patient may not be a suitable donor.

It should be remembered that tissues may be donated up to 72 h following death and are usually taken by the pathologist. The numbers of patients suitable for tissue donation is very large and unfortunately few families are offered this option. To know, for example, that corneal donation has restored someone's sight may give families much comfort following a death.

The number of patients on the waiting list for an organ transplant continues to grow and the numbers of organs donated remains static. Approximately 6500 patients in the UK are on the waiting list for a transplant ($\approx$ 75% kidneys) of whom about 10% will die per annum without a transplant. In the year to March 2005 there were 1783 kidney transplants in the UK of which 475 were living donors from a friend or family member, 143 from non-heart beating donors and 1565 from brainstem dead donors (figures from UK Transplant: http://www.ukt.nhs.uk). The ongoing shortage of donors has lead to a variety of strategies to increase donation. 'Elective ventilation', otherwise known as the 'Exeter Protocol', involved the ventilation of patients who had suffered massive strokes, not in the hope that it may do them any good, but on the expectation that they would become brain dead and would therefore be possible candidates for organ donation. This was estimated to have the potential for increasing kidney donation by 50% in the UK. However, it is a fundamental principle of organ donation that no living patient should come to harm due to the requirements of potential organ recipients. In the Exeter Protocol, harm was done when artificial ventilation was initiated because death was often postponed, especially since some patients would not proceed to brain death due to the reduction in intracerebral pressure by artificial ventilation, allowing the potential for the patient to survive in a brain-damaged state. If a patient has not consented to a treatment that is then carried out, and judged not to be in their best interests, this could constitute an assault. This may particularly apply to the case of elective ventilation, since the possibility exists to actually do harm, by leaving the patient in a brain-damaged state, when it may have been in their interests to be allowed to die without intervention. In 1994, the Department of Health effectively prohibited use of elective ventilation because of these concerns and also stated that whilst an advance directive could be used to withhold treatment that the patient did not want, it could not be used to demand treatment (in this case ventilation for the sole purpose of facilitating organ donation) that was not in that patient's best interests (Law Commission 1995).

Whilst numerous studies have shown that 90% of the public are in favour of organ donation as a concept, relatives' refusal rate for donation stands at around 45%. Reasons for refusal include feelings that the patient has been through enough, not wanting surgery to the body and not knowing the wishes of the deceased. Several proposals to change the law relating to donation have been proposed to increase donation, in particular 'presumed consent' where the patient is presumed to want to be a donor after death, unless they specifically opted out of doing so whilst alive. This remains the case in several European countries but in the UK remains controversial. If ever introduced, significant repeated opportunities would have to be given to people to opt out, (e.g. whilst taking out a driving licence or passport, etc.) and concerns would remain that some people had simply never been offered the chance or the information to make such a decision and this would not be respecting their autonomy. The counter argument is that this legislation would be to the benefit of society (distributive justice). A fairer system might be to insist that during one's life one had to make a decision and have this ratified at intervals, e.g. during passport renewal. The current situation remains that one may express one's view by joining the organ donor register (Tel: 0845 60 60 400) and it would be expected that if one had not done so one's relatives would make this decision after death, based on their perception of the patient's wishes.

RESEARCH IN CRITICAL CARE

Issues of consent and non-maleficence are vitally important in research to do with critically ill patients as the patient may not benefit directly from the proposed treatment and cannot consent to treatment since they are unconscious. Fundamental to the understanding of the ethics of research is the appreciation that the primary aim of research is the generation of knowledge to help the treatment of future patients in similar situations.

In the critical care setting, research subjects are usually unable to give their own consent. It has been argued that all research conducted must be in the patient's best interests but this may be hard to establish. In particular, there is an expectation that any drug administration should be expected to have a beneficial action that is likely to outweigh any expected adverse effects. The European Union Clinical Trials Directive was introduced in 2001 and specifically addresses issues such as research in the incapacitated adult. It states that if the patient is incapacitated and cannot consent to involvement in a research study, particularly involving the administration of a drug, then consent should be sought from the legal representative for that patient. This would normally mean the next of kin or first degree relative, but in the emergency situation theoretically could mean a professional independent of the study. This person would be called a professional legal representative. However, at the time of writing this concept has not yet entered clinical practice. This is an area of rapid change and will also be affected by the Mental Capacity Act which comes into force in 2007, regulating actions taken on behalf of incapacitated subjects, including research. Consideration is currently being given to allow incapacitated subjects to be involved in research as long as the consent of the legal representative (and subsequently the patient) is sought as soon as possible and the patient withdrawn immediately if either refuse consent.

This is a time of significant changes in the law in this area and the hospital ethics, research and development departments should be consulted if any research is to be conducted on unconscious patients. In Scotland, such a proposal would need to be reviewed by MREC Scotland. In general, any drug administered should have the expectation of a beneficial effect, as determined by studies in other groups of patients who have given informed consent, or non-drug studies comparing differing treatments where neither is known to be superior. In general, novel or invasive treatments cannot be used unless extremely well established in animal models. As with any research, ethical committee approval is mandatory.

RELIGION

In virtually all cultures, morality is guided by religious principles, and the ethical framework derived from these therefore varies according to prevailing religious beliefs. However, legal principles are established in relation to the prevailing religion in a particular country and this may lead to potential conflict in specific cases, e.g. the acceptance of brainstem death criteria. There are fewer actual conflicts between different religions in terms of end-of-life or extraordinary treatment decisions than one might suspect. For example, all the major religions accept organ transplantation in principle, including Muslims. The concept of medical futility is also generally accepted, with the possible exception of Orthodox Judaism where every minute of life is regarded as precious and God-given. Most Jews, however, are not orthodox and end-of-life decisions are rarely very different in practice.

Jehovah's Witnesses believe that to receive blood or derived products is wrong and their soul will be damned. The strength of this belief, however, is variable. For some this includes their own blood and they will not accept pre-operative autologous blood donation. On the other hand, others will accept this as well as human albumin, fresh frozen plasma and intra-operative cell salvage. It is important to discuss an individual's views on such matters, which should be recorded and signed by the patient, doctor and a witness. As discussed before in this chapter, one of the prerequisites for informed consent and autonomous decision making is to ensure that the individual makes an informed decision without outside coercion from the medical profession, family, friends or members of a religious community.

CONCLUSIONS

Medical ethics is based on the morality and values of society, which therefore changes with time and across cultures. Difficult ethical decisions will arise on a regular basis, particularly with evolving technology and the changing ethical framework within which we live. If in doubt, advice should be sought from experienced colleagues and difficult cases taken to the hospital clinical ethics committee, specifically established to deal with such situations. Equally the clinical ethics committee of the BMA will issue advice in difficult situations. It should also be remembered that there is continuous access to hospital legal advice and the medical defence societies and that legal rulings may be obtained at any time in particularly difficult situations.

The success of intensive care is not, therefore to be measured only by the statistics of survival, as though each death were a medical failure. It is to be measured by the quality of lives preserved or restored; and by the quality of the dying of those in whose interest it is to die; and by the quality of human relationships involved in each death.

(Dunstan 1985)

CASE 15.1

A 10-year-old girl refuses consent to have her bat ears corrected. Her parents insist that this should be performed as she will be the subject of bullying and this will damage her psychologically. Will you take parental consent?

Answer
In general terms a minor cannot overrule treatment that both her parents and medical staff agree is in her best interests. She may be Gillick competent at 10 years old, however this only relates to a minor consenting to treatment, not refusing it. You could theoretically therefore proceed.

However the proposed treatment is merely cosmetic and you do not know the psychological effects on the girl of proceeding as it may even alter the way she perceives herself. You need to explore the reasons for her refusal. If this cannot be resolved at the time, it may be more sensible to delay surgery and allow her and her parents time to discuss the options and why she does not want surgery, and even in difficult cases, seek the opinion of a child psychologist. Remember that although a child cannot refuse treatment which her legal guardian and medical staff agree is in her best interests, in practice, this usually relates to potentially life-saving or enhancing treatment. Court orders may be required in difficult or high-risk situations.

CASE 15.2

A 76-year-old man with disseminated carcinomatosis is admitted to hospital with a chest infection. He and his family insist on full treatment including CPR if he arrests. What will you do?

Answer
This patient cannot demand treatment that is not in (his) best interests and it would seem that CPR is not in his best interests. You need to decide why he wants CPR and this may involve speaking to him and his family, occasionally separately. A common misconception is that if a patient is not for resuscitation, then this means that they will not receive medical treatment. Having discussed this with him and ensuring that he understands what CPR actually involves, what the chances of full recovery are and that this does not alter any form of ongoing care, such as in the critical care unit, then you need to decide whether you think a DNR order is appropriate. If you think the patient has full understanding, then one would normally err on the patient's side. If you disagree with the patient, then you must seek a second opinion and inform senior staff that there is a disagreement over proposed medical management. Either way you need to document in the notes the reasons for this decision and that the patient understands that this decision does not affect any other treatment.

CASE 15.3

A 36-year-old man is assaulted and is ventilated on the critical care unit with a severe head injury which you think is a non-survivable injury. The police explain that there will be a murder enquiry if he dies. Is treatment withdrawal appropriate under such circumstances?

Answer
If it is the opinion of all the staff caring for this man that the outlook is universally fatal and that treatment withdrawal has the full agreement of

the next of kin, then it should be carried out. Often in such situations, brainstem death develops and patients should be stabilized to allow certification by brainstem testing as this may help the family to understand that death has occurred. It has been ratified in case law that if medical treatment is withdrawn because of futility, then the primary pathology remains the cause of death.

REFERENCES AND FURTHER READING

Airedale NHS Trust v Bland (1993) 1 All ER 821

Bonner S M, Pace N 2000 Witholding and withdrawing life saving treatment in intensive care. British Journal of Intensive Care 10:123–129

Branthwaite M 2000 Law for doctors. Royal Society of Medicine Press, London

Buttigieg M, Pace N 2004 Neuromuscular blockade during withdrawal of life support and the principle of double effect. CPD Anaesthesia 6(2):85–87

Conference of Medical Royal Colleges 1976 Diagnosis of brain death. Conference of Medical Colleges and their faculties in the United Kingdom on 11 October 1976. BMJ 2:1187–1188

Conference of Medical Royal Colleges 1979 Diagnosis of death. Conference of Medical Royal Colleges and their faculties in the United Kingdom. BMJ 1:322

DoH 2001a 12 key points on consent: the law in England. Department of Health, London

DoH 2001b Witholding and withdrawing life prolonging medical treatment: Guidance for decision making, 2nd edn. BMJ Books, London

Dunstan G R 1985 Hard questions in intensive care. Anaesthesia 40:479–482

Dyer C 2004 Doctors need not ventilate baby to prolong life. BMJ 329: 995

Dyer C 2005 Judge overrules earlier decision on Charlotte Wyatt. BMJ 331: 985

Ethox 2001 Clinical ethics support in the UK; a review of the current position and likely development. Nuffield Trust: London

European Convention on Human Rights. http://www.official-documents.co.uk/document/hoffice/rights/annex.htm

Gillick v West Norfolk & Wisbech Area Health Authority (1985) 2 BMLR 11, HL

Gillis J 1997 When lifesaving treatment in children is not the answer. BMJ 315:246–247

Glass v UK (2004) 61827/00

Gok M, Buckley P, Shenton B et al 2002 Long-term renal function in kidneys from non-heart-beating donors: a single-center experience. Transplantation 74(5):664–669

Intensive Care Society 2004 Management of the adult potential organ donor. Intensive Care Society, London. http://www.ics.ac.uk

Law Commission [1995] 4 WEB JCLI webjcli.ncl.ac.uk/articles4/rodgers4.html

Ms B v An NHS Hospital Trust [2002] EWHC 429 (Fam)

Pace N, Mclean S 1996 Ethics and the law in intensive care. Oxford University Press, Oxford

Portsmouth NHS Trust v Wyatt [2004] EWHC 2247. http://www.bailii.org/ew/cases/EWHC/Fam/2004/2247.html

Prendergast T J, Luce J M 1997 Increasing incidence of witholding and withdrawing life support from the critically ill. American Journal of Respiratory and Critical Care Medicine 155:15–20

Rachels J 1986 The end of life. Oxford University Press, Oxford

R v Adams [1957] Crim L R 365

R v Arthur (1981) 12 BMLR 1

R (on the Application of Burke) v General Medical Council [2004] EWHC 1879 (Admin)

Ridley S, Biggam M, Stone P 1994 A cost-utility analysis of intensive therapy. Anaesthesia 49:192–196

Ridley S, Plenderleith L 1994 Survival after intensive care. Comparison with a normal matched population as an indicator of effectiveness. Anaesthesia 49:933–935

Royal Liverpool Children's NHS Trust and North West Wales v Luke Winston-Jones and Rith Winston-Jones 2004

Sidaway v Board of Governors of the Bethlem Royal Hospital [1985] AC871, [1985] 1 All ER 643, HL

Turner J S, Michell W L, Morgan C J et al 1996 Limitation of life support: frequency and practice in a London and Cape Town intensive care unit. Intensive Care Medicine 22:1020–1025

UK Clinical Ethics Network. http://www.ethics-network.org.uk

Index

Page numbers ending in b, f, and t refer to boxes, figures and tables respectively

Index

O

P

Q

R

S

T

Urinalysis, acute renal failure, 240b
Urinary pH, altering, 282, 282t

V

Valsalva manoeuvre, 120
Variable flange tracheostomy tubes, 341
Variable performance devices (VPDs),
    oxygen delivery, 19–21
Variceal haemorrhage, 224–7
Varicella zoster virus (VZV), 200
Vascular injury, spinal cord, 213–14
Vasculitis, systemic, 246f
Vasoconstriction, sepsis, 78–9
Vasodilators, 7
Venlafaxine poisoning, 294–5
Venous distention, cardiac tamponade, 109
Venous thromboembolism, 151
Ventilation
    acute left ventricular failure, 102
    invasive see Invasive ventilation
    neuromuscular blocking agents, 371
    non-invasive see Non-invasive
        ventilation
    poisoning, 277
    withdrawal, 380–1
    see also Oxygen delivery
Ventilation/perfusion (V/Q) scan, 154, 154f
Ventilatory failure, 132

Ventricular ectopic beats, 97
Ventricular septal defect (VSD), 97, 104f,
    106
Ventricular tachycardia (VT), 98, 98f,
    122–3
Ventricular threshold, 128
Venturi mask, 19, 134f
Verapamil, 121
Vertebral column, 322f
Video-assisted thoracoscopy (VATS), 165
Viral meningitis, 199–200
Voluven, 37

W

Warfarin, 156
Water's circuit, 22
Wegener's granulomatosis, 239f, 269–70
Wenkebach phenomenon, 98
White cell activation, fluid loss, 31
Wolf-Parkinson White syndrome (WPW),
    122
Wriggler's sign, 219, 219f

X

Xanthochromia, 184, 185f